New Perspectives in Public Health

Second Edition

Edited by

Siân Griffiths
Professor of Public Health
Director, School of Public Health
The Chinese University of Hong Kong

and

David J Hunter
Professor of Health Policy and Management
and Director, Centre for Public Policy and Health
School for Health, Durham University

Foreword by

Sir Kenneth Calman
Vice-Chancellor
Durham University

Radcliffe Publishing
Oxford • Seattle

D1340750

Radcliffe Publishing Ltd
18 Marcham Road
Abingdon
Oxon OX14 1AA
United Kingdom

www.radcliffe-oxford.com
Electronic catalogue and worldwide online ordering facility.

British Library Cataloguing in Publication Data

A catalogue record for this book is available from the British Library.

ISBN-10: 1 85775 791 2
ISBN-13: 978 185775 791 0

Typeset by Lapiz Digital Services, Chennai
Printed and bound by Alden (Malaysia)

Contents

Foreword

It is tempting in writing a Foreword for *New Perspectives* to look back and compare these perspectives with the past. However, the landscape and environment have changed so much that it is almost impossible to do so even if it was thought to be worthwhile. Perhaps it is more important to look at functions and see how things have evolved. The fact that a few years after the first version of this book a second edition is published recognises how much has changed and how the scope of public health has developed. This slightly philosophical introduction must therefore begin with an examination of the function of public health and what all this activity is for.

The function of public health is to maintain and improve the health of populations. This is carried out by a series of practitioners but must also include communities themselves, organisations, politicians, individual members of the public, single issue groups, social movements and a whole host of other actors. The first lesson from this book therefore is that restricting action to a few qualified practitioners will have limited value, and this is well illustrated throughout the book.

The second issue is more complex. Is health a means or an end? Does improving the public health mean that all should have 'good' health and if this is to be the case, are there limits? How far do we go to improve the health of each individual, if this is at the expense of others? This is an issue which is touched on in many of the chapters and needs a full consideration. For example, if a pill to reduce obesity becomes available how will it be used, who will get it and who will pay for it? This is not a fanciful vision but one which will happen. Would it not be better to help people to eat less and take exercise than prescribe a pill? This implies of course that evidence exists to support the value of other interventions, hence the crucial issue of the evidence base for developing public health actions. This is a key issue. Politicians, community groups, patients and each of us would like to know how best to tackle lifestyle and socio-economic issues. In several of the chapters, and in one specific chapter, the matter of evidence is dealt with in detail. The need for evidence is urgent if we are to improve the health of those who are disadvantaged, deprived and where inequalities persist.

One of the most interesting issues in the book is the range of topics dealt with. Public health is all pervasive and it touches many aspects of life, if not all, and covers a huge area of public policy. Where are we to find the people with the capability and capacity, and indeed the vision to cover this range of subjects? Part of this must be in conveying to those in training that being involved in public health matters, is exciting, and that change can occur to the health of people and communities. This also means positively encouraging people to join the specialty. Another important issue is to ensure that in the organisation of the public health function, at whatever level in the population, a wide range of skills and expertise is available. This implies the development of teams. It will also mean a sharing of expertise, effective mentoring and working together. This is where leadership matters and this is covered in several chapters.

One issue which is not specifically covered, though is addressed in many parts of the book, is that of ethics. This surely is an area worthy of consideration. Most of the decisions made by practitioners will be related to uncertainty and issues of risk. Most will need to consider the rights of the individual against the needs of the wider public and link these to the duties individuals and groups have to society. Some of these decisions will relate to the allocation of resources and others to issues surrounding legal issues and the curtailing of choice and freedom for some people. The recent, and welcome, ban on smoking in Scotland, and now England and Wales, would be an example of that. However, such judgements are the day-to-day work of the public health practitioner and such professionals need to be clear about the scientific and socio-economic basis of the problem, be able to recognise the moral issue, be able to consider the arguments for and against the ethical dilemma, and have the ability to make decisions and be able to justify them. This is one reason why public health is such a topical and exciting specialty to be involved with. Managing risk and uncertainty at the level of the population is a major responsibility and this book will go a long way to help to prepare effectively all those who have that task.

There are many definitions of public health. My favourite is a simple one. It is any method for improving the quality of life of individuals or populations. What a great thing to be able to do, to help in the process of healing and improving health. It is not easy and it is necessary to show humility and recognise that we do not know all the answers and indeed may be far from achieving our goals; hence the importance of research and development. This is not a sterile activity designed to produce publications or support the research ratings of the academic unit. For public health practitioners it is a fundamental activity to improve health.

Sir Peter Ustinov, when Chancellor at Durham University, used to say that 'doubts unify, certitudes divide'. We need to be open to new ideas, be prepared to doubt, to be curious and always try to improve what we do. If we know we are right, the certitude of Sir Peter, we are likely to miss opportunities and be blind and unresponsive to new ventures and ideas. This is a positive message to all concerned with improving the quality of life; things can and will change if we harness all the energy, skills and expertise which we have for the greater good of others.

Sir Kenneth Calman
Vice-Chancellor
Durham University
August 2006

About the editors

Professor Siân Griffiths OBE, MB BChir, FFPH, FRCP, FHKCCM, FDSRCS(Eng) is currently Professor and Director of the School of Public Health at The Chinese University of Hong Kong. She is the immediate past president of the Faculty of Public Health. Prior to this she was Co-Chair of the Association of Public Health and played a key role in its merger with the Public Health Alliance to create the UK Public Health Association (UKPHA). She has practical experience at local and national level as regional and district Director of Public Health, as well as a long-term commitment to teaching and research. She continues to advise governments on health policy, most notably as adviser on *Choosing Health*, as Co-Chair of the Hong Kong Special Administrative Region (SAR) government's enquiry into the SARS (severe acute respiratory syndrome) epidemic and as a member of the National Health Authority for Qatar. Among national appointments she was a founding Board member of both the Health Protection Agency and the Postgraduate Medical and Education Board. Now based in Hong Kong she is following her interest in public health in China as well as keeping in close touch with her UK roots.

David J Hunter has been Professor of Health Policy and Management at Durham University since 2000. Prior to that he occupied the same chair at the University of Leeds where he was director of the Nuffield Institute for Health from 1989 to 1997. At Durham, he is director of the Centre for Public Policy and Health at the School for Health in the Wolfson Research Institute. David is Chair of the UK Public Health Association and was formerly Co-Chair of the Association of Public Health, one of the organisations which formed the UKPHA. David is a member of various committees, including the Healthcare Commission's Public Health Expert Reference Group, and the National Institute for Health and Clinical Excellence's Research and Scientific Advisory Group. He is a member of the External Advisory Group of the Glasgow Centre for Population Health. David is a special adviser to the World Health Organization and a former Board Director and President of the European Health Management Association. He is the author of several books and numerous journal articles. He is currently writing a book called *Managing for Health* to be published by Routledge. David is an Honorary Member of the Faculty of Public Health and a Fellow of the Royal College of Physicians of Edinburgh.

List of contributors

Fiona Adshead
Deputy Chief Medical Officer, Department of Health

Ken Aswani
General Practitioner, Leytonstone;
NE London PEC Chair, Waltham Forest PCT;
National PEC Chair Lead, NHS Alliance

Helen Bevan
Director of Service Transformation
NHS Institute for Innovation and Improvement, University of Warwick
(formerly, Director of Service Improvement, NHS Modernisation Agency)

Yinglen Butt
Nurse Advisor, Public Health, Department of Health

Anna Coote
Head of Engaging Patients and the Public, Healthcare Commission

Paul Corrigan
Health Adviser to the Prime Minister

Edward Coyle
Consultant in Public Health, National Public Health Service, Wales

Caroline Davey
Policy Manager, Family Planning Association

Peter Donnelly
Deputy Chief Medical Officer, Scottish Executive

Chris Drinkwater
Professor of Primary Care and Head of Centre for Primary and Community Care
Learning, University of Northumbria

Tony Elson
Head of Public Health, Department of Health;
Freelance consultant

Daragh Fahey
Health Improvement Directorate, Department of Health, London

Steve Feast
Clinical Improvement Director (Primary Care), NHS Modernisation Agency

Neil Goodwin
Chief Executive, Greater Manchester Strategic Health Authority

Diane Gray
Consultant in Public Health

Muir Gray
Programmes Director, UK National Screening Committee;
Director of Clinical Knowledge, Process and Safety for the National Programme for IT

Selena Gray
Professor of Public Health, University of the West of England

Scott L Greer
Member of The Constitution Unit, University College London;
Assistant Professor of Health Management and Policy, University of Michigan School of Public Health

Kit Harling
Head of Occupational Health and NHS Plus, Department of Health

Andrew J Hayes
Programme Director, SmokeFree London

Nicholas R Hicks
Director of Public Health, Milton Keynes Primary Care Trust

Lord Hunt of King's Heath
Parliamentary Under Secretary (Lords)
Minister of State, Department for Work and Pensions
Former Parliamentary Under Secretary of State for Health (Lords)

Tony Jewell
Director of Clinical Services and Public Health, Norfolk, Suffolk and Cambridgeshire Strategic Health Authority

Paul Johnstone
Regional Director of Public Health, Yorkshire and Humber Regional Directorate for Public Health

Lionel Joyce OBE
Chair, Mental Health Providers

Michael P Kelly
Director, Centre for Public Health
National Institute for Health and Clinical Excellence

Mark Kroese
Consultant in Public Health Medicine, Public Health Genetics Unit
Cambridge/Greater Peterborough Primary Care Partnership

Tim Lang
Professor of Food Policy, City University London

Paul Lincoln
Chief Executive, National Heart Forum

Mark McCarthy
Professor of Public Health and Honorary Consultant in Public Health Medicine,
University College London

Martin McKee
Professor of European Public Health, London School of Hygiene and Tropical
Medicine

Angus Nicoll
The Health Protection Agency UK and the London School of Hygiene and
Tropical Medicine

Sara Osborne
Director of Policy, British Dental Association

Jean Penny
Head of Learning, NHS Institute for Innovation and Improvement, University of
Warwick
(formerly, Head of Improvement Development, NHS Modernisation Agency)

Rowena Pennycate
Senior Policy Officer, British Dental Association

Geof Rayner
Visiting Research Fellow, City University London

Paul Redgrave
Director of Public Health, Barnsley Primary Care Trust

Harry Rutter
Deputy Director and Head of Impact Assessment, South East Public Health
Observatory

Simon Sanderson
Clinical Lecturer in Primary Care Genetics, University of Cambridge

Allison Thorpe
Networks Development Manager, Thames Valley Strategic Health Authority

Derek Wanless
Author of *Securing Our Future Health: taking a long-term view* and *Securing Good Health for the Whole Population*

Anne Weyman
Director, Family Planning Association

Jane Wilde
Director, Institute of Public Health in Ireland

John Wilkinson
Director, North East Public Health Observatory, Durham University Queen's Campus

Jude Williams
Head of Public Health, Healthcare Commission

Jenny Wright
Director, Public Health Resource Unit, Oxford

Ron Zimmern
Director, Public Health Genetics Unit, Cambridge

Acknowledgements

In undertaking this book, involving so many authors, we have relied greatly on the support of Christine Jawad. We are very grateful to her for all her efforts in liaising with the contributors and publisher. We would not have managed without her.

DJH

I would like to thank my daughter, Allie Chu, for her patience and support as well as invaluable help in preparing the manuscript.

SG

Introduction

Siân Griffiths and David J Hunter

The preventive health services of modern society fight the battle over a wider front and therefore less dramatically than is the case with personal medicine. Yet the victories won by preventive medicine are much the most important for mankind. This is not so only because it is obviously preferable to prevent suffering rather than alleviate it. Preventive medicine, which is merely another way of saying collective action, builds up a system of social habits that constitute an indispensable part of what we mean by civilisation. (Nye Bevan)

The time is now right for action. At the start of the 21st century England needs a new approach to the health of the public, respecting the freedom of individual choice in a diverse, open and more questioning society but also addressing the fact that too many groups have been left behind or ignored. (*Choosing Health*, Secretary of State for Health 2004)

In 1999 when we published the first collection of essays with the title *Perspectives in Public Health* (Griffiths and Hunter 1999) the new Labour government was still in its first flush of enthusiasm. Having been elected in May 1997 following 18 years of Conservative administration, New Labour, as the government came to be known, was impatient to make its mark on public policy, including health. The UK public health community, in the midst of recovering from a turbulent period of almost continuous organisational and managerial change in the running of health services, was hopeful of great things in terms of improving the public's health and moving the policy agenda away from a preoccupation with healthcare and acute care in particular. It was eagerly awaiting publication of what turned out to be the first of two public health white papers Labour would produce – *Saving Lives: our healthier nation* (Secretary of State for Health 1999) – and to greater engagement in the wider determinants of health promoted as a priority by the first Minister for Public Health, Tessa Jowell.

With her arrival and with the support of the Secretary of State for Health, Frank Dobson, a renaissance in public health seemed about to happen. In her Foreword to the first edition, the Minister highlighted the importance of addressing health inequalities: *'health inequality is unacceptable in a civilised society and we must bend our efforts to a long-term haul to reduce them'* (Jowell 1999). She also stressed the key role of partnership: *'the new public health is about partnership and mutual responsibility at all levels of society and between all levels of society – individual, community and national'*. And in stating that the new public health *'is as much about wider socio-economic and environmental policies as it is about those policies that fall within the portfolio of the Department of Health'*, she acknowledged the importance of the cross-government agenda. Indeed, 'joined-up' government was an early theme of the Labour government.

We published the first edition in a spirit of optimism. Were we justified in doing so? What, if anything, has changed? And what about those things that have not changed? As Derek Wanless (2004) observed, we are not short of reports and lofty rhetoric full of good intentions. Since our edited collection appeared, the

1

intervening period has witnessed a steady flow of government reports concerned with, or relevant to, public health together with parliamentary select committee reviews, and an overall increase in media reporting of public health issues all denoting a growing public interest in health. It is now some 8 years after that initial heady mix of optimism and hope and a new future. But perhaps we were expecting too much. While progress has undoubtedly been made, in England (though not elsewhere in the UK) major structural change is once again imposing its burden on the public health system as the National Health Service (NHS) undergoes its third reorganisation since 1997 and its 12th since the first major restructuring in 1974. Specialists are once again buffeted by job insecurity and local communities bemused about how they can engage with shifting structures. Health Action Zones and Healthy Living Centres have been replaced by social marketing and health trainers. Just as the delivery plan for implementing *Choosing Health* was published, the new consultation on primary and social care was announced. It gave rise to a new white paper published in early 2006, *Our Health, Our Care, Our Say: a new direction for community services* (Secretary of State for Health 2006). Avoiding the pitfalls of many government documents it explicitly builds on the legacy of the previous white papers, although many observers are critical of whether it was actually necessary at all. It does not say anything that is not already familiar or part of current policy. For decades, despite periodic attempts, successive governments have failed to bring about the necessary shift in either resources or attitudes. Once again, the white paper acknowledges that the NHS '*which channels people into high-volume, high-cost hospitals – is poorly placed to cope effectively*' with the burden of ill health. The real challenge, as Derek Wanless recognised, remains one of effective implementation and of ensuring that the requisite resources and political commitment exist to enable the desired changes to occur. Without these, this and other white papers will remain largely aspirational and risk going the way of previous attempts to shift the balance from healthcare to health. Maybe it will be different this time with the white paper's assertion that '*there has to be a profound and lasting change of direction*'. But, at the time of going to press, the jury is out.

Our Health, Our Care, Our Say tasks primary care organisations with prevention and health promotion as well as developing community care in its widest aspects. At the same time they are once more embracing the purchaser–provider separation with primary care in the driving seat, albeit using the language of practice-based commissioning. This is against a backdrop of growing social inequalities, especially in respect of the widening income gap between social groups. Continuing social injustice is well documented by, among others, the Institute for Public Policy Research (Paxton and Dixon 2004), which highlights that progress has been faltering, inconsistent and generally disappointing in terms of the pace of change envisaged in the early years. But, as Marmot has commented, this is not entirely surprising since addressing health inequalities is both a long-term initiative and also one which will be achieved through government-wide policy not just health sector action: '*to change social inequalities in life expectancy means both important social changes and translating these differences into changing disease rates*' (Department of Health 2005a). What remains uncertain is the degree to which a government that is in thrall to markets and anxious not to appear as the 'nanny state' is prepared to act tough when it comes to exercising leadership in the pursuit of health goals. Those concerned with improving public health are aware that we need to achieve the step change or paradigm shift that Wanless and others have insisted is essential if we are to make progress towards implementing what he termed *'the fully engaged scenario'* (Wanless 2002, 2004). If weak implementation and delivery have been stumbling blocks in the past they remain so now as the government acknowledged in its second public health white paper, *Choosing Health* (Secretary of State for Health 2004). Indeed, the government seems to share the sense of unease and frustration evident in, and perhaps provoked by, Derek Wanless's trenchant critiques of policy in the area of health as distinct from healthcare. Above all else, it is his reports that have made policy makers sit up and take note. Despite already having a health strategy in the shape of the 1999 white paper, the government used the occasion of the second Wanless report in 2004 to launch a major public consultation on public health and the respective roles of individuals and government in its pursuit. The outcome of this exercise was a new public health white paper published in late 2004 which also reflected a different philosophy concerning the merits or otherwise of government action as opposed to empowering individuals to act for themselves. *Choosing Health* refocused the emphasis on improving health through individual action to make healthier lifestyle choices, tipping the balance away from government-led interventions. In fact, as the two quotes cited at the start of this Introduction nicely illustrate, whereas in its first white paper the government extolled the virtues of healthy public policy with government offering a clear lead, by 2004 the government's thinking about public sector reform in general (not just in health) had moved significantly in the direction of market-style solutions based on the exercise of choice and personal engagement in determining outcomes (Hunter 2005). Government's role is to facilitate the exercise of choice by providing information to enable informed healthier choices to be made. The chapter by Paul Corrigan (Chapter 8), adviser to two health secretaries between 2001 and 2005 and now health adviser to the Prime Minister, offers a clear statement of the government's approach to public service reform which began to emerge during its second term of office.

Many other contributors to this second edition also pick up on these issues in their respective chapters. But a major factor in the lack of progress in advancing public health objectives remains, as in many other parts of the world, a preoccupation with the healthcare sector and its increasing cost. While the government entered office in 1997 committed to delivering a public health policy, it was not long before it inevitably became embroiled in micro-managing the NHS and setting it on a new course. Perhaps inevitably, the government came to the conclusion that the financial and managerial problems plaguing the NHS were of such severity that before it could turn its attention to upstream issues, the modernisation of healthcare downstream had to be the priority during its first term in office. In return for injecting significant sums of new money, the government wanted to be assured, and to reassure the electorate, that the investment would result in real change and not be absorbed by a system that was clearly failing its users. Indeed, the Prime Minister had staked his personal reputation on improving the NHS and ensuring that it was fit for the 21st century. Perhaps inevitably, therefore, the familiar story of hospitals, beds, waiting lists, access to care and budgets all came to dominate the policy agenda both nationally and locally.

It would be wrong to imply there has been insignificant progress in improving health or in developing public health policy. Death rates for coronary heart disease have fallen as services have improved. When primary care trusts (PCTs) were introduced in England in 2002 they were given a clear remit to improve the health of their local communities. Achievement has been patchy largely because the focus of attention from their inception has been on delivering improvements in healthcare provision. Initially the performance management regime and target culture proved to be biased towards achieving gains in the priority areas of reducing waiting lists and strengthening capacity to treat more people quicker. But in the summer of 2004, following the appearance of the second Wanless report, the NHS Chief Executive felt able to say with confidence that the modernisation of the NHS was well underway and with key targets being hit there was now an opportunity for the NHS to lift its gaze and take heed of the wider health landscape and its role in contributing to health improvement (Department of Health 2004). Many PCTs engaged with their local authority and other colleagues to create initiatives which addressed the wider determinants of health such as play spaces, exercise referral and healthy schools initiatives.

But with the NHS in the midst of another major restructuring (*see* below), with familiar financial problems once again looming large as it heads for a deficit approaching £1 billion by the end of the 2005–6 financial year, and with the new investment the NHS has enjoyed in recent years coming to an end in 2008, doubts are being expressed about how far, and for how long, the NHS will truly embrace a public health agenda as opposed to retreating into the familiar territory of acute services – a dilemma Wanless was quick to identify in his first report (Wanless 2002).

Of course not all changes in the profile of public health are the result of planned policy or can even be foreseen or anticipated. Events such as 9/11, the outbreak of SARS (severe acute respiratory syndrome) in 2003, and the devastation of New Orleans following Hurricane Katrina dramatically highlighted the need for national public health infrastructures across the world. As the Institute of Medicine for the US so clearly stated:

> *the glare of a national crisis highlighted the state of the infrastructure with unprecedented clarity to the public and policy makers: outdated and vulnerable technologies; a public health workforce lacking in training and reinforcements; lack of epidemiological systems; ineffective and fragmented communications, incomplete domestic preparedness and emergency response capabilities; communities without access to essential public health services.* (Institute of Medicine 2003, p.3)

These words were echoed in reports following SARS (Naylor, Chantler and Griffiths 2004), acting as the stimulus to review and develop public health systems to be better able to respond not only to crises but to meet the demands of fulfilling *'society's interest in assuring conditions in which people can be healthy'*. In Canada, a new national agency, the Public Health Agency of Canada (www.phac-aspc.gc.ca) has been established with the mission of promoting and protecting the health of Canadians *'through leadership, partnership, innovation and action in public health'*. Stimulated by their experiences, the government in Hong Kong has established the Centre for Health Protection (www.chp.gov.hk). Sweden has also produced a new public health strategy, and Stockholm is to host the new European Observatory on Health Systems and Policies (www.who.dk/observatory).

Addressing inequalities

Internationally, the words may differ but solutions to reducing disparities in health as a result of social and economic differences are sought in many societies. The World Health Organization (Murray *et al.* 2002), Kickbusch (2004, 2005) and Strong *et al.* (2005) have described the gross inequalities between developing and developed nations and the potential of prevention in respect of tackling chronic disease. For example, by the year 2020 there will be nine million deaths caused by tobacco compared to almost five million now; five million deaths attributable to overweight and obesity compared with three million now, many of these in countries with rapidly developing economies such as China. At the same time, 110 million healthy life-years will be lost by underweight children, lower than the current 130 million but still unacceptably high. An estimated 40% of the world's burden of disease is caused by 20 risk factors, many of them preventable (World Health Organization 2002). Underlying factors influencing the disease burden from both communicable and non-communicable disease include the need for clean water and air, food, literacy, and an adequate income. Basic services are still needed in many parts of the world. Three quarters of the world's children are being reached by essential vaccines but only half the children in sub-Saharan Africa have access to basic immunisation against common diseases such as measles, tuberculosis (TB), tetanus and whooping cough. In poor and isolated areas of developing countries only 1 in 20 children may be reached. In contrast, parents in the UK have the luxury of debating the science and evidence of the MMR (measles, mumps and rubella) vaccine and its attendant risks. Faced with these challenges, public health cannot merely sit on the sidelines and observe and commentate but must engage in positive action.

Notwithstanding our earlier comments on the lack of sustained attention accorded public health, important progress on raising its profile and developing policies to address inequalities has been made across the UK. In line with the early commitment of the new government in 1997, the prominence of inequalities as a major national health issue has been addressed through mainstream policy. The independent inquiry into health inequalities by Sir Donald Acheson published in 1998 made 40 recommendations ranging from poverty, income, tax and benefits, education and employment to mothers, children and families and ethnicity (Acheson 1998). Indeed, only three were specifically concerned with the NHS thereby illustrating the breadth of both the problem and the policy response required. The English health strategy *Saving Lives: our healthier nation* (Secretary of State for Health 1999) and the accompanying report *Reducing Health Inequalities: an action report* (Department of Health 1999) appeared in July 1999. While *Saving Lives* emphasises the need to focus on major threats to health and to engage individuals, communities and governments in improving health, the action report set out what was needed to address the inequalities through actions across government to tackle the underlying causes of ill health, including socio-economic factors. Building on these reports, prevention and inequalities were put firmly on the agenda in the *NHS Plan* (Department of Health 2000) which set out expectations of the NHS both in terms of service delivery and expectations of partnership working by the NHS with, and through, other agencies. Local targets for reducing health inequalities were set and then underpinned further by the creation of national health targets. The strategy laid out in *Tackling Health Inequalities: a programme for action* (Department of Health 2003) targeted resources to:

- supporting families, mothers and children
- engaging communities and individuals
- preventing illness and providing effective treatment and care
- addressing the underlying determinants of health.

Progress on these targets will be monitored through the government-wide public service agreement (PSA) targets which were agreed in the 2004 Spending Review and which expect action and progress in reducing geographical inequalities in life expectancy, cancer, heart disease, stroke and related diseases. Faster progress in reducing the gap is expected in the most deprived fifth of areas with the worst health and deprivation indicators. They receive extra resources based upon local authority areas that are in the bottom fifth nationally for three or more of five indicators:

- male life expectancy at birth
- female life expectancy at birth
- cancer mortality rate in under-75s
- cardiovascular disease mortality rate in under-75s
- Index of Multiple Deprivation 2004 (local authority summary).

These indicators help them tackle the many wide-ranging factors that need to be addressed but the challenge of reducing inequalities is not to be underestimated. Without commitment at all levels and at all strata inequalities will persist.

Developing capacity

Another area in which there has been progress is in the infrastructure of public health. Multidisciplinary specialist practice was given impetus by *Saving Lives: our healthier nation*. The specialist public health profession has moved forward and specialist skills are now becoming competency based, and dependent on ability rather than on a designated professional qualification. Directors of Public Health (DsPH) no longer need to be medically qualified and nor is professional development confined to the NHS. Yet, as we have already described, one of the problems facing public health delivery is that the public health workforce is continually under threat, or in the throes, of structural change. Indeed, at the time of writing and in little under 2 years since its last major reorganisation, the NHS is facing another period of major upheaval and organisational churn. Whatever the merits of the outcomes of such engineering, they come at a heavy price in terms of staff morale and an increasingly disenchanted and disengaged workforce. The price paid is high in terms of a diversion of managerial energy and effort from dealing with the direction of the organisation and its outcomes to its internal operations and processes. Arguably, such organisational rejigging amounts to a huge distraction from the business of securing improved health. In an atmosphere of constant change – a feature of the NHS since 1974 which has intensified in recent years with shorter periods between major changes – it becomes extremely difficult to plan and achieve objectives, especially those in public health which generally have a long lead time to prove themselves. The partnerships necessary across many professions and organisations need a stable environment to succeed and these become more vulnerable if personnel and organisations change frequently. The nature of the position of the Director of Public Health (DPH), for example, means he or she is closely associated with managing and organising healthcare services and since the management structures seem to be in constant, rapid evolution if not revolution there are inevitable effects on jobs and careers and on the stability of the partnerships they are expected to nurture and work within. This instability leads us once again to call for a public health system (Griffiths, Jewell and Donnelly 2005) which places the health of populations at its heart rather than the structural demands of the English healthcare system. Examples from the Celtic countries making up the rest of the UK demonstrate the benefits of stability and also recognise, rather than pay lip service to, the strengths of networks and clearly identified expertise, as described in Chapters 1, 3 and 4. The commitment in *Our Health, Our Care, Our Say* to redefining and strengthening the role of DsPH and the support for joint appointments between primary care organisations and local government is welcome although we urgently need evidence on whether the introduction of joint posts is effective. The signs are promising but, at present, there is only anecdotal evidence to support such a move. If it can be demonstrated that joint posts are an important means to secure lasting change across organisational boundaries, then such support needs to be translated into action. It will be important to ensure, too, that the important progress made in opening up PCT DPH appointments to non-clinicians is preserved in future when there will be far fewer PCTs in existence.

But can we learn from constant change? In 1998 the structure of the English public health system was based on a network with regional and district nodes. Ninety district health authorities had DsPH with departments of ranging strengths and sizes, linked to university departments in various ways and collected into regional units. The sudden announcement of *Shifting the Balance of Power in the NHS* (Department of Health 2001a) by the then health secretary, Alan Milburn, in April 2001 led to the rapid dissolution of these departments without a clear plan for the future delivery of public health in the newly proposed PCTs. It was over 6 months before the acting Minister of Public Health, Lord Hunt, a good friend of public health, announced in his November speech to the Faculty of Public Health (Department of Health 2001b) that it was proposed there should be a DPH for each of the 300 PCTs and that such individuals would not be required to be medically qualified. It represented a breakthrough for the wider public health and a recognition of the skills of those working in public health from backgrounds other than medicine.

> *The engine of public health delivery will be at the front line around the primary care trust. Every primary care trust will have a director of public health and support team. These directors of public health will be board level appointments working at the heart of the new organisations. The focus of their activity will be on local neighbourhoods and communities leading and driving programmes to improve health and reduce inequalities. They will also play a powerful role in forging partnerships with, and influencing, all local agencies to ensure the widest possible participation in the health and health care agenda.*

> *The director of public health will not be a remote, strategic figure – she or he will be well known, respected and credible with local people – particularly those in the most deprived communities, local authorities, general practitioners and other local clinicians.*

A new wider role for regional public health was envisaged shifting the focus from the NHS to influencing the wider determinants such as environment, housing, transport and employment. To quote the Hunt speech again:

> *The new role of the regional director of public health is an exciting one. They will be uniquely placed to address the wider determinants of health in their regions, working with other government departments and local strategic partnerships. They will also have a lead role for health protection and will have some responsibilities in relation to the NHS, accounting for these links to the new regional directors of health and social care.*

Confusion remained about how this would work out, particularly since the public health role at strategic health authorities was left unclear and the regional responsibilities in the health system somewhat confused. To further confound the capacity problems of extending the specialist profession in this welcome but unplanned way, the Chief Medical Officer's (CMO) report, *Getting Ahead of the Curve*, was published in January 2002 (Department of Health 2002), proposing the establishment of the Health Protection Agency (HPA) in April 2003. Stimulated by events such as 9/11 and outbreaks of new diseases such as Ebola and West Nile Fever and the risk of an avian flu pandemic, the strategy proposed the creation of a new national agency to combine responsibility for communicable disease control and services to protect people's health from infectious diseases, poisons, chemical and radiation hazards. While the creation of the HPA undoubtedly adds to the strength of the public health infrastructure, it further highlights the capacity problems of the public health community. Public health specialists in health protection are no longer employed and working alongside their generalist colleagues in the local NHS public health departments, thereby increasing fragmentation and stretching already scarce resources. Inevitably, tensions have resulted in some localities, overcome through good will, common sense and high-quality professional practice supported by local agreements or memoranda.

Continual change is not reserved for local level practice. At national level, new structures created in one white paper have been changed by the next – for example, the Health Development Agency (HDA) established in *Saving Lives* was merged into the National Institute for Health and Clinical Excellence (NICE) in *Choosing Health* (Secretary of State of Health 2004). But such changes are not unique to public health. The Healthcare Commission was no sooner established, having replaced the Commission for Health Improvement, than it was told it would be joining with the Social Care Inspectorate. The Modernisation Agency, Leadership Centre and NHS University proposed in the NHS Plan have metamorphosed into the NHS Institute for Innovation and Improvement. The upside of recent change is the inclusion of public health in the mainstream and its place near the top of the health policy agenda. The downside is the anxiety about the capacity to deliver while absorbing the ever-changing roles, structures and expectations.

But capacity can be increased not just by more of the same but by working differently – a clear lesson to emerge from the Modernisation Agency and Leadership Centre. The NHS and local government sectors are now working much more closely together, utilising tools such as local planning mechanisms and common targets. The boundaries are increasingly blurred between local government and the NHS with new opportunities for developing models of co-commissioning and co-delivery and for joint appointments of DsPH between local authorities and primary care organisations. This model of joint posts, universal in Wales, is generally welcomed if it allows the true nature of multidisciplinary public health to be developed. Joint working with Regional Development Agencies and Regional Government Offices at regional level offers opportunities to promote health through tackling the wider determinants. The increasing focus on health is also reflected in healthcare organisations with a requirement that they take public health seriously. However, these new ways of working raise not only a capacity issue but a capability one. Public health practitioners, wherever they are located, require the necessary skills for working in complex and often highly political organisational contexts. It is arguable whether the appropriate leadership and management development skills have been provided in sufficient quantity and quality to equip people to take on the new jobs in public health. Indeed, many practitioners feel ill-equipped for the tasks expected of them (Brocklehurst *et al.* 2005; Hunter and Goodwin 2004). However, there are signs that these deficits are both recognised by the Department of Health and being addressed (Hannaway, Plsek and Hunter 2005).

Another area of weakened practice under review is the academic sector, particularly its relationship with service public health. While joint working between the NHS and academia is recognised as essential, collaboration between academic and service public health remains problematic in many areas. Local issues perceived as relevant to primary care organisations may be inappropriate areas for academic departments who are often involved in work related to national and international priorities with their greater value in the Research Assessment Exercise which drives the priorities and policies of universities. Moves are now being made to redress this tension through developing mutual understanding and engagement in the national health research strategy (Department of Health 2005b).

In compiling this second edition of *Perspectives*, we have sought to reflect these and other contemporary themes and issues in UK public health. Much of the contribution is England focused but we believe that most of the issues raised here are generic to public health systems elsewhere. We have sought to include coverage of recent structures, policy and practice. We invited each of the chapter authors to reflect on recent history, to identify current issues, and to highlight challenges for the future. We have not sought to produce a totally inclusive volume covering all aspects and angles of public health – but the themes selected will enable the reader to gain a sense not only of current public health issues but of progress over the last few years and future challenges. We have not repeated Ashton's historical account from Liverpool (Jowell 1999). Instead, we open the book with a lecture given there by Sir Derek Wanless. Some authors have updated their previous contributions; others are new. We hope we have succeeded in our objective of providing a new perspective in public health that both updates the first edition and shows how ways of thinking about public health, especially the focus on individuals and choice, have caused shifts in policy that were certainly not fully anticipated in the late 1990s.

References

Acheson D (1998) *Independent Inquiry into Inequalities in Health*. London: The Stationery Office.

Brocklehurst NJ, Hook G, Bond M and Goodwin S (2005) Developing the public health practitioner workforce in England: lessons from theory and practice. *Public Health*. **119** (11): 995–1002.

Department of Health (1999) *Reducing Health Inequalities: an action report*. London: The Stationery Office.

Department of Health (2000) *The NHS Plan: a plan for investment, a plan for reform.* Cm 4818. London: HMSO.

Department of Health (2001a) *Shifting the Balance of Power in the NHS.* Speech by Alan Milburn, Secretary of State for Health, 25 April 2001.

Department of Health (2001b) *The Future of Public Health.* Speech by Lord Hunt to Faculty of Public Health Medicine, 13 November 2001.

Department of Health (2002) *Getting Ahead of the Curve: action to strengthen the microbiology function in the prevention and control of infectious diseases.* London: Department of Health.

Department of Health (2003) *Tackling Health Inequalities: a programme for action.* London: Department of Health.

Department of Health (2004) *Caring in Many Ways. The NHS Modernisation Board's Annual Report 2004.* London: Department of Health.

Department of Health (2005a) *Tackling Health Inequalities: status report on the programme for action.* London: Department of Health.

Department of Health (2005b) *Best Research for Best Health: a new national health research strategy.* London: Department of Health.

Griffiths S and Hunter DJ (eds) (1999) *Perspectives in Public Health.* Oxford: Radcliffe Medical Press.

Griffiths S, Jewell T and Donnelly P (2005) *Public Health in Practice: the three domains of public health. Public Health.* **119**: 907–13.

Hannaway C, Plsek P and Hunter DJ (2005) *Framework for the Leadership for Health Improvement Programme.* York: North East Yorkshire and North Lincolnshire Strategic Health Authority.

Hunter DJ (2005) Choosing or losing health? *Journal of Epidemiology and Community Health.* **59** (12): 1010–12.

Hunter DJ and Goodwin N (2004) Public health – coming of age. *Public Health News.* **21 May**: 8–9.

Institute of Medicine (2003) *The Future of the Public's Health in the 21st Century.* Washington DC: The National Academies Press.

Jowell T (1999) Foreword. In: S Griffiths and DJ Hunter (eds) *Perspectives in Public Health.* Oxford: Radcliffe Medical Press.

Kickbusch I (2004) The end of public health as we know it: constructing global public health in the 21st century. *Public Health.* **118** (10): 463–9.

Kickbusch I (2005) Action on global health: addressing global health governance challenges. *Public Health.* **119** (11): 969–73.

Murray C *et al.* (2002) *World Mortality in 2000 – tables for 191 countries.* Geneva: World Health Organization.

Naylor CD, Chantler C and Griffiths S (2004) Learning from SARS in Hong Kong and Toronto. *JAMA.* **291**(20): 2483–7.

Paxton P and Dixon M (2004) *The State of the Nation: an audit of injustice in the UK.* London: Institute for Public Policy Research.

Secretary of State for Health (1999) *Saving Lives: our healthier nation.* Cm 4386. London: HMSO.

Secretary of State for Health (2004) *Choosing Health: making healthier choices easier.* Cm 6374. London: The Stationery Office.

Secretary of State for Health (2006) *Our Health, Our Care, Our Say: a new direction for community services.* Cm 6737. London: The Stationery Office.

Strong K, Mathers C, Leeder S and Beaglehole R (2005) Preventing chronic diseases: how many lives can we save? *The Lancet.* 5 October.

Wanless D (2002) *Securing Our Future Health: taking a long-term view. Final report.* London: HM Treasury.

Wanless D (2004) *Securing Good Health for the Whole Population. Final report.* London: HM Treasury/Department of Health.

World Health Organization (2002) *The World Health Report 2002 – reducing risks, promoting healthy life.* Geneva: World Health Organization.

Setting the agenda for public health

Derek Wanless

Sir Derek Wanless has been a major influence on the direction of health policy in general and public health development in particular through his two major reports to government. Since 2002 he has become a critical and valued friend to public health. His analysis leads him to stress the need for a step change in practice, involving a revolutionary not evolutionary approach. His chapter synthesises the key elements of his reports and gives a critique of the response by government as set out in Choosing Health. His message is both clear and unequivocal – there is no need for further analysis and policy but for action at both government and individual levels. Action needs to be taken in a long list of areas which include an increase in the capacity of the skilled workforce, in self-care, in the engagement of healthcare professionals in preventive approaches. Workplaces, both within the NHS and across other sectors, need to focus on improving the health of their employees. This is not just an agenda for government but for individuals, and efforts are needed to improve health literacy and develop social marketing. Primary care organisations and their local public health consultants/specialists need to be engaged in ensuring local engagement particularly with local government partners, with whom coterminosity is desirable. New organisations such as NICE face a challenging agenda. Better use of information technology and enhanced research to promote evidence of cost-effective interventions are urgently needed along with better management of prevention.

My report for government in 2004 opened with a quote from Dr Elizabeth Blackwell. Born in 1821, she was our first woman doctor and she caught the spirit I wanted to convey. *'We are not tinkers'*, she said, *'who merely patch and mend what is broken … We must be watchmen, guardians of the life and health of our generation, so that stronger and more able generations may come after'* (Wanless 2004).

Now is a fascinating time for public health, full of opportunity but also of danger that the opportunity will be missed. To capitalise successfully on the opportunity will be complex, requiring patience to do the groundwork for the substantial shifts needed to build a physically and mentally healthier population in the UK.

There are vital roles for government – national and local – in public health across many major determinants of health. But what we do not need is simply a list of frenetic and uncoordinated short-term activity, which can be stopped as easily and quickly as it began. Rather, we need sustained, coordinated and well-evaluated efforts which will make a difference to the population's health.

My first report for the Treasury in 2002 sought to answer the question: 'what resources will be needed in 20 years' time to provide high quality health services in the UK?' (Wanless 2002).

Taking as a starting point a vision of what we thought people might want and the UK might need, we consulted widely, received strong support, and then drew up three scenarios to capture some significant uncertainties.

- *Slow uptake* – which was a very unattractive view of the future where little changed from the UK's historic path.
- *Solid progress* – which essentially meant succeeding with announced plans while enhancing productivity. Life expectancy was assumed to improve to 80.0 for men by 2022 and 83.8 for women.
- *Fully engaged* – which assumed further life expectancy improvements (81.6 and 85.5 for men and women) and significant further improvement in levels of engagement in prevention. For example, smoking by 2010 was assumed to fall to 17% of adults, against 27% and 24% in the other two, less-attractive scenarios. These were not marginal shifts.

What was the state of healthcare in 2001? Compared with many other developed countries in terms of outcomes, the UK was not doing well. This was understandable given the history of relative under-investment demonstrated by too few doctors, nurses and other professionals, too many old and inappropriate buildings and late and slow adoption of medical technologies. On the positive side, there was scope for more productive use of resources, particularly by more appropriate use of ICT (information and communications technology), further skill-mix shifts and better use of money and information flows to enhance decision making at delivery level. We consulted on a range of issues (*see* Box A).

Box A Key issues from consultation and analysis

- Patients would want more choice in future, although the immediate issue was access to services.
- There was a desire for choice in non-clinical issues rather than in clinical matters.
- Ageing was an important factor driving up healthcare costs though not the main factor over the coming two decades.
- The main pressures were forecast to be medical technologies, including drug costs, and the costs, direct and indirect, of more staff.
- Primary care would play a proportionately bigger role.
- Productivity rates and the success of prevention were major uncertainties.

To cost health services in 2022, we needed to capture some major uncertainties, in particular how successful we will be in preventing ill health and in improving productivity of our use of resources.

In all three scenarios, we concluded that significantly more money was needed. However, money would not solve the problems without radical reform. The three scenarios we modelled illustrated the huge prize to be gained from higher productivity on the supply of health services, and from greater public engagement and healthier lifestyles on the demand side.

The 'C' word that dominated the first report was *capacity* rather than choice! Without adequate capacity, much of the debate about options, about the possible pace of change, and about the practical implementation of opening up choice cannot in practice be contemplated.

The headline-grabbing conclusion in 2002 was that the difference in spending between the worst scenario – 'slow uptake' – and the best – 'fully engaged' – was £30 billion per year in 2022. Not, as often claimed by overzealous public health practitioners and by lazy journalists, £30 billion from prevention but £30 billion from better prevention and higher productivity.

The first report encouraged government to think more about healthcare system standards and the processes it controlled. The second report, published in early 2004, looked at public health and in particular sought to address the question: 'How could we get on track for the "fully engaged" scenario?' It set out essential changes in approach if we want to move towards full engagement. It requires high productivity in public health as well as healthcare; adequate workforce capacity, with appropriately broad skill mixes expanded by self-care and imaginative use of the knowledge and time of patients and of those with particular risks; revolutions in the use of technology and information handling; redirection of resource to areas of proven effectiveness; enhanced research programmes; and better measurement tools. The report sought to put forward recommendations which would enable the key determinants of our future health to be tackled. They were by no means all for government. And they were not intended to be a 'pick and mix' list but an attempt to tackle all the most important reasons for our past failures.

The existing definition of public health – *'the science and art of preventing disease, prolonging life and promoting health through the organised efforts of society'* – seemed to me inappropriately narrow. It may well be valid where protection at a population level is what we need and where much of the great public health of the past has its focus. But it fails to describe what *preventive* public health should become in the early 21st century.

The definition should be debated and changed to include the need to operate not simply through 'the organised efforts of society' but rather 'through the organised efforts and informed choices of society, organisations, public and private, communities and individuals', recognising that population health is primarily affected at present by issues and organisations outside the health sector. As the 2004 white paper, *Choosing Health*, states:

> Public health was often seen as something that was done to the population, for their own good, by impersonal and distant forces in Whitehall and the public bodies and professionals that it directed, with varying degrees of success.
> (Secretary of State for Health 2004)

Examining smoking, obesity, salt consumption, physical activity and health inequalities illustrated the conceptual muddle. We found inconsistencies in ambition, realism and timescales in the setting of targets. From back of the envelope over a weekend to wild ambition based on dubious international comparators. For none of the major determinants did the target-setting process encourage a belief that resource management was remotely near optimal. No wonder targets historically have not helped to mobilise engagement.

We *do* need national objectives – short and medium term – for all the major determinants. To inform resource planning and priority setting and to drive action, to enable us to measure progress, and to feed back new knowledge and information.

Research, analytic thinking and consensus building are needed. Sub-groups – for example children, ethnic groups and the economically deprived – will often need separate objectives.

I concluded that public health objectives require more ambition if we are to become 'fully engaged' and that the white paper would need to show how objectives, plans, budgets and research programmes would be ratcheted up to a different level in order to create an irreversible momentum for change.

Public health targets set in 2004 after I reported still appear tentative and not adequately ambitious to be considered 'fully engaged'. Nor is there transparency in the process by which they were reached. Objectives for all the key determinants should be based on independent advice, medical and managerial, and that advice should be published.

Government should fix the objectives to help mobilise activity by many types of organisation, public and private, national and local. It is locally that the design of networks to tackle local issues will happen. National objectives should inform local decisions but should not lead to the imposition of centrally calculated targets on local organisations. Passing out smoking cessation targets to PCTs has probably been the worst example of that sort. We need better management than that.

Local networks know best their own local problems, priorities and complex trade-offs. Much planning and delivery will be local, for example in tackling activity levels or availability of healthy foods; national action, such as resource allocation and the design of financial and information flows, objective setting, performance management and audit, must not distort decision making nor cause unjustifiable spending to achieve marginal gain. Crude bureaucratic administrative systems corrode professionalism but well-coordinated and directed central efforts can add value.

We have failed in the past, too, because the evidence base about cost-effectiveness is so weak. Lack of funding of public health intervention research has contributed; so has very slow acceptance of economic perspectives within public health; so has the lack of a clear, coherent set of government priorities for research. The future research programme will be technically very demanding and will require greater resource and greater expertise and depth in core disciplines. I called on the government to tell us how such a research programme will be delivered. The white paper increases central funding for public health research from April 2006 and establishes a welcome new public health research initiative backed by projects focusing on effective health interventions and the National Prevention Research Initiative.

We have also failed because of the related problems about the adequacy and usefulness of the information base; often it is not telling us in sufficient detail what is happening or why.

All those thinking about use of resources need to have access to, and understand, a consistent cost-effectiveness framework. Such a framework would allow the comparison of the cost-effectiveness of different public health interventions within and across both risk factors and disease areas, including those directed towards the wider determinants of health. It would be most useful if there were to be substantially enhanced information, nationally and locally.

Meanwhile, the need for action is too pressing to allow a lack of comprehensive evidence to excuse inertia. Activity underway, albeit haphazard, should help build the evidence base quickly. It must be drawn into a comprehensive research programme with an agreed framework for evaluation. The sound me being developed by NICE should be the base, forcing consideration of benefits (exceptionally difficult to assess, partly because they are so difficult to conceptualise) and introducing techniques to involve 'real' people in making difficult assessments of value. NICE has done that well. The decision to abolish the Health Development Agency (HDA) and put its functions into NICE was risky. It threatens both to slow down NICE's traditional work at a time when that work also needs expansion, and to disrupt the useful work the HDA had underway. Nor should it produce public health assessments even more skewed towards clinical care. The need for a long-term view in assessing benefits is crucial, as is the rate of discount. QALYs (quality-adjusted life years) are a good sensible start but the quality component must reflect people's views.

The announcement of an Executive Director for Health Improvement by NICE and additional resources for NICE are a start but there is a lot to be done to deliver the necessary service to sufficient quality and volume.

There are roles for government and its agencies nationally. Only they can set national objectives, create the framework, use economic instruments and allocate resources. They can ensure information is adequate and good practice is shared. They need to get feedback from the population and to ensure that a research strategy and the capacity to undertake it are there.

But much action needs to be local. The white paper agrees. It makes the commitment that local authorities and PCTs will have more flexibility to develop local targets through local partnerships in response to local needs. Local area agreements (LAAs) will be piloted in 21 areas and PCTs will develop targets to meet the needs of people in their area that are agreed with local partners to help us meet national targets. The words read well but all who work locally will need to ensure they become much more than words.

In the past, capacity problems, the impact of repeated organisational changes and the lack of alignment of performance-management systems have limited achievement. PCTs have spread resources thinly yet are vital in making new mechanisms – such as new contracts – work to advantage rather than becoming a bureaucratic nightmare and a diversion away from sound professionalism towards opportunistic point-scoring.

Our well-developed network of primary care providers could provide a unique resource for evaluation and health promotion. If the NHS is to be 'the best insurance policy in the world', it must start to think like an insurance company and manage risks.

Pooling of resources between PCTs and local authorities should be closely reviewed to see if it produces the expected benefits. Coterminosity should be examined carefully to see if it brings benefits. The white paper promises to give PCTs the means to tackle health inequalities and improve health through funding to give greater priority to areas of high health need and it promises development of new tools to help PCTs and local authorities jointly plan services and check on progress. So again there are some useful promises but it will be necessary to make sure they are followed through and that the research lessons are identified and learnt for everyone's benefit.

Workforce capacity planning needs much more attention, including assessment of the significant skill shifts needed. It must develop to encompass the wider public health workforce and the social care workforce. Planning this, and delivering the accreditation likely to be required, is a massive task. It will need to incorporate new types of advisory and support roles and must include recognition of the need to create effective teams capable of sharing and using information.

There is, in one respect, a crucial gap in related government policy. Failure to integrate thinking about healthcare and social care is a massive weakness which must be tackled. All work in this area is incomplete without it. However, it will open up difficult issues about choice and funding and it will throw an even sharper focus on the role of local authorities. All involved should use their various influences to encourage integrated thinking and use their experience to inform the thinking when it happens.

The capacity planning will need to take a long-term view, taking into account the way delivery is likely to develop; for example, as primary care transforms. The opportunity which is opening up to consider what primary care should become over the next couple of decades must be taken. How will knowledge of genetic make-up and of individual risk assessment influence personalised health promotion and disease prevention?

Information technology (IT) will drive change, and marketing techniques will be facilitated and will find their place. A key message is: 'Bring in the marketing professionals.' Beware in the future the way medical models have tended to dominate in the recent past. Again there are hopeful signs. My own instinct, for example, is that the recent smoking adverts concentrating on the psychological problems of quitting are more likely to have an impact on key audiences than the medically orientated adverts of the past. But the lack of good information bases and the inability yet to mobilise modern communication techniques mean that obvious tricks are being missed.

Huge commitments being made to improve technology will have, as part of their justification, identification of personalised risk profiles. But also government must address the threat to public health research arising from the difficulty of obtaining access to data. Debate is needed about the balance between individual confidentiality and the public policy benefit of enhanced knowledge.

A well-structured pilot in the provision of personalised risk management and prevention could pay huge dividends in teaching us what works. But a revolutionary and not an evolutionary approach is called for. So far, instead, we have, for example, loose proposals for personal trainers, which do not seem well rooted in evidence or particularly clearly thought through. They will have to prove they are effective and not gimmickry. If they are seen that way, they will not survive and will discredit the public health function.

Primary care will only be one support. Many organisations need to be shown the business case, the self-interest, in helping their employees, members, insurees and so on to engage. The potential for employers to help their employees engage is under-used. Some examples are emerging. 'Investors in health', for example, is a concept with a chance of catching on.

I said in my report that the NHS as an employer should be showing the way. It is very welcome to see the white paper set out what the NHS will do to become a 'model employer'. There are 1.3 million people following that commitment closely and they should make sure it is delivered.

Private sector organisations can help too by creating and developing markets to deliver products and services which will be built taking full account of individuals' preferences, their choices. Individuals' concerns about their and their families' future health will change their buying patterns. Such organisations work in the long term not just by pushing product but by recognising the pull from customers. They should be encouraged not vilified.

Government's role extends across all departments. A Cabinet member, the Secretary of State for Health in my view, should ensure action across government is having its public health impact assessed and that coordinated action is tackling the wide-ranging objectives for the determinants of health. We must do better than those limited assessments in the past, for example of agricultural or built environment policies, which have led to situations so difficult to resolve, even in the long term.

It is necessary to correct systemic, socio-economic failures in public health which influence decision making at the individual level. These include a lack of information about preventive action across the population, the inability of individuals always to take account of the wider costs to society of their behaviours, and failures in the social and environmental context which contribute to poor health and to health inequalities.

Information failures are understandable. Much health information is ultimately about probabilities and risks. It is scientific and difficult to digest and people's understanding of risk may be inadequate to assess options. Their 'health literacy' may not be sufficiently well developed. Those seeking to change people's behaviour need to ask regularly whether their messages have reached the public. Indeed, have they always reached the health professionals?

Health literacy is an important precondition for success. The language used and the medium must be right. Research should regularly be undertaken to identify what forms of intervention best improve health literacy and how messages should be targeted at sub-groups, including those with low health literacy, where the prevalence of chronic diseases is often high.

People's understanding of the health and social consequences, both costs and benefits, of their behaviour needs to be considered by policy makers on the evidence available. Each individual has primary responsibility for their own and their children's health. But many need help. Given the failures outlined, individuals are often not living in circumstances which encourage healthy behaviour. Interventions will generally be needed if we are to reach the outcomes sought. Those objectives need to be set and reset on a regular basis as successes and failures become apparent, here and internationally, and as the value of behaviour changes becomes clearer. There needs to be continual reassessment of how far 'fully engaged' can go. What will be acceptable and achievable? 'Fully engaged' will ultimately need to mean the maximum attainable shift in behaviour and attitudes.

The report suggests principles to govern the government's choice of actions to determine when its various levers, information or taxation or subsidies or regulation or deregulation might be justified to help individuals make informed choices; not, generally, to impose choice but rather to inform choice and to encourage changes which make healthy choices easier. Those principles, I said, should also govern government's actions to help overcome the lack of information and confusion of messages, for example in food labelling; to check whether messages have been received, believed and understood; to ensure people take account of the wider costs of their behaviours; to help shift social norms, a legitimate activity for a government when it has worked through and gained commitment for objectives for behaviour change; to find out what works at acceptable cost, even those programmes which worsen inequalities in isolation provided they are accompanied by programmes addressing the resulting inequalities; and to report on progress annually. The white paper commitment from 2006, through the public health observatories, to publish new reports for local communities and a national composite report will help, provided the reports are tailored to their users.

Leadership will be the difference between success and failure. Recognising that individuals are ultimately responsible for their own and their children's health but they need information and support. And their right to choose does need to be balanced against any adverse impacts those choices have on the quality of life of others. In our society, strong, persuasive leadership is most likely to be effective, nationally and locally, by establishing aggressive goals, building widespread consensus, encouraging action by the self-interested as well as by the community conscious and driving through voluntary engagement. And powerful feedback from local deliverers needs to be heard, loud and clear, by all those fixing national policy, resource and information planning. Public health practitioners must make their voices heard.

I was pleased that the government reacted to my report with its consultation and a white paper. The consultation period gave an opportunity to build consensus and shared priorities for action. That and the white paper are welcome but certainly not in themselves enough to guarantee success. As the white paper states:

> *The time is now right for action. At the start of the 21st century, England needs a new approach to the health of the public. Respecting the freedom of individual choice in a diverse, open and more questioning society but also addressing the fact that too many groups have been left behind or ignored.*

My report was designed to establish a checklist against which the government's responses can be judged. There is, in summary, much to applaud in the white paper. My judgement is that most of the recommendations have survived and have chances of being taken forward. The issue for me in the white paper's plans is pace and, longer term, the issues will be persistence, rigour and the need for continued commitment to local solutions in local situations. There are too many signs of tentative attitudes and a lack of openness or logic to give either full confidence or an unequivocal welcome. A crucial element still not well enough developed is the assessment of the value of outcomes.

But, just as the government's response to my report can be judged and debated, so can the responses of all those others who have parts to play if we are to achieve the prize of full engagement. And what *is* clear is that a 'fully engaged' solution does lie in many hands.

References

Secretary of State for Health (2004) *Choosing Health: making healthier choices easier.* Cm 6374. London: The Stationery Office.

Wanless D (2002) *Securing Our Future Health: taking a long-term view. Final report.* London: HM Treasury.

Wanless D (2004) *Securing Good Health for the Whole Population. Final report.* London: HM Treasury/Department of Health.

Part I

The UK, Europe and international

Introduction

Our first edition was published before the impact of devolution on UK public health. In this edition we have asked five authors to comment on country-specific public health issues and developments, and Scott Greer to comment on a UK perspective. Mark McCarthy describes the European dimension, and Martin McKee highlights some of the global issues facing public health.

For Scotland, devolution has provided opportunities to introduce primary legislation on important public health issues. The Scottish Parliament has had the freedom to lead on changing legislation to ban smoking in public places and to promote breastfeeding as well as initiate protection for sex workers through zones of tolerance. Open discussion within the Scottish Parliament has promoted democratic discussion, underpinned by the Scottish Executive's strategy of focusing on health in early years, during teenage transition, health in the workplace and community development. The strong public sector ethos and structural stability of public health within Scotland has also promoted a climate in which public health is integral to decision making by health boards supported by national structures.

In England it is, however, a less stable story. In contrast to Scotland, constant change in organisational structures and national bodies is once again destabilising the public health delivery system. This is not to deny the policy progress in the last 5 years in developing a greater public health presence at national and local levels across health-sector policy. The understanding of the impact of socio-economic determinants on health, the importance of addressing health inequalities, the Wanless reports, and the most recent white paper, *Choosing Health*, are all testament to an increasing mainstream presence. However, shifting structures amid the introduction of payment by results, practice-based commissioning, patient choice, the reintroduction of the commissioner–provider separation, and the complexities of plurality of provision, including foundation trusts, could either contribute to or, as critics believe, undermine some of the progress in developing joint work with local authorities. Progress such as joint appointments of Directors of Public Health and developing a multidisciplinary specialist profession needs to be nurtured as does the focus on local performance management against national standards which are now inclusive of public health.

Wales has taken a different route again, and the development of the National Public Health System supported by the Wales Centre for Health is a model which is being closely observed across the UK. Welsh public health heroes such as Archie Cochrane and Julian Tudor Hart remind us of the importance of research for effective interventions and the need to seek solutions to challenges posed by, for example, the industrial legacy of high levels of permanent sickness in the valleys. Although the Welsh Assembly does not have the autonomy of the Scottish Parliament there is a distinctive feel to Welsh public health policy, focusing as it does on a systematic approach to community-wide action. Coterminosity with local government has helped to underpin the population base.

Jane Wilde's chapter reminds us of the progress being made in Ireland. While the Republic of Ireland and Northern Ireland are two separate structures for government, administration, finance, healthcare systems and priorities, the Institute of Public Health straddles the two entities as a unifying force for public health. Recent history underscores the importance of political leadership and the increasing climate of cooperation and stability. North and South are now learning and sharing together how best to address the public health problems they jointly face.

As Scott Greer's analysis of the devolved systems within the UK shows, it is not surprising that there has been substantial divergence in public health policy making in the first decade of devolution. Each of the devolved governments is responsible for the dedicated public health function in its area. In drawing out the differing characteristics of the four systems he contrasts the policy emphasis on hospitals and healthcare in England with the Northern Irish history of local organisational autonomy. Further contrast is evident in the Welsh commitment to reducing inequalities which has polarised the debate between determinants and services, while the most successful public health system appears to be in Scotland with its long tradition of professional leadership.

At the same time as these developments in public health and healthcare systems across UK, the relevance and importance of the European dimension of public health has grown. Public health in Europe is both the sum of public health within its member states and also their collective action, both between countries and by all countries working together. Networks such as the World Health Organization (WHO)-sponsored *Healthy Cities* movement allow the exchange of best practice in developing community-based approaches to promoting health. But, as McCarthy points out, while the WHO and EU (European Union) play key roles, public health and healthcare services remain under the control of national governments and are subject to national legislation. So within the EU, while governments may have similar objectives, the structures and practices they develop will differ. The recent expansion of the EU coincided with the development of the three programme themes for health: preventing diseases and injuries (including mental illness, cancer, cardiovascular diseases, rare diseases and accidents); improving cooperation between health systems (including patient safety, transnational specialist centres and cross-border care); and developing structures for emergency preparedness and threats. These themes will be the focus for discussion and collaboration for member states, along with action flowing from environmental charters on transport, air and water. The UK Presidency of the EU during the second half of 2005 saw an emphasis placed on action to reduce inequalities in health culminating in a major health summit held in London in October. Two expert reports specially commissioned for the summit respectively described the substantial inequalities in health which persist and reviewed the various public policy goals and targets being set in different countries.

We are aware that there are many aspects of global public health that we could have included, not least the challenges of the Millennium Goals, the growing awareness of the problems of non-communicable disease as well as the threats of avian flu. The basic public health problems of clean water and sanitation remain challenges in many parts of the developing world. Tobacco companies continue to extend their markets, and obesity rates continue to reach epidemic proportions. The impact of political changes has led to the demise of public health systems in Eastern Europe and China, where privatisation of healthcare systems and a focus on high-tech medicine rather than basic prevention has led to growing inequalities and in some instances falling life expectancy. HIV/AIDS (human immunodeficiency virus/acquired immune deficiency syndrome) rates are rising not only in sub-Saharan Africa but also in countries such as Ukraine and India.

Aware of these multiple issues and the public health challenges they pose, the final chapter in this part of the book by Martin McKee emphasises what we are increasingly aware of, that no government acts alone. The forces of globalisation are evident walking down the high streets of any city or town across the world. The same goods are available, the same fast-food outlets, the same tobacco and other brands. The WHO's framework convention for tobacco control is an example of the awareness of the need for global action and for governments to act for the benefit of their populations' health, not just to support corporate profit or economic success. McKee focuses his analysis on the adverse impact of US neoconservatism, and the need for solidarity and sustained efforts rather than self-interest in addressing the global health challenges of the 21st century.

Chapter 1

Public health in Scotland: the dividend of devolution

Peter Donnelly

Scotland's challenge

For many years Scotland has been known in public health circles as 'the Sick Man of Europe'. Scotland's high prevalence of smoking and alcohol misuse became the stuff of comic caricature. Its diet was almost legendary in its alleged awfulness. What other country could have invented the deep-fried Mars bar?

Yet such a tabloid and populist representation of Scotland's health challenge is a partial story. A more balanced and intellectually rewarding account is given by Leon *et al.*(2003) in their careful study which suggests a number of things about Scotland's health. First, Scotland's health is improving but not at the rate of some of its European counterparts. Second, the shortfall in terms of health improvement performance is relatively recent in that it has only occurred since around 1950, before which Scotland's health was improving on a par with others. The third observation is that the health deficit in Scotland is not due to problems at the extremities of life. Neonatal and perinatal mortality are unremarkable and the old are just as likely to become very old in Scotland as elsewhere. Rather, Scotland's health deficit is focused upon men and particularly women of working age who die before their time from largely preventable conditions such as ischaemic heart disease, stroke and chronic obstructive pulmonary disease. Finally, this burden of ill health and premature mortality is disproportionately borne by those in lower socio-economic classes.

The opportunity of devolution

Unlike other parts of the UK, the devolution settlement presented Scotland with a Parliament with primary legislative powers. Furthermore, as a result of a separate question in the Devolution Referendum it also has tax-raising powers of plus or minus three pence in the pound. Thus far these tax-varying powers have not been utilised but the primary legislative powers certainly have been and what is more they have been used in the field of public health.

To understand fully why this has happened, one has to consider the make-up of the Scottish Parliament. Its partially proportionate system means that coalition government is always likely and that parties who may not gain representation in an exclusively first-past-the-post system do have members in the Chamber. Thus, for example, in the current Parliament (2003–7) the Green Party has seven representatives and the Scottish Socialist Party has six, and the coalition in this Parliament as with the last Parliament (1999–2003) is a Labour/Liberal Democrat one. The most numerous opposition party is the Scottish Nationalist Party (SNP). Unlike many nationalist parties in other parts of Europe, the SNP is not of the right, with most political commentators considering it to be slightly to the left of the ruling coalition, although not as far to the left as the Scottish Socialist Party. The opposition from the right in terms of the Scottish Conservative and Unionist Party is numerically smaller.

The single-chamber nature of the Scottish Parliament, and a prevailing ethos at the time of devolution which placed great store upon involving the public, has given rise to a number of interesting procedural consequences. For example, any member of the public can start a petition and if they are successful in obtaining the requisite number of signatures have a right to present this to the Petitions Committee and to be heard. The single-chamber nature of the Parliament means that considerable effort is put into the Committee stages of legislation and at Committee stages an emphasis is placed upon fact finding and discussion, rather than overtly party political argument.

The legislative response

It is instructive, given the above background in terms of Scotland's ill health and the devolution of powers, to examine a number of pieces of actual or proposed public health legislation and to compare and contrast what motivated their proposal and what has governed their progress. These three pieces of legislation are the Breastfeeding Act, the Bill which bans smoking in all enclosed public spaces in March 2006, and finally the Private Members' Bill which has not yet reached, and indeed may never reach, the Statute Books but which argues for the creation of prostitution tolerance zones. The first Bill on breastfeeding makes it illegal for any café owner, publican or hotelier to stop a woman in Scotland breastfeeding her child. It was a popular measure politically and met with little opposition and its importance was in sending a very firm signal of national intent on an important public health issue. Arguably it could have been pursued in other ways, although the very process of proposing and achieving legislative change brought a great deal of attention to this crucial but underexplored area of public health policy.

The second Bill relates to smoking. Here again it is probably easier in Scotland to make progress than in certain other parts of the UK, partly because of the make-up of the Parliament as described above. Indeed, of the parties mentioned above, only the Scottish Conservative and Unionist Party opposed the legislation, arguing instead for a voluntary code with, for example, the retail publican trade. Such opposition as there has been has come from outside of the Parliament in the form of the organised retail publican trade as well, of course, from predictable sources such as the Tobacco Manufacturers' Association. At the time of writing the Bill has successfully progressed through Parliament and very recently received Royal Assent and so is now law, becoming effective in March 2006.

The decision to pursue this course of action in Scotland is distinct from that which is being pursued in other parts of the UK at present. In particular it goes further than the initially proposed policy in England. A number of factors may be responsible for this, including the aforementioned parliamentary balance of power. Another factor may be the realisation that Scotland's needs were greater and that it needed to make its own policy and follow its own course in this regard.

Some would see the asynchronous political cycles as also being relevant with a Scottish election being at least 2 years further on than the date of the UK general election.

Commentators might also argue that this was a test of devolution. What better issue for Scotland to do something different than on smoking when so much of its poor health record is tobacco related? At the time of writing, it seems less likely that the issue of legislation on prostitution tolerance zones will be seen as such a public health touchstone. The Bill has been championed by the former SNP, now Independent MSP (Member of the Scottish Parliament), Margo Macdonald and seeks to create a legislative basis that would empower local authorities if they wished to create 'zones of toleration' within which street prostitutes would not be prosecuted by the police. Those who argue for such an approach say that it would facilitate the concentration of health and social services on a highly vulnerable group of women and it could at least remove the additional stigma and disadvantage brought about by criminalisation. Those who are against have adopted this position for a number of reasons. Some are simply morally repelled by any suggestion of condoning or tolerating prostitution. Another group sees any form of prostitution as abuse and any toleration of such as condoning abuse. A third strand driven by residents is focused upon where such zones would be sited and their opposition is largely one of location and the avoidance of considerable inconvenience and unpleasantness.

The parliamentary system has at the very least allowed this difficult and sensitive issue to be thoroughly rehearsed and a wide variety of different pieces of evidence gathered. Whether it finally results in legislation creating 'zones of toleration', or whether it simply better informs the de facto zones that already exist in some cities as a result of police forces exercising their discretionary powers of non-pursuance and non-prosecution, remains to be seen.

Overall however, it appears heartening that a relatively new devolved administration can find parliamentary time to debate, discuss and progress issues as diverse as breastfeeding, smoking in enclosed public places, and prostitution tolerance zones.

The policy response

Of course Scotland's policy response to its challenging health status goes beyond legislation. Before describing this it is perhaps first worth rehearsing what has not been done because that is equally important. In particular, and in marked contrast to England, there has not been a series of system-wide reorganisations. The NHS in Scotland, and indeed local government, has over the immediate past period been fairly stable. Scotland for many years has had 15 geographically defined health boards. Following consultations about one of these being integrated with neighbouring boards there are now 14 health boards. However, this occurred for specific local reasons rather than because of a policy shift. These geographically defined boards have become unified in that they are once again responsible for the operational running of what previously were NHS trusts. However, this change has been achieved with the minimum of fuss, has been seen as popular, and has brought in many people's eyes the 'NHS family' back together. Scotland is also blessed with strong national agencies in terms of Health Protection Scotland (formerly known as the Scottish Centre for Infection and Environmental Health), Health Scotland (an amalgamation of the former Health Education Board for Scotland and the Public Health Institute for Scotland), and the Information and Statistics Division of NHS National Services Scotland, which provides much of the nation's health and health services intelligence. Box 1.1 illustrates the organisation of the Scottish public health system. Scotland also has a culture of strong professional engagement and professional influence with policy makers. In his comparison of devolution arrangements across the UK and analysis of growing health policy divergence, Greer indeed picks out the importance of professional influence within Scotland (Greer 2001).

Box 1.1 Scotland's public health system (2005)

Tier 1
Community health partnerships between one and five per unified board. Have a leading role in health improvement and tackling health inequalities – generally coterminous with local authorities and technically sub-committees of the 15 boards.

Tier 2
Fourteen unified health boards combine strategic and operational responsibilities with there being no separate trusts. The Director of Public Health and their departments remain key, with responsibilities for health protection, health improvement and public health input to service planning and service quality.

Tier 3
The 14 boards are grouped into three regional networks. Much of the emphasis is on the commissioning of specialist services. However, formal mutual aid arrangements exist between public health departments and appropriate topic-specific cooperation occurs.

Tier 4
National agencies have an important role and interface with both the policy centre and territorial boards. They include:

- NHS Health Scotland
- National Services Scotland including the Information and Statistics Division, Health Protection Scotland and Quality Improvement Scotland
- NHS Education Scotland.

Tier 5
Scottish Executive Health Department public health leadership comes from the responsible Civil Service Policy Group headed by a board-level appointee and from the Chief Medical Officer discharged via one of two Deputy CMOs and his Public Health Professional Group.

Scotland's response to the Leon *et al.* (2003) analysis is encapsulated in the *Challenge* document (Scottish Executive 2003). It talks about four pillars of endeavour, namely: early years, teenage transition, health at work, and community development (*see* Box 1.2). It also has a special focus upon sexual health, diet, exercise, alcohol and mental health (*see* Box 1.3). Each pillar was an attempt to address different aspects of the Scottish Challenge. First, early years was seen as an important time when children could be given the best start in life through breastfeeding, delayed introduction of solid food, immunisation, good parenting, etc. The teenage transition was seen as important in terms of smoking, alcohol, drugs, sexual health, diet and exercise. The focus upon health at work seemed a logical response to the observations of Leon *et al.* (2003), and the Scotland's Health at Work Programme has successfully driven forward occupational health and concepts of health improvement within workplace settings. The fourth pillar of community development was seen as essential in helping the others remain sustainable over time and also in terms of helping communities and individuals grow in confidence to help them in terms of improving their life circumstances and lifestyles in a way which would avoid risk factors for premature mortality.

Box 1.2 Scotland's health improvement challenge – the four pillars

- Early years.
- Teenage transition.
- Workplace health.
- Community development.

Source: Scottish Executive (2003).

Box 1.3 Scotland's health improvement challenge – special focus programmes

- Healthy eating.
- Smoking.
- Alcohol.
- Mental health and wellbeing.
- Health and homelessness.
- Sexual health.

Source: Scottish Executive (2003).

These pillars are supported by a number of National Demonstration Projects. For example, the Starting Well National Demonstration Project focuses greatly enhanced social and healthcare support for young children upon socio-economically challenged areas within Glasgow. The Healthy Respect National Demonstration Project focused upon teenage sexuality and in particular upon reducing unplanned teenage pregnancies and reducing incidents of sexually transmitted diseases. It is seen as an important contribution to the teenage transition pillar. The Have a Heart Paisley National Demonstration Project contributed to the health at work and community development pillars through exploring ways of reducing risk factors for ischaemic heart disease in one of the areas of Scotland with the poorest record for morbidity and premature mortality from these causes.

In one of these special focus areas, a lengthy and inclusive piece of work culminated in the publication of a National Sexual Health Strategy early in 2005 (Scottish Executive 2005). In his presentation to Parliament the then Health

Minister, Mr Andy Kerr MSP, pledged his personal commitment to taking this difficult and sensitive area of work forward.

Scotland's diet has also received much attention. The success of the breastfeeding legislation has been followed by a highly innovative and much-praised programme entitled 'Hungry for Success' which laid out for the first time acceptable standards of salt and fat content for contractors providing school meals. This much-praised and now much-copied initiative has been endorsed by the World Health Organization and even the celebrity chef Jamie Oliver (2005) has said that it is 'light years ahead' of anything he has seen elsewhere. Interestingly, Mr Oliver's comments received considerably more press coverage than those of WHO! In terms of exercise, programmes such as Sporting Chance in primary schools have been very successful at engaging participation and the challenge now is to keep active children involved as they move forward in secondary school and into adulthood.

In that regard, working with the Countryside Information Network, Scotland is keen to explore the use of its beautiful and accessible countryside for exercise and mental health promotion. That field of mental health promotion is another one in which Scotland is seen as playing a leading role. Much effort has been put into suicide prevention and in particular into removing the stigmatisation that often occurs of those who have suffered serious mental ill health. A ministerial group on alcohol is working closely with professional voluntary and industry concerns to try and reduce the adverse impact that alcohol undoubtedly has upon Scottish society.

The future

Turning to the future, there is clearly a need for additional capacity building within public health and recent progress in terms of building multidisciplinary capacity through the employment of public health practitioners and public health colleagues within local authorities will be further progressed. There also will be a challenge as to how Scotland can maintain positive momentum in terms of health improvement, while at the same time balancing it with further improvements in health service delivery. Targeting simple, proven and effective therapies upon parts of the population who do not currently come forward for them, often from socio-economic deprived areas as part of a chronic disease ascertainment and management programme, may be one important area of overlap and mutual interest between these two areas of activity. There is a growing feeling that this may be an effective measure in the short to medium term to reduce inequalities (as opposed to simply improve health) and the effective control of high blood pressure, cholesterol, smoking and alcohol seem likely to remain a focus of activity. Current trends give some reason for optimism. For example, among Scotland's three big killers considerable reductions in under-75 death rates have been achieved in the last 10 years. Cancer deaths are down by 14.8%, coronary heart disease deaths down by 43.6% and stroke deaths down by 40.0%.

In summary, Scotland has woken up to the scale of the challenge that it faces in terms of changing the health trajectory of its population. The Scottish Executive has utilised its new devolved status and parliamentary capacity for primary legislation. It is tackling smoking and diet. Its mental health promotion programme is innovative. There is a realisation that alcohol abuse now requires further attention and that the targeted secondary prevention of the big killers of ischaemic heart disease, cancer, stroke and chronic obstructive airways disease is going to be important.

Scotland thus remains a challenging but highly rewarding place in which to study, learn and practise public health. The additional powers conferred by the devolution settlement have been important in allowing appropriate policy divergence and innovation.

Note

The author has since February 2004 been Deputy Chief Medical Officer at the Scottish Executive. However, these views are personal and do not necessarily reflect current or proposed Scottish Executive policy.

References

Breastfeeding Act: www.scottish.parliament.uk/business/bills/15-breastfeeding/b15s2-introd.pdf.

Greer S (2001) *Devolution and Health: a four way bet*. UCL. www.ucl.ac.uk/constitution-unit/unit-publications/106.html.

Have a Heart Paisley National Demonstration Project: www.show.scot.nhs.uk/publicationsindex.htm.

Healthy Respect National Demonstration Project: www.scotland.gov.uk/Publications/2005/04/07105005/50064.

Hungry for Success: www.scotland.gov.uk/library5/education/hfs-00.asp.

Leon D *et al.* (2003) *Understanding the Health of Scotland's Population in an International Context.* London School of Hygiene and Tropical Medicine and Public Health Institute of Scotland. www.phis.org.uk/projects/network.asp?p=ff.

Oliver J (2005) Comments in *Scotsman*. 31 March 2005. http://news.scotsman.com/health.cfm?id=339092005.

Private Members' Bill on Prostitution Tolerance Zones: www.scottish.parliament.uk/business/research/briefings-04/sb04-10.pdf.

Scottish Executive (2003) *Improving Health in Scotland: the challenge*. Edinburgh: Scottish Executive. www.scotland.gov.uk/library5/health/ihis-00.asp.

Scottish Executive (2005) *Respect and Responsibility – Scotland's strategy for sexual health*. www.scotland.gov.uk/library5/health/shst-00.asp.

Smoking Bill: www.scottish.parliament.uk/business/bills/33-smokingHealth/b33bs2-aspassed.pdf.

Starting Well National Demonstration Project: www.gorbalslive.org.uk/data/community/cgroups/startingwell.htm.

Chapter 2

Public health in England

Fiona Adshead and Allison Thorpe

Public health issues have become regular headline features in England, as elsewhere. In 2001, national newspapers ran 30 stories with the word 'obesity' in the headline. In 2004, the number exceeded 400. This is an exponential rise, which indicates the growth in public interest. We live in a consumer society where the cultural obsession with celebrity has been used to highlight issues which had previously been almost invisible to the public consciousness. To take just one example, Jamie Oliver's campaign on school dinners had delivered the kind of profile to a public health issue which activists have dreamed about in vain for years. It provided people with a vehicle and a voice for expressing their concerns collectively and demanding positive action for the health of their children. It demonstrates the way in which people are becoming more attuned to the health debate, and shows that they are more interested in the development of their own health. Public health is once more becoming the 'organised efforts of society' (Acheson 1988).

For us, as public health professionals, the challenge could not be more explicit: we need to capitalise on this increased awareness and willingness to respond and use it opportunistically to promote and support long-term behavioural changes which will in turn nurture and sustain the health of the population.

This chapter, which will focus on health improvement, will look at how public health in England is rising to this challenge.

The policy context

The practice of public health is, and always has been, shaped by the political and cultural context. Changing paradigms of the appropriate levels of responsibility and involvement for the state, the individual and the community provide a context for delivery (Beaglehole *et al.* 2004). In the 19th century, when the focus was on infectious diseases, legislation was a first-line response to effect change. Today, the focus in on chronic diseases. While our response has evolved to reflect a position where promoting health is moving to the centre of the political and professional agenda, the tools and the context have also changed considerably.

Since the election of the Labour government in 1997 there has been a shift in the context for public health, with an explicit recognition of health inequalities in policy documents and national targets. *Saving Lives: our healthier nation* (Secretary of State for Health 1999), which built on the *Health of the Nation* (Secretary of State for Health 1992), highlighted three complementary levels of action to improve health:

- individuals and their families taking action for themselves
- communities working together in partnership
- government action to address the major determinants through policy on areas such as jobs, housing, education.

The *NHS Plan* and subsequent papers such as *Tackling Health Inequalities: summary of the 2002 cross cutting review* (Department of Health 2002) and *Tackling Health Inequalities: a programme for action* (Department of Health 2003) have continued the process of mapping out the cross-government, community and civic responsibilities for tackling health inequalities. However, despite this policy recognition, criticisms in the past have suggested that the NHS and its resources are too focused on the downstream 'patient' at the expense of the upstream prevention agenda, with Wanless (2002, 2004) in particular highlighting the need to invest in reducing demand by enhancing the promotion of health and prevention of disease.

Policies such as the *NHS Plan* (Department of Health 2000), the *NHS Improvement Plan* (Department of Health 2004c), *Choosing Health* (Secretary of State for Health 2004) and the *Choosing Health* delivery plan (Department of Health 2005) provide a blueprint for the future, and begin to answer this criticism. They articulate the need to focus on people, connecting with their lives and empowering them to develop as the engine for their own health and behavioural changes. *Choosing Health* explicitly highlights three key principles to support this process:

- *supporting informed choice*: people want to make their own health decisions, but they expect the government to help by creating the right environment
- *personalisation of support to make healthy choices*: building information, services and support around people's lives and ensuring they have equal access to them
- *working in partnership to make health everybody's business*: health needs are complex and real lives do not fit neatly into the boundaries of individual organisations or government departments and organisations.

Promoting health has to fit in with other aspects of people's lifestyles and aspirations. Services need to cater for the individual. Smoking, for instance, is known to be the single biggest preventable cause of the socio-economic gradient in infant mortality and life expectancy. However, reducing the numbers who smoke requires engagement of more than just the NHS, as the clear co-delivery agenda with local government set out in *Choosing Health* recognises. *Choosing Health*'s proposals to shift the balance in favour of smoke-free environments, and the new measures on tobacco which will help smokers to give up, require engagement of external partners, and 'joined-up' action at many levels (governmental, national, regional, local and multisectorally), working with the population, if they are to work.

The *Choosing Health* consultation received more than 150,000 responses, confirming the high levels of interest people have in their health, and expressing a need to tie delivery to the local level and connect with people's lives. Responses showed that people wanted to take responsibility for their own health, but within a supportive climate, which provided information people could clearly understand and trust, and support for making and taking the choices available to them. The policy recognition of this request for self-determination is strongly articulated throughout *Choosing Health*, which emphasises the need for a broader social contract between the state and individuals, with choice and civic action being key to this process. The responsibility of the state is to provide the right environment and enabling conditions for this to take place.

Action to support health improvement is ongoing, and increasingly part of the mainstream corporate government agenda. Across government, there are:

- public service agreement (PSA) targets which commit government departments to improving health outcomes
- a Cabinet Sub-Committee, chaired by the Deputy Prime Minister, which coordinates action across departments
- a commitment to wider action to improve the health of the most disadvantaged and tackle health inequalities (e.g. through action on housing, fuel poverty, and employment).

This is in addition to the very specific targets of the Department of Health itself, and its role in supporting delivery in other departments, e.g. through the NHS getting people back to work.

Tackling health inequalities is a multi-agency, cross-government agenda, with local authorities and PCTs being the key partners for change at the local level. As England strives to improve the health of its population a priority must be given to tackling health inequalities so that all groups in society benefit from improvements in public health. The overall approach to this is pragmatic, embedding health inequalities into mainstream systems and targeting money and other resources towards areas and groups with the highest need. *Delivering Choosing Health* (Department of Health 2005), which was published in March 2005, gives a comprehensive overview of the ways in which delivery will be resourced across the 170 commitments made in *Choosing Health*, with specific commitments for the spearhead areas – the 70 local authorities, and the 88 PCTs which map to them – which make up the worst fifth of areas for health and deprivation indicators. These commitments include developing and delivering on health trainers, school nurses and Health and Wellbeing Equity Audits.

The Delivery Plan reflects a pragmatic partnership approach to driving delivery at the national, regional and local levels, which recognises that driving the agenda forward needs more than bilateral relationships. Joined-up action across multiple agencies is a fundamental requirement for success.

Partnerships between the NHS and local government, working with voluntary, private and public sectors, are fundamental building blocks for creating a delivery system for public health priorities which will ensure action at the local level. Key to the success of the system will be the ability to translate policies into operational contexts, embedding health improvement in the wider health and social context leading to practical actions. Local authorities and PCTs already have explicit shared responsibilities for co-delivery of national priorities and targets, identifying local needs and achieving local targets and commissioning and delivering services. Partnerships need to cross over the traditional boundaries to engage in shared working around key objectives with clear expectations of delivery. But they need support – both at a national level and from public health leaders within the system – and constant dialogue if they are to achieve the optimum results.

Local area agreements (LAAs) are an important part of this new system, marking a radical change in central and local relationships, simplifying funding streams from the centre and engaging key partners in developing locally responsive strategies and targets for health inequalities issues. With the extension of the scheme to a further 66 local authorities and their partners, and a promise that all top-tier authorities will be engaged by 2007, they offer a huge opportunity to encourage action across the public sector, supported by a system which works to align resources, performance management, standards and regulations, e.g. through the Healthcare Commission.

Systems for supporting delivery

One of the challenges such a broad approach creates is the need to equip all those with an interest in developing public health skills with the necessary opportunities to develop these skills and to support them in effecting change.

Recent work by the Faculty of Public Health and the Association of Directors of Public Health conceptualised public health as part of a system, with three distinct, but interrelated, domains of practice – health protection, health improvement, and health and social care quality (Griffiths, Jewell and Donnelly 2005). Each domain needs to be supported by public health intelligence and information, by academic research and by a clear strategy for developing the workforce – as *Choosing Health* recognises. This approach, which was supported strongly by the specialist workforce (Griffiths, Thorpe and Wright 2006), provides a coherent framework for describing both the services to be delivered and the different roles and responsibilities of those delivering them. In particular, it provides a vehicle for recognising and developing the core skills, knowledge and competencies that are needed to deliver across the entire agenda at each of the levels of practice. As long ago as 1987, Levin's article on the 'School of the New Public Health' suggested that:

> *The public health establishment as we know it represents the most available and appropriate resource with which to begin the task of building the necessary infrastructure for health promotion.* (Levin 1987, p.91)

The three-domains approach, which focuses on public health as a system, provides a vehicle for delivery which recognises that public health is not just about specialists, and provides a formalised context within which skills at the other levels of practice can be developed. Delivery on the complex and challenging health-improvement agenda, both in trusts, local government and in the wider environment, as *Choosing Health* recognises, needs more than just public health professional and technical engagement if we are to succeed in our goal of improving people's health. It requires engagement from the whole health-improvement workforce and indeed the public themselves – in Wanless's words 'a fully engaged scenario'. There is increasing recognition that achieving long-term sustainable health improvement requires a new conceptualisation of the health-improvement workforce, which enables everyone who can contribute to do so. This is both explicitly and implicitly linked to ensuring the sustainability of the NHS by building health into every contact, thereby increasing its overall productivity.

Many of the levers to support this wider view of the role of the workforce have been put in place at policy level for the health service. *Choosing Health* supported a proactive skills escalator approach to workforce development for public health in England, which recognises that achieving the expected benefits will require all NHS employees to have some understanding of their health-improvement role. Many who could contribute currently are latent, as opposed to active participants in health improvement – some because their roles are not recognised, others because they have been unable to achieve, or have not been supported in achieving, access to the necessary opportunities to develop the relevant skills and support in effecting change. Proactive workforce development plans – such as the inclusion of public health within NHS induction programmes, *Modernising Medical Careers* (Department of Health 2004b) and *Agenda for Change* (Department of Health 2004a) – provide a framework (Department of Health 2004d) to build on within the NHS. But tackling health inequalities is not just the prerogative of the NHS – it is a dynamic agenda with multiple partners engaged in its delivery.

The broad-based social marketing strategy outlined by *Choosing Health* supports this process, by focusing on engaging individuals, organisations and broader society in action on health, and provides help to deliver key messages for and to the public on how to improve and protect their health. It provides a stronger basis for understanding and using 'people intelligence', supporting better use of public health intelligence by linking it to better communications strategies.

Shifts in the overall models of assessment within the health system reflect the key role of the Healthcare Commission in driving improvements across the full spectrum of healthcare. The inclusion of public health within the seven domains independently assessed by the Commission ensures a consistency in approach across the country, enabling healthcare organisations to identify the steps required to meet the standards and allowing monitoring of progress. It also ensures that all organisations are addressing the same priorities. The new role of NICE in producing guidance and recommendations for public health will be a key element of this process.

The role of the public health specialist and practitioner

As this chapter has stressed, many of the prerequisites for the development of the holistic public health system are already in place. *Choosing Health* has provided a framework for designing future service provision with reference to accurate knowledge and data-collection practices, and with true collaboration between people and practitioners – but it is up to public health specialists and practitioners to support the people in realising the full potential of this model for their own health, and to support other members of the workforce in achieving their own potential contribution to the agenda.

Take, for example, the hospital trust. Acute trusts, by definition, have traditionally had a treatment focus to their agenda, but from the seminal work of the Chief Medical Officer, Sir Liam Donaldson, to the more recent reports from the Faculty of Public Health (2004) and *Choosing Health*, a wide range of activities has been identified within the acute sector which would benefit from public health support and enable hospitals to achieve a more holistic health-promoting role. Public health has a wide range of skills to offer in the trust setting, with a key role in promoting and facilitating evidence-based practice (*see* Box 2.1).

Choosing Health formally required hospital trusts to contribute to health improvement in the local community. To do this effectively, the trust will need support in recognising its role and learning to work across organisational and sectoral boundaries, which can and would be supported by the skills of public health specialists and practitioners.

Box 2.1 The public health role in trusts

- To promote evidence-based clinical policy.
- To promote the development of clinical governance, creating the culture, system, support and facilitation to improve quality of care, assure quality of care and improve safety.
- To promote high-quality information systems, particularly trying to make these systems more population based.
- The appraisal of health technology.
- The reduction of infection.
- The prevention of disease.
- To develop pharmaco-epidemiology.
- To promote the role of the NHS as a corporate citizen.
- Health services research.
- To re-energise the sustainability agenda, with green hospitals and the greening of hospitals.

Source: Sir Liam Donaldson, speech to Faculty of Public Health (FPH) workshop, 3 April 2003.

There are many challenges to be faced and overcome if the *Choosing Health* agenda is to be delivered:

- workforce capacity
- role of performance management
- alignment of regulation
- money
- culture: it is almost counter-cultural for us to think about health rather than sickness
- restructuring services to cater for the individual – ongoing listening, ongoing flexibility and responsiveness
- understanding what works.

Public health specialists and practitioners have a key role in helping others to understand and respond to these challenges effectively. Leadership, advocacy, and the ability to provide moral and professional support to others are all key skills which public health professionals have practised over the years – the challenge is to bring them to bear in ways which provide practical support, leading, coordinating and promoting partnerships working in support of individuals and communities. Public health specialists and practitioners have a great deal of experience to offer in supporting and designing a fit-for-purpose public health system, using and developing skills in ensuring effective community action, promoting partnership working and pragmatism in delivering on the health-improvement agenda. They are supported in this by the shift in the system to reflect the drive towards standards of quality and care across the full spectrum of healthcare acting as the key national driver for improvements, with independent assessment of progress carried out by the Healthcare Commission informing performance ratings from April 2005. Supported by the new role of NICE in public health evidence, we are well positioned to develop a robust and sustainable delivery system for health and healthcare, which recognises the role of reliable research in assuring delivery of 'what works'.

In conclusion

Legislation, campaigns and structural changes have all made, and will continue to make, valuable contributions to the public health arsenal, but only in so far as they support a long-term culture change which is driven by the needs and aspirations of individuals and their communities. Achieving health improvement and delivering *Choosing Health* requires pragmatic action from both the professional public health workforce and the wider workforce who may not, as yet, wholly recognise their essential input. The white paper, *Your Health, Your Care, Your Say*, published by the Secretary of State in February 2006, builds on this approach, calling for public engagement in the design of a *'twenty-first century health service outside hospitals'* (Secretary of State for Health 2006). This call to action is equally applicable to those of us in the public health workforce. It offers a huge potential to position ourselves *with* other partners to facilitate the development of a fit-for-purpose system to support health improvement and reduce inequalities. It is a challenging agenda – but it is a shared agenda. And it is one which the public health workforce in its widest sense in England is uniquely capable of delivering, via a co-delivery model, which takes a functional, pragmatic – but nevertheless evidence-based – approach.

If we can keep up the momentum, and lean on each other's expertise, vision and tenacity, and if we keep listening and responding to people and tailoring the services to meet their needs, it's within the realm of possibility that we could create what our successors might look back on in another hundred years' time and think of as the true Golden Age for Public Health.

References

Acheson D (1988) *Independent Inquiry into Inequalities in Health: Report*. London: TSO.

Beaglehole R, Bonita R, Horton R, Adams O and McKee M (2004) Public health in the new era: improving health through collective action. *The Lancet*. **363**: 2084–7.

Department of Health (1988) *Public Health in England*. Report of the Committee of Inquiry into the Future Development of the Public Health Function. London: Department of Health.

Department of Health (2000) *The NHS Plan*. Cm 4818. London: HMSO.

Department of Health (2002) *Tackling Health Inequalities: summary of the 2002 cross cutting review*. London: Department of Health.

Department of Health (2003) *Tackling Health Inequalities: a programme for action*. London: Department of Health.

Department of Health (2004a) *Agenda for Change: final agreement*. London: Department of Health.

Department of Health (2004b) *Modernising Medical Careers: the next steps. The future shape of foundation, specialist and general practice training programmes*. London: Department of Health.

Department of Health (2004c) *The NHS Improvement Plan*. London: Department of Health.

Department of Health (2004d) *NHS Knowledge and Skills Framework and Development Review Guidance*. London: Department of Health.

Department of Health (2005) *Delivering Choosing Health: making healthy choices easier*. London: Department of Health.

Faculty of Public Health (2004) *Public Health in Trusts Workshop Report.* London: Faculty of Public Health.

Griffiths S, Jewell T and Donnelly P (2005) Public health in practice: the three domains. *Public Health.* **119**(10): 907–13.

Griffiths S, Thorpe A and Wright J (2006) Public health in transition: views of the specialist workforce. Submitted to *Pub Health Med.*

Levin LS (1987) *The School of the New Public Health: a proposal, health promotion.* Oxford: Oxford University Press. **2**(2): 91–4.

Secretary of State for Health (1992) *Health of the Nation.* London: HMSO.

Secretary of State for Health (1999) *Saving Lives: our healthier nation.* London: HMSO.

Secretary of State for Health (2004) *Choosing Health: making healthy choices easier.* Cm 6374. London: The Stationery Office.

Secretary of State for Health (2006) *Our Health, Our Care, Our Say: a new direction for community services.* Cm 6737. London: The Stationery Office.

Wanless D (2002) *Securing Our Future: taking a long term view.* London: HM Treasury.

Wanless D (2004) *Securing Good Health for the Whole Population.* London: HM Treasury/Department of Health.

Chapter 3

Public health in Wales

Eddie Coyle

Public health – everybody's business

Improving health has been a key concern for Welsh society and responsibilities for public health have been shared between central and local government and the National Health Service.

Administrative devolution was introduced in the 1960s with the establishment of the Welsh Office. The Welsh health minister's brief included public health and influence could be exerted over other areas of the Secretary of State's powers, such as transport, agriculture and environment. Local public health services were centred on local government until the 1974 reorganisation. Since then, local government in Wales has remained an active partner in directing public health policy and delivery of services. The key to this effective collaboration in public health has been coterminosity and alignment between the NHS and local government within the jurisdiction of the regional tier of government.

The Welsh people, through their keen sense of community and organised groups, have always played a key role in action to improve health and wellbeing. Archie Cochrane's seminal epidemiological studies in the Welsh valleys were only achieved through high response rates (over 90%!) and Julian Tudor Hart (1988) led the development of community-based primary care from his practice in Glyncorrwg with the overwhelming support of his patients.

Recent developments in public health policy and organisation

Since 1997, considerable changes have occurred in policy and organisations delivering public health services in Wales.

The 1997 report of the Chief Medical Officer (CMO) in Wales identified a significant health deficit, with death rates higher and life expectancy shorter in Wales than in most European countries. It noted substantial inequalities in health between communities in Wales. It recognised that health policy in Wales, with high levels of permanent sickness from its industrial legacy, could never be disconnected from its social and economic determinants. The CMO report provided the context for ensuing policy and coincided with the new UK government policy focus to address inequalities in health.

Public health policy: Better Health – Better Wales 1998

The new public health policy *Better Health – Better Wales* (Welsh Office 1998a) was produced for consultation by the Welsh Office in 1998 and was based on the analysis of the CMO report. Collaboration and partnerships with communities and groups were given a particularly prominent role. *Better Health – Better Wales* was published at the same time as the English green paper *Our Healthier Nation* (Dobson 1998). Tackling inequalities in health linked to the wider determinants of health was the dominant theme of both policies.

The consultation was followed by *Better Health – Better Wales Strategic Framework* (Welsh Office 1998b) which matched the English white paper, *Saving Lives: our healthier nation* (Department of Health 1999). The *Strategic Framework* emphasised working with local government through health alliances and building linkages with social policies to address poverty and unemployment, through connecting with community programmes and workplace health. A key recommendation was to establish the Wales Centre for Health to support public health policy development. *See* Table 3.1.

Table 3.1   Public health policies in Wales and England

Date	Wales	England
1998	Better Health – Better Wales (Welsh Office 1998a)	Our Healthier Nation (Dobson 1998)
1998	Better Health – Better Wales Strategic Framework (Welsh Office 1998b)	Saving Lives (Department of Health 1999)
2002	Well Being in Wales (Welsh Assembly Government 2002)	
2003	The Review of Health and Social Care in Wales (Welsh Assembly Government 2003a) 'Dai Wanless'	Securing Good Health for the Whole Population (HM Treasury 2004) Wanless 2
2004	Health Challenge Wales (Welsh Assembly Government 2004a)	White paper – Choosing Health (Department of Health 2004)
2005	Health Challenge Wales – national and local programme	White paper – Choosing Health Delivery Plans

Public health and devolution

The National Assembly for Wales was established in 1999, following the Government of Wales Act 1998 and a closely won referendum.

The first Assembly administration (1999–2003), known from 2000 as the Welsh Assembly Government, used the *Strategic Framework* as the basis for its public health policy.

Devolution brought no new powers to those held by the Welsh Office. The health and social services ministerial portfolio remained responsible for approximately 40% of a total budget of £10 billion.

The first administration of the Welsh Assembly Government set out its overall strategy – *Better Wales.com* – which identified equal opportunities, tackling social disadvantage and sustainable development as its core themes.

The new Health and Social Care Minister commissioned Peter Townsend, the joint author of the Black report, to target health policy around addressing inequalities in health.

The first Welsh Assembly Government (1999–2003) worked closely with UK government policy to address inequalities and social justice. It participated in Sure Start (Welsh Office 1999) and launched the Communities First programme.

The Communities First programme was targeted on improving communities in the 100 poorest electoral areas in Wales and worked closely with the similar English programme.

Wales, with relatively low GNP (gross national product) within the then European Union of 15 states, benefited from Objective 1 funding to develop the socio-economic and community infrastructure for its most deprived areas.

Putting health at the heart of public policy

In 2002, *Well Being in Wales* was published (Welsh Assembly Government 2002), which built on *Better Health – Better Wales*. It set out the policy expectations for health in all parts of the Welsh Assembly Government responsibilities, including transport, housing, culture and rural affairs. For example, it defined how transport policy could encourage walking and cycling and reciprocally identified areas where the NHS could engage with the sustainable development policy.

The second Welsh Assembly Government (2003–2007) set out its strategic vision in *Wales: a better country* (Welsh Assembly Government 2003b), in which improving health was identified as a high-level cross-cutting theme.

Wanless and Wales

Wales's health policy has followed closely common themes with the UK government. This is illustrated by the work of Derek Wanless in setting the long-term vision for the health sector in the UK. He was commissioned by the Treasury and the Prime Minister to consider the long-term sustainability of the health system in the UK and then to identify the implications required to achieve the 'fully engaged' scenario, whereby the population was maximally engaged in health-promoting behaviour. Between these reports (HM Treasury 2002, 2004), he reviewed health and social care in Wales and concluded that its current system was unsustainable. He recommended fundamental changes to the health and social care system. The report, nicknamed 'Dai Wanless', indicated that Wales was presently nowhere near achieving the 'fully engaged' scenario and more preventive action was needed.

The English white paper and Health Challenge Wales

The English white paper on public health followed the second Wanless report, *Securing Good Health for the Whole Population* (HM Treasury 2004). In response, the Welsh Assembly Government (2004a) announced the *Health Challenge Wales* campaign whereby the Welsh First Minister challenged organisations, including his own government and its ministers, statutory organisations, communities and individuals to take action to improve their health.

Public health structures following devolution

The Welsh Office, which had supported the Welsh Secretary of State, adapted to the requirements of the new constitutional circumstances without an explicit organisational development project. With the notable exception of the Welsh Health Planning Forum, the Welsh Office had rarely developed an independent health policy capacity, 'topping and tailing' policy letters from Whitehall departments.

Some preparation within the health portfolio was made through an internal report by Sir Graham Hart which recommended that the CMO become a divisional head to manage public health and the functions of the Health Promotion Authority of Wales which had been brought into the Welsh Assembly Government.

Reorganisation for local delivery

Public health structures were reorganised as a consequence of the new *NHS Plan* in 2001. The NHS Plan recommended, to some surprise of its widely consulted stakeholders, the abolition of the five health authorities and the establishment of 22 local health boards (LHBs). These were to be coterminous with the unitary local authorities that were established in 1996 and representing average populations of 130,000 (range 70,000 to 300,000).

The statutory LHBs had over 20 members and were strongly representative of community-based interests, with four representatives of the local authority, including elected members. Each LHB produced a *Health, Social Care and Wellbeing Strategy* with its local partners to direct local programmes to improve health in their communities. To ensure appropriate technical and professional support for public health, the National Public Health Service for Wales (NPHS) was established. The NPHS was formed from the staff of the five public health departments in abolished health authorities and the units of the Public Health Laboratory Service based in Wales. The NPHS was to ensure that each LHB and local authority received public health services, coordinated by a local Director of Public Health. The NPHS aimed to provide a locally delivered public health service to the LHBs and specialised services which need a concentration of expertise in areas such as specialised commissioning and the environment, which in England would be carried out by public health networks. The NPHS did not employ all staff connected with public health delivery, with some programmes being delivered through a range of partnerships with local government and community organisations based on time-limited funding, such as healthy living centres.

These structural changes were announced at the same time as *Shifting of the Balance of Power* in England (Department of Health 2001b), whereby the English health authorities were abolished and public health services were divided between primary care trusts and the Health Protection Agency. The Health Protection Agency was established following *Getting Ahead of the Curve* (Department of Health 2001a) as an England and Wales body for advisory purposes with local service delivery in Wales occurring through the NPHS. The changes in Wales were implemented 1 year after the English 'D-day' on April 2003.

Key support to public health policy development and delivery

The public health academic sector in Wales has broadened from its traditional base in the College of Medicine, due to the establishment of new clinical schools in Swansea and Bangor and the inclusion of other disciplines as a consequence of multidisciplinary public health. Cardiff University School of Social Science, for example, hosts units in the field of health impact assessment and health and ethics.

The Welsh Local Government Association has established a Health Unit to coordinate their members' input to LHBs with designated public health capacity.

Wales has a strong network of voluntary groups and non-governmental organisations (NGOs).

As in England, Wales has seen an expansion in community-based health-improvement services, supported by short-term funding such as the Healthy Living Centres (lottery funded) and the Inequalities in Health Fund, which was established following the Townsend report.

Coordination at the regional tier of government

Strategic coordination of the public health system has occurred at the all-Wales level through the Chief Medical Officer within the Welsh Assembly Government, who holds the service level agreement for the NPHS, is the sponsor division for the Wales Centre for Health and maintains the interfaces with the Health Protection Agency, Department of Health and joint England and Wales arm's-lengths bodies such as NICE, and with arm's-lengths agencies in Wales whose remit links to public health such as the Environment Agency and Food Standards Agency in Wales.

The *Better Health – Better Wales Strategic Framework* recommended the establishment of the Wales Centre for Health as a statutory body under the Health (Wales) Act 2003, which would become an Assembly Sponsored Public Body on 1 April 2005. It was recommended that the Wales Centre for Health will coordinate core public health functions on information, research and training and public engagement.

The new body reports to the National Assembly for Wales's Health and Social Service Committee which acts like a parliamentary select committee in holding ministers to account. This scrutiny is a significant development in strengthening democratic accountability for health to the public at the regional tier of government.

Perspectives

Policies affecting public health in Wales have been adapted to its population's needs, but have matched the core themes of the UK government policies to address inequalities in health. Policy differences regarding NHS policy have occurred, notably the rejection of private finance initiatives and the retention of community health councils in Wales.

The powers of devolution to set different public health policy have not yet been tested and will only happen when the UK and Welsh governments are led by different political parties.

Devolution is already manifesting some significant changes in the delivery of public health. Public health in Wales is led by the regional tier of government, coordinating NHS, local government and other bodies in equal partnership.

The Welsh Assembly Government has set out a policy to establish a core public service for Wales. The current proposal does not involve the NHS, but the potential for public health to be based within a Welsh public service is not only feasible, but potentially desirable.

Such developments would require some preparation. A first step would be a review of the respective roles of the National Public Health Service, the Wales Centre for Health and the health promotion and research functions within the Welsh Assembly Government, 3 years on from the implementation of the Chief Medical Officer's Public Health Review in 2002.

Assessment of current public health capacity in Wales should include the health-improvement initiatives which have been funded by time-limited funding, including for example the Healthy Living Centres, Inequalities in Health Fund, Health Alliances and health promotion grants to the voluntary sector. Wales, like England, faces considerable challenges to integrate the effective components of these programmes into core services once funding ends.

The primary aim would be to specify a core template of effective public health programmes needed by a Welsh public service at the all-Wales and local level. The implementation of the *Health Challenge Wales* programme provides an opportunity to refresh and enhance arrangements for public health delivery. It has started with a major national marketing exercise, local delivery is being driven through LHBs' *Health, Social Care and Wellbeing Strategies*, and the Wales Centre for Health has established a Health Challenge Wales Network to coordinate the programme.

In recent political debates about the health service in Wales, much has been made of the strength of its public health system, within Wales and by external reviewers. These assertions need to be formally assessed by a structured comparison between public health delivery in Wales and England, delivered at regional government tier. Comparative performance of public health delivery at the level of the regional tier could be assessed using the development framework to be used by the Healthcare Commission integrated with the regional indicators for public health that have been developed by the Association of Public Health Observatories working to a standard audit methodology.

This would be timely as the implementation of the English white paper may see the performance for public health delivery between England and Wales receiving the same scrutiny as has recently occurred for waiting lists for hospital care.

Wales, through its Welsh Office of Research and Development (WORD), needs to coordinate its considerable public health research capacity through a funded public health research stream that strengthens the contribution of research to policy and evaluation of public health delivery.

The new statutory body, the Wales Centre for Health, could lead the coordination of applied public health research in Wales, drawing on European models of Institutes of Public Health which are close to but independent of ministries of health in government.

Wales needs to maintain and strengthen its links with UK and European developments in public health. However, Wales's geography and service use by its population make its relationship to England of particular importance. Public health law is made by the England and Wales constitutional entity, as is the census through the Office for National Statistics. Key public health advisory functions are provided by England and Wales bodies, such as NICE (until April 2005) and the Health Protection Agency. Devolution's opportunities for public health will be best realised if Wales maintains and strengthens its close links with scientific and professional capacity in England.

Wales has worked with UK initiatives to develop a multidisciplinary public health workforce through a UK voluntary register. Wales has strong links with local government and is in a position to lead the development of local government-based sponsorship for public health specialist and practitioner training.

The emergent plans for a common public service in Wales provide an important opportunity to develop a multidisciplinary public health training workforce outside of the NHS.

Wales has a track record in taking innovative and radical steps in public health, though often struggling to sustain the trail it has blazed. An area where Wales could lead for the UK is in developing a modern legislative basis for public health, linking an explicit framework of public health ethics to citizenship in the community. The innovative work commissioned by the Nuffield Trust on the case for a new Public Health Act could be tested in Wales. It could test accountable methods to engage the public as citizens and build on early steps to make public health more democratically accountable through the Health (Wales) Act 2003. This work could contribute to the next review of Welsh Assembly Government powers in 2010.

In conclusion

Devolution has seen relatively little divergence in policy between England and Wales, but significant changes in the delivery of public health services. The emerging differences in the implementation of common public health policies in England and Wales represent an important experiment whose rigorous study would be of value not just for Wales, but to aid the development of regional policy for public health in England.

References and further reading

Acheson D (1998) *Independent Inquiry into Inequalities in Health: report*. London: The Stationery Office.

Cardiff Institute of Society, Health and Ethics: www.cf.ac.uk/socsi/cishe/ (accessed 29 March 2005).

Cochrane A and Blythe M (1989) *One Man's Medicine*. Cambridge: Cambridge University Press.

Department of Health (1999) *Saving Lives: our healthier nation*. London: The Stationery Office.

Department of Health (2001a) *Getting Ahead of the Curve: a strategy for combating infectious diseases (including other aspects of health protection)*. London: The Stationery Office. www.dh.gov.uk/PublicationsAndStatistics/Publications/PublicationsPolicyAndGuidanc e/PublicationsPolicyAndGuidanceArticle/fs/en?CONTENT_ID=4007697&chk=t0v3Uu (accessed 29 March 2005).

Department of Health (2001b) *Shifting the Balance of Power: securing delivery*. London: The Stationery Office.

Department of Health (2004) *Choosing Health: making healthier choices easier*. London: The Stationery Office.

Dobson F (1998) *Our Healthier Nation: a contract for health*. Consultation paper presented to Parliament by the Secretary of State for Health by Command of Her Majesty. Cm 3852. London: The Stationery Office.

Great Britain (1998) *Government of Wales Act*. Chapter 38. London: HMSO.

Great Britain (2003) *Health (Wales) Act 2003*. Cardiff: The Stationery Office.

Greer S (2004) *Four Way Bet: how devolution has led to four different models of the NHS*. London: UCL Constitution Unit.

Hall R (1998) *Welsh Health: annual report of the Chief Medical Officer*. Cardiff: Welsh Office.

HM Treasury (2002) *Securing Our Future Health: taking a long-term view*. London: HM Treasury. Available from: www.hm-treasury.gov.uk/Consultations_and_Legislation/ wanless/consult_wanless_final.cfm (accessed 29 March 2005).

HM Treasury (2004) *Securing Good Health for the Whole Population. Final report*. Norwich: HMSO.

Hunter DJ, Wilkinson J and Coyle E (2005) Would regional government have been good for your health? *BMJ*. **330**: 159–60.

Monaghan S, Huws D and Navarro M (2003) *The Case for a New UK Health of the People Act.* London: Nuffield Trust.

National Assembly for Wales (2000) *Better Wales.com.* Cardiff: National Assembly for Wales. Available from: www.wales.gov.uk/themesbetterwales/pdf/strategicplan_e.pdf (accessed 29 March 2005).

National Assembly for Wales (2001) *Targeting Poor Health: Professor Townsend's report of the Welsh Assembly's National Steering Group on the Allocation of NHS Resources Vol. 1.* Cardiff: National Assembly for Wales. Available from: www.cmo.wales.gov.uk/content/work/townsend/targeting-poor-health-e.pdf (accessed 29 March 2005).

National Public Health Service for Wales. Available from: www.wales.nhs.uk/sites/home.cfm?OrgID=368 (accessed 29 March 2005).

Office of the Deputy Prime Minister. *Supporting Communities.* Neighbourhood Renewal Unit, Office of the Deputy Prime Minister. Available from: www.neighbourhood.gov.uk/page.asp?id=4 (accessed 20 March 2005).

Osmond J (1999) *Devolution: 'a dynamic settled process'.* Cardiff: Institute of Welsh Affairs.

PHA Cymru: http://www.ukpha.org.uk/activities/regions/phacymru/default.asp?region_id=1&page_id=98 (accessed 29 March 2005).

Tudor Hart J (1988) *A New Kind of Doctor.* London: Merlin Press.

Welsh Assembly Government (2001a) *Improving Health in Wales: a plan for the NHS with its partners.* Cardiff: NHS Wales. Available from: www.wales.nhs.uk/Publications/NHSStrategydoc.pdf (accessed 29 March 2005).

Welsh Assembly Government (2001b) *Social Disadvantage – communities first.* Cardiff: Welsh Assembly Government. Available from: www.wales.gov.uk/themessocialdeprivation/content/comfirsthome_e.htm (accessed 29 March 2005).

Welsh Assembly Government (2002) *Well Being in Wales. Consultation document.* Office of the Chief Medical Officer. Cardiff: Welsh Assembly Government.

Welsh Assembly Government (2003a) *The Review of Health and Social Care in Wales. The report of the project team advised by Derek Wanless.* Cardiff: Welsh Assembly Government. Available from: www.wales.gov.uk./subieconomics/hsc-review-e.htm.

Welsh Assembly Government (2003b) *Wales: a better country. The strategic agenda of the Welsh Assembly Government.* Cardiff: Welsh Assembly Government. Available from: www.wales.gov.uk/themesbettercountry/index.htm (accessed 29 March 2005).

Welsh Assembly Government (2004a) *Health Challenge Wales.* Cardiff: Welsh Assembly Government. Available from: www.wales.gov.uk/subihcw/index-e.htm (accessed 29 March 2005).

Welsh Assembly Government (2004b) *Making the Connections.* Cardiff: Welsh Assembly Government. Available from: www.wales.gov.uk/themespublicservicereform/content/Making_Connection_Eng.pdf (accessed 29 March 2005).

Welsh European Funding Office (2000) *Objective 1 Funding.* Available from: www.wefo.wales.gov.uk/default.asp?action=page&ID=238 (accessed 29 March 2005).

Welsh Health Impact Assessment Unit: www.whiasu.cardiff.ac.uk/ (accessed 29 March 2005).

Welsh Local Government Association (1998) *Working Together for a Healthy Wales: the local government role.* Cardiff: WLGA.

Welsh Local Government Association: http://www.wlga.gov.uk/index3e.htm (accessed 29 March 2005).

Welsh Office (1998a) *Better Health – Better Wales. A consultation paper presented to Parliament by the Secretary of State for Wales by command of Her Majesty.* Cm 3922. London: The Stationery Office.

Welsh Office (1998) *Better Health – Better Wales Strategic Framework.* Cardiff: Welsh Office.

Welsh Office (1999) *Sure Start; a programme to increase opportunity for very young children and their families in Wales.* Cardiff: Welsh Office Circular 21/99. Available from: www.wales.gov.uk/subichildren/content/circulars/start/start-e.htm (accessed 29 March 2005).

Chapter 4

Public health in a changing Ireland: an all-island perspective

Jane Wilde

This chapter describes the state of health of people on the island of Ireland[1] and identifies some of the main opportunities and challenges for public health against a backdrop of remarkable social and political change.

Background

The two jurisdictions of the Republic of Ireland and Northern Ireland (part of the United Kingdom) differ markedly with separate structures of government, administration, financing systems and, in many cases, priorities. Economic growth (the 'Celtic Tiger') and dramatic reductions in levels of absolute poverty in the South, and falling unemployment in the North have contributed to improvements in aspects of health status (Hillyard, Rolston and Tomlinson 2005). Other major changes include an ageing population and a rise in the numbers of people who are refugees or seeking asylum (Central Statistics Office 2003; National Council on Ageing and Older People 2005). Despite increasing economic standards, South and North, levels of relative poverty and child poverty are high and the 2003 World Development Report describes levels of income inequality in Ireland second only to the USA among OECD (Organisation for Economic Co-operation and Development) countries (Hillyard *et al.* 2003; United Nations Development Programme 2003).

Health services on the island have developed quite differently. In the South an 'extraordinary symbiosis' has developed between private and public medicine, and means tests or income limits have been used to determine access to health services (Barrington 1987). For example, people with income above a defined level are directly charged for primary care services.

In the North, debates and policies often 'read across' from Britain and while the health service differs in some important ways from other parts of the United Kingdom, for example health and social services have been integrated since 1973, it tends to have common features (McLaughlin 2005). The Northern Ireland Assembly, formed as a result of the 1998 Good Friday Agreement, has had little opportunity to stamp its own mark on local policies due to its repeated suspension (Northern Ireland Office 1998).

The Agreement also changed significantly the relationship between Britain and Ireland, allowing for greater cooperation across the border and breaking the 'icy silence' of the years following partition (Arthur 2000). As well as important

---

[1] For clarity the term Ireland is used to describe the geographical entity of the island, and the terms North and South to describe the separate parts of the island.

changes in relation to human rights and equality, six cross-border bodies were set up, including one in the area of food safety, as well as a general clause support-ing cooperation in health.

A picture of health?

Life expectancy is increasing in both parts of the island with falling death rates from major chronic diseases such as heart disease, respiratory disease and some cancers (Department of Health and Children 2004; Report of the Chief Medical Officer for Northern Ireland 2004).

But many challenges remain. Mortality rates from chronic diseases, including heart disease and cancers, are higher than in most western European countries (*see* Boxes 4.1 and 4.2).

Box 4.1 Mortality on the island

During the period 1989–1998 mortality on the island compared unfavourably to Europe. After adjusting for age, mortality rates for the main causes of death including circulatory and respiratory diseases were greater on the island than they were for the (combined) EU-15 countries. This was true for both the North and the South.

Source: Institute of Public Health in Ireland (2001).

Box 4.2 Cancer incidence, mortality and survival for the island of Ireland, 1998–2000

- Breast, colorectal, lung, lymphoma and oesophageal cancer incidence and mortality rates for women in Ireland are significantly higher than rates for women in the EU.
- Colorectal, oesophageal and prostate cancer incidence and mortality rates for men in Ireland are significantly higher than for men in the EU.

Source: Northern Ireland Cancer Registry and National Cancer Registry, Ireland (2004).

The most recent surveys of health and lifestyle, South and North, show adult smoking rates of 26% and 27%, respectively, and the health of young people is threatened by high levels of smoking, unhealthy nutrition, unsafe sex and dan-gerous drinking. Estimates suggest that more than 300,000 children on the island are overweight or obese, with the annual number growing by 10,000. Lifestyle surveys show wide differences in levels of smoking, drug misuse, suicide, and obesity between different socio-economic groups. No clear social class gradient is reported for alcohol use (Department of Health and Children 2005; Health Promotion Agency 2005; Kelleher *et al.* 2003).

Recent reports also highlight growing concern about the rise in sexually trans-mitted diseases including chlamydia (Communicable Diseases Surveillance Centre

2003; National Disease Surveillance Centre 2003). One in ten adults suffers from mental health problems and there is concern about the rise in suicide among young men (Crowley, Kilroe and Burke 2004). The ageing population means a frailer population with more chronic disease.

Inequalities in health on the island

A particular public health challenge is the wide gap in the health of rich and poor. In 2000 a report, based on nearly half a million deaths during 1989–98, describing age, gender, regional and occupational class differences in mortality for 65 causes of death, established the pervasiveness and magnitude of occupational class inequalities on the island (Balanda and Wilde 2001). A steep occupational class gradient running across all social groups was present for circulatory diseases, cancers, respiratory diseases, and injuries and poisonings (*see* Box 4.3).

Box 4.3 Inequalities in mortality on the island

All-causes mortality rate in the lowest occupational class was 100% to 200% higher than the rate in the highest occupational class. This was evident for nearly all the main causes of death, including cancers, respiratory diseases and accidents and poisoning. Excess mortality among males was also striking, with the all-causes mortality rate for males 54% higher than it was for females.

Source: Institute of Public Health in Ireland (2001).

A more recent study explored systematically the complex relationships between demographic and socio-economic characteristics, and five measures of perceived health (general health, limiting long-term illness, general mental health, satisfaction with health, and quality of life). Significant demographic and socio-economic inequalities were apparent for all the measures of perceived health used, with the nature of the inequalities depending on the particular measure of perceived health being considered. Indicators of social capital were also found to have significant independent effects on perceived health (Balanda and Wilde 2004).

Summary reports South and North highlight inequalities in infant and perinatal mortality, childhood accidents, and in rates of low birth-weight births as well as long-standing illness and disability (Barry *et al.* 2001; Burke *et al.* 2004; McWhirter 2004). Groups experiencing reduced life expectancy include travellers, a distinct minority group of Irish people with their own lifestyle and culture.

North–South differences reflect the tragic effects of the conflict in the North and greater levels of inequalities in access to and use of health services in the South, but the general picture is that people from both parts of the island face similar public health challenges including appalling levels of inequalities in health (Wren 2003).

Policy responses

This brief review looks at the different ways in which the South and North handle policy on public health and poverty, while acknowledging that a much wider range of policy responses is needed to address the wider determinants of health. Growing levels of cooperation on the island are also described.

South

In the South the most recent health strategy, *Quality and Fairness – a health system for you*, has three themes – access, quality and equity – identified to respond to wide concern about standards and geographical inequalities. It states that '*Equity will be central in developing policies (1) to reduce the difference in health status currently running across the social spectrum in Ireland; and (2) to ensure equitable services based on need*' (Department of Health and Children 2001). The strategy contains 121 recommendations, and notes which agencies are responsible. It commits to a broad population health approach and identifies a wide range of strategies to tackle key challenges including heart disease, mental health, alcohol, drugs, cancer and accidents. The latest aims to tackle obesity.

The recent Health Services Reform Programme has brought all health services together, within one overarching Health Services Executive (HSE) with a population health directorate responsible for health protection, health intelligence, health promotion and policy (Department of Health and Children 2003).

The Irish government has a long-standing commitment to a national anti-poverty strategy. In 1997, the National Anti-Poverty Strategy (NAPS) was published, the first anti-poverty strategy adopted by any European government detailing the causes and consequences of poverty and setting key targets for poverty reduction. While health issues were outlined in NAPS no specific health targets were set. In 2000, the government's Programme for Prosperity and Fairness committed to reviewing the original targets and setting new ones. A series of NAPS working groups was established, one with the remit to develop health targets and an associated implementation and monitoring framework. Targets were set to reduce gaps in premature mortality, and low birth-weight rates and life expectancy for travellers (*see* Box 4.4) (Institute of Public Health in Ireland 2001). The government has adopted these targets and the NAPS plan as '*the most appropriate framework for concerted action in addressing health inequalities*'. Each government department reports progress to the Office for Social Inclusion which coordinates work on behalf of a cabinet sub-committee headed by the Taoiseach (Prime Minister).

Box 4.4 National Anti-Poverty Strategy health targets, Ireland

- To reduce the gap in premature mortality between the lowest and the highest socio-economic groups by at least 10% for circulatory diseases, cancers and injuries and poisoning by 2007.
- To reduce the gap in low birth-weight rates for children from the lowest and highest socio-economic group by 10% by 2007.
- To reduce the gap in life expectancy between the traveller community and the whole population by at least 10% by 2007.

Source: Government of Ireland (2002).

North

In the North, *Working for a Healthier People* is one of five key themes of the Northern Ireland Assembly's Programme for Government (Office of the First Minister and Deputy First Minister 2001). It reflects the public health strategy, *Investing for Health* (IfH), which takes a broad social approach, with a central focus on tackling inequality (Department of Health, Social Services and Public Safety 2002). The strategy, sponsored by the Ministerial Group on Public Health which includes all ten government departments, sets two broad goals and a series of targets and objectives, aimed at improving the wider determinants of health (*see* Box 4.5). The programme includes a mix of interventions involving all government departments and the services they provide. These cross-departmental actions constitute the programme for action to tackle inequalities in health. Follow-up included setting up Investing for Health partnerships led by the health sectors and involving many organisations and community groups, and government funding for a community grants scheme and a research programme.

Box 4.5 *Investing for Health* goals, targets and objectives, Northern Ireland

Goal 1: To improve the health of our people by increasing the length of their lives and increasing the number of years they spend free from disease, illness and disability.

- Improve life expectancy by at least 3 years for men and by 2 years for women between 2000 and 2010.

Goal 2: To reduce inequalities in health between geographic area, socio-economic and minority groups.

- To halve the gap in life expectancy between those living in the fifth most deprived electoral wards and the average life expectancy for both men and women between 2000 and 2010.
- To reduce the gap in the proportion of people with a long-standing illness between those in the highest and the lowest socio-economic groups by a fifth between 2000 and 2010.

Objectives:

- To reduce poverty in families with children.
- To enable all people and young people in particular to develop the skills and attitudes that will give them the capacity to reach their full potential and make healthy choices.
- To promote mental health and emotional wellbeing at individual and community level.
- To offer everyone the opportunity to live and work in a healthy environment and to live in a decent affordable home.
- To improve our neighbourhoods and wider environment.
- To reduce accidental injuries and deaths in the home, workplace and from collisions on the road.
- To enable people to make healthier choices.

Source: Department of Health, Social Services and Public Safety (2002).

Following the recent Review of Public Administration, sweeping changes are proposed in the organisation of local government and bodies responsible for education and health (Northern Ireland Executive 2005). Recommendations from a separate Review of the Public Health Function include strengthening interdepartmental working within government, extending the health protection function and its links to the Health Protection Agency in England and Wales, combining health promotion and health intelligence function in one body, and increasing cooperation on the island (Department of Health, Social Services and Public Safety 2004).

In contrast to the South the North has yet to develop an anti-poverty strategy, although this is now underway following strong criticism that the programme, *Targeting Social Need* (TSN), set up to redress unequal social need experienced by Catholics, failed to address the structural determinants of inequality (Office of the First Minister and Deputy First Minister 2004).

North/South cooperation on the island

Cooperation between professional associations on the island has been a long-standing feature of health services, but until recently this has rarely developed into shared policies or programmes.

The CAWT (Cooperation and Working Together) initiative by the (then) four health boards adjoining the Irish border is an important attempt to overcome the complexities of cross-border working in providing services for people living on either side of the border. An extensive range of programmes has been developed, mainly with European funding (www.cawt.com/).

In 1999 a new Institute of Public Health in Ireland was set up to promote cooperation in information and surveillance, research, capacity building and policy advice. It is based on a belief that there are practical benefits from tackling similar public health problems together, exploring differences and ways they are tackled, and looking ahead to identify future public health concerns. Inequalities is the focus of its work, which includes an all-island leadership programme, research and evaluation, building capacity for health impact assessment (HIA) and the development of an all-island population health observatory (www.publichealth.ie/; www.inispho.org/).

There is also growing cross-border cooperation by other organisations, including research by the cancer registries, joint health-promotion campaigns and shared responses to health protection (Campo, Comber and Gavin 2004; Communicable Diseases Surveillance Centre 2003; National Disease Surveillance Centre 2003). The Health Research Board in Ireland and the Research and Development Office in Northern Ireland are funding cross-border research, and the nursing profession has a well-planned strategy including building leadership, developing all-island databases and sharing good practice (DHSSPS and DOHC 2003).

Outside government the newly formed Public Health Alliance in Ireland and the re-emergence of the Northern Ireland Public Health Alliance provide a home for multidisciplinary groups and individuals from all sectors to add their voice to efforts to improve health and the recent move to form an all-island Public Health Alliance acknowledges a desire to tackle common public health challenges together (www.nipha.org; www.publichealthallianceireland.org).

Challenges and opportunities for public health on the island of Ireland

Responding effectively to the wide and varied nature of public health challenges on the island raises critical issues, many of which feature internationally (Allin *et al.* 2004; Beaglehole 2003). In Ireland the most important are political leadership and policy coherence; support for policy implementation including a widely shared agenda and sustainable public health system; and building knowledge.

Political leadership and policy coherence

Government policy, South and North, espouses a strong vision for public health, highlighting the importance of broad determinants and joining up government policies. But policy coherence is often lacking with policy makers in 'sectoral silos' failing to consider how their actions affect health.

There is a constant preoccupation with economic success. Debates on 'health' are dominated by waiting lists and when attention does turn to public health it is often divisive, concentrating on arguments about individual and collective responsibility.

This is illustrated by the introduction of the ban on smoking in public places in the South where the Minister of Health and government acknowledged the importance of state action in protecting health, and their leadership in standing up to economic arguments about widespread job losses and the destruction of the 'Irish pub' was widely praised (Howell 2004). But the pendulum swings and state interventions to reduce alcohol use or obesity are now more often billed as the 'nanny state'.

The challenge is to encourage and convince politicians and opinion formers of the central idea of public health, the need for collective responsibility and action.

From policy to implementation

The strongest policies will do little good if not implemented. Examples from South and North illustrate the importance of understanding what is needed to put policy into practice, and providing realistic levels of support. The health strategy in the South was developed with a strong public health approach but the lack of an implementation plan and insufficient support has so far left many commitments unmet. And in the North funding for community development projects to support the IfH strategy was withdrawn just as evaluation was showing signs of success.

Effective implementation needs a widely shared agenda with a well-supported community sector, cross-sectoral partnerships, a skilled workforce and relevant and timely information and surveillance system. Policies, South and North, see the value of the community sector in shaping and sustaining implementation yet pioneering community development initiatives are having to survive on a shoestring.

There are multiple cross-sectoral community health partnerships. In the North they include Health Action Zones, Healthy Living Centres and Healthy Cities, as well as the recent Investing for Health Partnerships, and in the South a wide range also exists providing important opportunities for a widely shared public health effort.

The argument is now accepted, South and North, that public health needs a skilled and multidisciplinary workforce; the challenge is to ensure support for training needs and career development.

In the South a new national body, the Health Information and Quality Authority (HIQA), is expected to tackle some of the long-standing difficulties with health information and there are moves South and North to establish responsibility for population health intelligence and improved knowledge management. A new all-island Population Health Observatory, linked to similar initiatives in the United Kingdom and internationally, is an exciting initiative which responds to calls for all-island comparative data (www.inispho.org/).

Evidence and learning: what works?

No single organisation in Ireland has the remit to develop the evidence base for public health and capacity for policy research and systematic reviews in public health is limited. The main emphasis is using evidence generated elsewhere, making it accessible and finding appropriate and locally sensitive ways of implementing it. Awareness and access to evidence needs to be promoted, highlighting where evidence is lacking and continuing exploration of innovative ways to get evidence into practice (Boydell and Wilde 2006). An important aspect is ensuring that high-quality evaluations are carried out including cost-effectiveness studies which will increasingly be required as health services and public services come under even greater pressure.

Although much has been invested in evaluating local projects, research into public health delivery is almost non-existent. Evidence is fragmentary or inconclusive, with no systematic database to which practitioners can turn for information. Often project evaluations are ignored, and new projects set up regardless, and those projects which do not demonstrate high-profile 'success' are often stopped just as they are showing signs of development.

Understanding more clearly how policy is implemented South and North offers real opportunities for learning. Networks are growing but further support is needed to encourage multidisciplinary research and cooperation between researchers, policy makers and practitioners.

Looking ahead: working across borders

In Ireland, South and North, we now have considerably more knowledge about the extent and causes of poor health, and inequalities in health. Research and advocacy have been influential in shaping some policies in directions favourable to public health and reducing inequalities. But to ensure implementation we need to grasp the opportunity of change to move from tentative and often ineffectual approaches to robust systems and effective networks for public health which tackle the social and economic determinants of health.

Across the island different social and economic policies and health structures created as a result of 80 years of back-to-back development have been serious barriers to cooperation, and differing health and information systems have complicated comparisons between the two jurisdictions.

The Good Friday Agreement has been the stimulus for a changed relationship between the two jurisdictions and cooperation has increased dramatically. There is a level of stability and cooperation, unrecognisable even 10 years ago, reflecting ways in which the 'three solitudes' (Arthur 2000) around Belfast, Dublin and London are being challenged and overcome, with growing interest in common responses, and a realisation of the potential of all-island approaches.

Building cooperation and crossing organisational, sectoral, professional and geographic boundaries is crucial in addressing the many pressing public health problems in Ireland.

There could not be a more convincing case for governments, South and North, to break from the past and demonstrate they are truly interested in transforming the lives of people in Ireland than by placing health at the top of the political agenda.

References

Allin S, Mossialos E, McKee M *et al.* (2004) *Making Decisions on Public Health: a review of eight countries.* Copenhagen: European Observatory on Health Care Systems.

Arthur P (2000) *Special Relationships – Britain, Ireland and the Northern Ireland problem.* Belfast: The Blackstaff Press Limited.

Balanda K and Wilde J (2001) *Inequalities in Mortality 1989–1998.* Dublin/Belfast: The Institute of Public Health in Ireland.

Balanda K and Wilde J (2004) *Inequalities in Perceived Health. A report on the All-Ireland Social Capital and Health Survey.* Dublin/Belfast: The Institute of Public Health in Ireland.

Barrington R (1987) *Health, Medicine and Politics in Ireland 1900–1970.* Dublin: Institute of Public Administration.

Barry J, Sinclair H, Kelly A *et al.* (2001) *Inequalities in Health in Ireland – hard facts.* Dublin: Department of Community Health and General Practice, Trinity College.

Beaglehole R (2003) *Global Public Health: a new era.* Oxford: Oxford University Press.

Boydell L and Wilde J (2006) Evidence on health inequalities: an evidence based approach to public health and tackling health inequalities in Ireland and Northern Ireland. In: A Killoran, C Swann and M Kelly (eds) *Public Health Evidence Tackling Health Inequalities.* Oxford and London: Oxford University Press/Health Development Agency/NICE.

Burke S, Keenaghan C, O'Donovan D *et al.* (2004) *Health in Ireland – an unequal state.* Dublin: Public Health Alliance Ireland.

Campo J, Comber H and Gavin A (2004) *All-Ireland Cancer Statistics 1998–2000.* Belfast/Dublin: Northern Ireland Cancer Registry/National Cancer Registry.

Central Statistics Office (CSO) (2003) *Population and Migration Estimates April 2003.* Dublin: CSO.

Communicable Diseases Surveillance Centre (NI) (CDSC (NI)) (2003) *Communicable Diseases. Provisional Summary 2003.* Belfast: CDSC (NI).

Cooperation and Working Together (CAWT): www.cawt.com/

Crowley P, Kilroe J and Burke S (2004) *Youth Suicide Prevention. An evidence briefing.* London: Health Development Agency and Institute of Public Health in Ireland.

Department of Health and Children (DOHC) (2001) *Quality and Fairness – a health system for you.* Dublin: DOHC.

Department of Health and Children (DOHC) (2003) *The Health Service Reform Programme.* Dublin: DOHC.

Department of Health and Children (DOHC) (2004) *Fourth Annual Report of the Chief Medical Officer: better health through prevention.* Dublin: DOHC.

Department of Health and Children (DOHC) (2005) *Obesity. The policy challenges. The report of the National Taskforce on Obesity.* Dublin: DOHC.

Department of Health, Social Services and Public Safety (DHSSPS) (2002) *Investing for Health.* Belfast: DHSSPS.

Department of Health, Social Services and Public Safety (DHSSPS) (2004) *The Review of the Public Health Function in Northern Ireland.* Belfast: DHSSPS.

Department of Health, Social Services and Public Safety (DHSSPS) and Department of Health and Children (DOHC) (2003) *From Vision to Action – strengthening the nursing contribution to public health.* Belfast/Dublin: DHSSPS and DOHC.

Government of Ireland (2002) *Building an Inclusive Society: a Review of the National Anti-Poverty Strategy*. Dublin: Stationery Office.

Health Promotion Agency (HPA) (2005) *Health and Lifestyle Survey for Northern Ireland 2002*. Belfast: HPA.

Hillyard P, Kelly G, McLaughlin E *et al*. (2003) *Bare Necessities: poverty and social exclusion in Northern Ireland*. Belfast: Democratic Dialogue.

Hillyard P, Rolston B and Tomlinson M (2005) *Poverty and Conflict in Ireland: an international perspective*. Dublin: Combat Poverty Agency.

Howell F (2004) Ireland's workplaces, going smoke free. *BMJ*. **328**: 847–8.

Institute of Public Health in Ireland (IPH): www.publichealth.ie/

Institute of Public Health in Ireland (IPH) (2001) *Report of the Working Group on the National Anti-Poverty Strategy and Health*. Belfast/Dublin: IPH.

Ireland and Northern Ireland's Population Health Observatory (INIsPHO): www.inispho.org/

Kelleher C, Nic Gabhainn S, Friel S *et al*. (2003) *The National Health and Lifestyle Surveys*. National University of Ireland, Galway; Department of Public Health Medicine and Epidemiology, University College Dublin, Galway.

McLaughlin E (2005) Governance and social policy in Northern Ireland (1999–2004): the devolution years and postscript. In: M Powell, L Bauld and K Clarke (eds) *Social Policy Review 17: analysis and debate in social policy, 2005*. Bristol: The Policy Press/Social Policy Association.

McWhirter L (ed.) (2004) *Equality and Inequalities in Health and Social Care in Northern Ireland – a statistical overview*. Belfast: Department of Health, Social Services and Public Safety.

National Council on Ageing and Older People (2005) *An Age Friendly Society. A position statement*. Dublin: National Council on Ageing and Older People.

National Disease Surveillance Centre (NDSC) (2003) *National Disease Surveillance Centre Annual report 2003*. Dublin: NDSC.

Northern Ireland Executive (2005) *The Review of Public Administration in Northern Ireland. Further consultation*. Belfast: Northern Ireland Executive.

Northern Ireland Office (NIO) (1998) *The Agreement Reached in the Multi-Party Negotiations on Northern Ireland*. Belfast and London: NIO.

Northern Ireland Public Health Alliance: www.nipha.org/

Office of the First Minister and Deputy First Minister (OFM/DFM) (2001) *Making a Difference – programme for government*. Belfast: OFM/DFM.

Office of the First Minister and Deputy First Minister (OFM/DFM) (2004) *Towards an Anti-Poverty Strategy: new TSN – the way forward: a consultation document*. Belfast: OFM/DFM.

Public Health Alliance: www.publichealthallianceireland.org

Report of the Chief Medical Officer for Northern Ireland (2004) *The Health of the Public in Northern Ireland*. Belfast: Department of Health, Social Services and Public Safety.

United Nations Development Programme (UNDP) (2003) *Human Development Report 2003. Millennium Development Goals: a compact among nations to end human poverty*. Oxford: Oxford University Press.

Wren MA (2003) *An Unhealthy State – anatomy of a sick society*. Dublin: New Island.

Chapter 5

Public health policy making in a disunited kingdom

Scott L Greer

The problem of making public health policy is the problem of bridging the gap between people who are concerned with good public health and politicians who make policy. The former are concerned with evidence-based interventions, with inequalities, with the wider determinants of health and with health protection. The latter can make important decisions but are not necessarily interested in public health, have radically different careers that might not benefit from work on public health, and generally lack the time and interest to engage in a topic that does not bring them identifiable political benefit. All the evidence base in the world will go to waste unless it can produce a policy – and getting that policy made requires looking at the policy makers.

This chapter looks at the forces that shape policies and the trajectories of public health in the UK since devolution. Other chapters discuss the policies enacted, their rationales, and the way they work; this chapter looks at the *politics* of public health. It looks first at what different UK governments can and cannot do in public health; it then looks at the major differences between the politics of England, Northern Ireland, Scotland and Wales and explains how they shape the kinds of public health policies that get made.

Scope to differ: the institutions

The constitution of the United Kingdom – the politics and policies it makes possible – might be one of the most important factors shaping public health and public health policy, but like most other political institutions it was not designed with good public health policy making in mind. Devolution was pragmatic from the start. It was, fundamentally, about solving immediate problems such as the intolerable pressure from Scotland and Wales for change in their constitutional status, and by the complex Northern Ireland peace process. It might look to future generations like a radical reform of the UK, but it is important to remember that history and particular problems shaped it and created the structure that governs public health policy today (Bogdanor 1999; for analyses of how devolution works, *see* Burrows 2000; Trench 2005, 2006).

The consequences of history for devolution are often forgotten. One of the most important is the simple fact that while the Northern Ireland Assembly, the National Assembly for Wales and the Scottish Parliament are new bodies in themselves, their administrations – the Northern Ireland Executive, the Scottish Executive and the Welsh Assembly Government – are much older. The newly elected devolved representatives inherited old administrations in the form of the spending departments known as 'territorial offices' that had been responsible for most policy in the three areas. The Scottish Office dates back to the 19th century, the (separate) Northern Ireland Civil Service is the last of a long line of Irish administrations, and the Welsh Office was established in 1964 (Carmichael 2002; Deacon 2002; Mitchell 2003).

The inheritance of the past had two consequences. One was that from the start it was a mistake to think of devolution as starting from a clean slate. The territorial offices already had distinct administrations, distinct 'policy communities' of advisers and technicians, and distinct styles of doing business. The political and technical realities – the pressures on Northern Irish, Welsh and Scottish policy makers – changed less with devolution than the amount of autonomy they had with which to respond differently (Greer 2004).

The other consequence, which increasingly matters, is that devolution has a loosely joined-up institutional structure (Greer 2006). This meant, for example, that the UK (almost uniquely among decentralised states) did not create a charter of social rights for all its people. It kept a crude block grant (the Barnett formula) that had previously been an in-house tool to allocate funds to the three territorial offices. There was no thought to channelling or constraining divergence, and, more worrisome, no thought to managing tensions and frictions.

Devolution is also highly 'asymmetric', meaning that the autonomy and size of the different parts of the UK varies enormously (Hazell 2006). England, with around 85% of the UK population, is ruled directly by the UK government. When an English voter chooses an MP (Member of Parliament), that voter is making a choice about health, education and other policies. A Scottish or Welsh voter is not; for them MPs are confined to UK issues such as defence. The result is a terminological minefield: the UK government, elected across the UK, governs the English health system (and indeed until fairly recently chose to make a Scottish MP the Secretary of State for Health in England, thereby making him responsible for English health but not health in his own Scottish constituency). Northern Ireland makes things more complicated as no major UK party campaigns there, and because its career as an autonomous devolved unit has been short and largely ineffective. When it is suspended, it is governed by 'direct rule', meaning the Secretary of State for Northern Ireland and a varying number of junior ministers, all of them UK government politicians.

The result of this institutional arrangement is that the UK is a very good environment for public health policy experimentation, with England, Scotland and Wales free to develop and adopt new policy ideas (and their motion makes Northern Ireland's comparative lack of change a distinctive trajectory in its own right).

It is not surprising that there has been substantial divergence in public health policy making in the first decade of devolution. Public health is an area with *comparatively* cleanly divided functions; the devolved governments are each responsible for the dedicated public health function in their areas, and the UK government for public health in England as well as regulatory functions that operate in more than England (such as the Food Standards Agency). The *issues* are of course often complicated and cross-border, but the *resources* and *powers* are comparatively cleanly devolved because responsibility for various tasks was already fitted to different agencies and offices, and they usually are clearly responsible to one devolved or UK minister. Insofar as there is a major structural constraint in what devolved public health policy makers can and cannot do, it is the developing public health competency of the European Union.

And insofar as there is a problem, it is that it includes neither coordination mechanisms nor an overall plan and coherent division of responsibilities for health protection. As in many other policy areas, the UK has relied for coordination and information flows on existing networks of professionals and officials (in public health, this means the professionals and their associations). This means that ideas flow between professionals – meetings of UK-wide professional societies are where they exchange the ideas that they then promote in their various systems. It also means that when real joint working is required – as in the case of preparations for a major communicable disease outbreak – the absence of serious formal networks will put informal ones under tremendous strain.

Reasons to differ: parties

Politicians live and die by parties. They are elected if their parties do well; they are promoted if they do things that their party leadership wants to reward. That means that when polities have different party systems, they produce different kinds of policy.

England has a three-party system organised primarily around 'left–right' debates between Labour and the Conservatives, with a strong Liberal Democrat party on the centre-left. The effect is that public health interventions are attacked on classic 'right' grounds (paternalism, big government) in England, by Conservatives, and Labour feels that it must adjust. The basic pattern of Labour fearing to intervene in lifestyles (such as through comprehensive bans on smoking in public places) or attacking economic underpinnings of health inequalities is one that is shaped by the electoral hazards it faces in England. It is notable, for example, that it is the UK government's fear of electoral consequences in England that has held back efforts to ban smoking in public places; both Northern Irish and Welsh policy makers would have liked to go further, but Wales could not because of legal issues, and Northern Ireland could not because it was under direct rule – i.e. rule by that same UK government.

Scotland has a far more fluid and complicated party system, with Labour and the Liberal Democrats in coalition, weak Conservatives, two parties well to the left of Labour (the Scottish Socialist Party and the Greens), and the largest opposition to Labour in the form of the separatist Scottish National Party. That means Scottish Labour makes health policy in a five-party system where four of the parties are somewhere to the left of Labour in Westminster, and three of them are formally committed to Scottish separation from the UK. The centre of gravity in Scottish politics lies far from the centre of gravity in English politics, and so therefore do the day-to-day political problems ministers face. This means, for example, that the Scottish Socialist Party and the Scottish National Party, with battle cry of 'free fruit in schools', both made school food an issue long before it emerged elsewhere.

Wales has a system with many features in common with Scotland, and similarly complex and distinctive politics. Again, Labour rules, in or on the edge of a coalition, and is faced with substantial opposition from a nationalist party. Its less-fragmented party system has only one Wales-only party, the nationalist Plaid Cymru. Wales lacks the left-wing 'anchor' of the two Scottish left parties, and Plaid might therefore have more space to change policies than the SNP. Nevertheless, Welsh government ministers constantly face attacks on the grounds that they do not do enough to defend distinctive Welsh interests.

Northern Ireland, finally, has a party system organised around attitudes towards the UK rather than health systems; the major Northern Irish parties scarcely campaign on health and have only poorly developed public health policies if they have any at all. Uniquely in the UK, Northern Ireland gives its politicians little reason to pay attention to health.

Policies

The policy communities of the four different UK health systems are the sources of most policy ideas – the professional leaders, officials, think-tankers, journalists and others who engage seriously with public health policy, advocate for ideas, and argue with each other about desirability and feasibility, evidence, costs and benefits. Their activity is local – being a known quantity in Cardiff Bay or Westminster is more important than many a publication. The participation of public health advocates in each of these communities varies, giving a different cast to public health policy and also shaping the extent of public health's achievements and policies.

In England, the policy community has a strong focus on health services, in part because public health is a poor fit with efforts to use managerial techniques to increase the throughput of health services. The English policy community contains a great deal of public health leadership and expertise, but in London policy debates public health is *comparatively* unrepresented compared to those who advocate for a focus on various aspects of health services. Compared to England past, the Labour government (with its focus on complex 'wicked issues') is extremely interested in public health and willing to accept it as a route to policy goals as diverse as an economically sustainable NHS and the reduction of incapacity benefit. Advocates of various schemes for joint working and local service integration have, given Labour's political environment, often had better luck than those arguing for regulation of markets or societies (such as those concerned with obesity).

Scotland, meanwhile, is the inheritor of a long tradition of professional leadership across health policy (Nottingham 2000; Woods and Carter 2003). This includes Scotland's public health policies, in which there is a long tradition of public health scholarship and leadership – and much closer connections with authority, dating back to the Enlightenment. Public health medicine bulks large in Scotland, and medicine bulks large in Scottish policy debates. The importance of professionals and professional organisations in shaping health policy debates in Scotland is such that a focus on public health can coexist with a great deal of attention to health services. Scotland, both in its efforts to reduce inequalities through large funding shifts and its willingness to regulate social behaviour, takes public health very seriously.

Northern Ireland's lack of headline policies, meanwhile, has the interesting consequence of creating a great deal of local organisational autonomy. The various components of the Northern Irish health and social services system are organisationally very stable by UK standards, and the central department has comparatively little control over them. This means that individual managers and leaders of all sorts are able to develop their own focuses, including in some cases a considerable interest in the wider determinants of health and in inequalities issues. The paralysis of high-level policy making means that there is not much serious public health policy making at the Northern Ireland level, but there is a great deal of local variation.

Finally, there is Wales. Wales at devolution (and still) lacked the dense and numerous professional leaders of Scotland and the health-services-orientated English policy community. Instead, when the National Assembly first convened it was a group of actors who are almost invisible in England who stepped forward to shape health policy and put a focus on public health. They are local government, unions, and public health professionals. Their argument was for a strong focus on the reduction of inequalities, on local integration of health and local government, and a great deal of investment in work on the wider determinants of health. This corresponded with their interests and skills as well as ideological conviction, and provided the outline of a distinctive, left, Welsh policy orientation. It involved trying to use NHS Wales as one of several tools to improve health outcomes, and a great deal of funding intended to reduce inequalities as well as a unified all-Wales public health body.

The problem in Wales is partly that there are severe structural problems with health *services* that turn any portfolio associated with health into a political albatross. More worrisome, the distinctive debate in Wales is based on an opposition. Welsh politics increasingly oppose public health and a long-term focus on the wider determinants of health *against* a short-term focus on making hospitals work better. The visibility and popularity of hospitals, doctors and nurses mean that, once such an opposition is created, public health measures become politically difficult to sustain. Such an opposition need not exist; it is, like most things in politics, a creation. There are other long-term issues that excite public interest – pensions and the environment, for example – and there are short-term benefits to investing in public health that can be trumpeted. Arguing simply that Wales has opted for a long-term solution to health at the expense of short-term waiting times is entering a fight public health will have a difficult time winning.

Conclusion: divergent public health policy making

In short, there are good structural reasons for public health policy divergence in the UK. Politicians live and die by their performance in party politics, and the party politics of England, Northern Ireland, Scotland and Wales are very different. And the 'policy communities' – the people advocating for public health measures – work best on the ground, offering their policy ideas. That means that the different debates in Belfast, Cardiff, Edinburgh and London – the different participants in the policy debates, the different traditions of public health – filter the ideas that get to those politicians. The result is a structural tendency to diverge.

It produces less of a tendency to learn and compare notes. The professional and official networks that tie together the UK are the ones who transmit ideas, and advocate for their chosen, and often evidence-based, policies in very different political environments. Only at the highest level do media and political agendas interact. It is much more likely that issues such as school food come on and off agendas at different times – public health advocates, the SNP and the Scottish Socialist Party put school food on Scottish political agendas long before television chef Jamie Oliver put it on the UK (English) agenda. The result is that Jamie Oliver's impact on English debates is significant, but is much less so in Scotland, where the debate is already moving in a different direction and partly resolved. It is not to the level of Oliver and prime ministers that we should look if we want to see the real interconnections.

While we can be sure that ideas will travel and be proposed – if not adopted – everywhere across the UK, there are grounds for concern at the formal interconnections between the four health systems. How well do the public health protection systems mesh? We have yet to see the post-devolution public health infrastructure tested in a crisis, but the combination of slow decay of working networks between officials and legal vagueness as to who does what is worrisome.

The result, finally, is that it is a mistake to regard England as a baseline. England is indeed much larger than the other UK health systems, and the London-based media capable of changing political agendas and debates around the UK in ways that the Edinburgh or Belfast – let alone Cardiff – media cannot. But that counts for surprisingly little. All politics, including the politics of public health, is local, and victories usually go to those who best create challenges and opportunities on the ground for politicians.

References

Bogdanor V (1999) *Devolution in the United Kingdom*. Oxford: Oxford University Press.

Burrows N (2000) *Devolution*. London: Sweet and Maxwell.

Carmichael P (2002) The Northern Ireland Civil Service: characteristics and trends since 1970. *Public Administration*. **80**: 23–49.

Deacon RM (2002) *The Governance of Wales: The Welsh Office and the policy process, 1964–1999*. Cardiff: Welsh Academic Press.

Greer SL (2004) *Territorial Politics and Health Policy*. Manchester: Manchester University Press.

Greer SL (2006) The fragile divergence machine: citizenship, policy divergence, and intergovernmental relations. In: A Trench (ed.) *Devolution and Power in the United Kingdom*. Manchester: Manchester University Press.

Hazell R (2006) *The English Question*. Manchester: Manchester University Press.

Mitchell J (2003) *Governing Scotland*. Basingstoke: Palgrave Macmillan.

Nottingham C (2000) The politics of health in Scotland after devolution. In: C Nottingham (ed.) *The NHS in Scotland: the legacy of the past and the prospect of the future*. Aldershot: Ashgate, pp.173–90.

Trench A (ed.) (2005) *Dynamics of Devolution*. Exeter: Imprint Academic.

Trench A (2006) *Devolution and Power in the United Kingdom*. Manchester: Manchester University Press.

Woods KJ and Carter D (eds) (2003) *Scotland's Health and Health Services*. London: The Stationery Office.

Chapter 6

European public health

Mark McCarthy

Europe is variously a geographical, politico-legal and cultural concept. We use the term to imply the land and states within the continent of Europe; or as political groupings, such as the European Region of the World Health Organization (52 states) or the European Union (25 states); or culturally, as Europe is tied through common traditions, and shares music, literature and art across a variety of languages. In the United Kingdom, Europe is often talked about as a separate entity, meaning 'those nearby countries where people are (a bit) different from us': perhaps that is why there is a separate chapter in this book for European public health. But public health in Europe is both the sum of public health within member states and also collective action, both between countries (for example, cooperation across the border between the UK and the Republic of Ireland) and by all countries together.

Public health and hygiene have a long tradition in Europe. For many centuries, quarantine was used routinely by port authorities, and by cities in time of plague. Laws to protect workers from accidents, and to provide financial insurance against sickness and unemployment, were developed in many European countries in the 19th century. As well as laws to protect property, states have legislated against child labour and provided support for the weak and destitute. Clean water and sanitation, education and adequate nutrition contributed to reductions in child mortality and longevity. Most European countries made the epidemiological transition from communicable diseases to non-communicable diseases during the first half of the 20th century.

Yet public health and healthcare services are controlled by national governments, and subject to national legislation; so, while governments may have similar objectives, the structures and practices they have developed differ. For example, the United Kingdom and Ireland draw on professional/academic bodies, the Royal Colleges and the Faculty of Public Health, to define standards for practice and to examine professional competence, while most other European countries devolve these arrangements directly to universities. Even the words 'public health' have different meanings between countries, with varying traditions for hygiene, health promotion and planning health services.

Health in Europe

The World Health Organization has made a major contribution to international public health by developing standard measures of health and health determinants. Age- and sex-specific mortality and morbidity rates are collected through well-established systems of death certification, while data are also increasingly collected about morbidity, health behaviours, health services, and broader health determinants. The European Regional Office of WHO coordinates these as the

Health for All Database of 600 items, which can be accessed and freely used (www.euro.who.int/hfadb).

European health indices improved overall in the second half of the 20th century, and are likely to continue to do so. Nevertheless, there have been differences between countries. France and Sweden, and Austria (from a lower base), have been among countries with the most consistent improvements in life expectancy. By the 1990s, a weaker trend was identified in Denmark, and this stimulated national debate on health behaviours and a new national public health programme. Eastern European countries, for example Poland, showed a slowing down in the later 20th century, and indeed a reversal at the beginning of the 1990s at the time of economic upheaval; more recently, health indices have been improving again. Countries further east emerged from the Soviet period with more difficulty, and indices have yet to return to earlier levels.

The picture also varies between health indices. Perinatal mortality did not deteriorate with the collapse of the communist regimes, partly because basic preventive health services continued. Birth rates have fallen in all countries, but have stabilised at different levels, partly related to immigration patterns. Disease-specific mortality rates reflect different patterns of health behaviour – smoking, drinking, vehicle use.

Mortality patterns also differ at local level, and within-country variations may be larger than those between-country. The European Atlas of Mortality suggests the historic impacts of industrialisation in Europe, for example in cities such as Glasgow, Barcelona and Milan, in comparison with rural areas. Industrialisation impacts through housing and limited availability of family support, as well as lifestyles including smoking and food. Interestingly, rural areas of central France are among those with the highest expectation of life, while having diets of good quality markedly different from the much-praised 'Mediterranean diet'.

WHO has described health systems and services of individual member states in the European Region, and publishes these through the European Health Observatory (www.euro.who.int/observatory). At the same time, there are specialist reports and publications across a wide range of topics. For individual countries, it is also possible to access information from national ministries of health (www.euro.who.int/countryinformation).

European health politics

European health politics has three broad groups of players: European-level public agencies (including WHO and European Union); national governments; and non-governmental organisations – which may be single-issue, single-industry or broad.

The WHO European Region has its main offices in Copenhagen, Denmark. As one of WHO's six regions, it is subject to broad policy of WHO Headquarters in Geneva, Switzerland. When WHO was established in 1948, the full Soviet Union was included in the European Region; so the Copenhagen office still covers peoples from the Atlantic to the Pacific, and includes the successor central Asian republics bordering on China and the Himalayas. Partly as a result of the opening up of these countries to greater international cooperation, partly because of their greater health needs, and partly because of the separate development of the EU health agenda, WHO EURO has faced eastwards in recent years. Initiatives on system reform, infrastructure development, human resources, and sanitation and water are particularly aimed at these countries.

The WHO European administration is quite small, and mainly staffed by public health experts. Some units are funded directly by national governments and are sited within their territory; for example, there are units for environment and health in Germany, Italy and Greece. Policy within the Regional Office is developed by long-term staff in association with national experts and ministries of health. The Regional Assembly of national ministers of health meets annually and approves the programme and budget. The strength and weakness of WHO is that, as a United Nations body, it can only work with the approval and engagement of each national ministry of health. While all ministers may approve a policy area, there is no sanction for weak or non-existent implementation.

This contrasts with the European Union, where there is more power for implementation but less professional expertise. The EU has broadly three interlinking structures: the Council of Ministers (which approves directives that are binding across member states), the European Commission (which proposes and implements policies) and the European Parliament (which comments on legislative proposals, mainly through sub-committees). Member states are responsible for translating directives into national laws (forming the body of European legislation, the *acquis communautaire*) and can be held accountable at the European Court of Justice. Broad changes in policy, for example expansion of members or changing structures, are enacted through formal treaties between the member states.

Apart from directives on member states, the EU also holds a budget from contributions from member states which is approximately 1% of the total GNP of all EU member states. Traditionally, almost half of this budget has gone to the common agricultural policy, and a third to regional and transport capital investment. These priorities reflect the origin of the EU in stabilising trade rather than internal development. Funds for social programmes are low on the list, and expenditure through the Commission's Health Directorate is only 0.05% of its total budget – estimated as 18 cents per European citizen per year.

During the 1980s, interest in health grew within the European Commission, including concern for health at work and prevention of HIV/AIDS and cancer.

The Treaty of Maastricht, signed in 1991 and ratified by member states in 1992, among other actions, first established a full European jurisdiction for health. Article 129 stated that '*The Community shall contribute towards ensuring a high level of human health protection by encouraging cooperation between the Member States and, if necessary, lending support to their action*'.

A new Directorate for Health and Consumer Affairs in the European Commission was established in 1994. The first two health commissioners, Paddraigh Flynn and David Byrne, were both from Ireland. Byrne, previously a barrister and politician, in particular took a strong position on banning cigarette advertising – against the entrenched positions of Germany and the United Kingdom – and also on obesity. Marcos Kyprianou, with a political background as finance minister in Cyprus, took over as Commissioner in 2004.

The EU Council of Health Ministers meets only once every 6 months (compare ministers of finance, who meet every week). The meeting is formally chaired by the minister of the country holding the Presidency of the full Council of Ministers (which rotates 6-monthly). The Chief Medical Officers of the member states also meet every 6 months for more informal coordination.

The agendas are prepared by officials over the preceding months, although handling contemporary issues, such as epidemics including BSE (bovine spongiform encephalopathy), SARS and avian influenza, may be prioritised at the meeting. The need for continued coordination between member states has been recognised by establishing specialised agencies for medicines (London), food safety (Helsinki) and controlled drugs (Lisbon); and the new Centre for Disease Control (Sweden) is a clearing house for information and coordination, especially for communicable diseases.

Action across Europe requires collaboration, and non-governmental organisations (NGOs) have readily learned this. NGOs are more influential in the EU than in WHO because of better access. They can talk either to European Commission staff, or to the Parliament (and Parliamentarians' staff). Brussels is a focus for lobbying and influence, both political and financial. The NGOs either take up single issues, or provide a broad framework for multiple input. Parliamentarians particularly benefit from this process, as it puts them in touch with national perspectives they might otherwise not know of, without needing to go formally through the national government. Similarly, European Commission staff can harness local opinion, sometimes called 'civil society'. An example is the Health Forum set up by the European Commission's Health and Consumer Safety Directorate: this is a body of about 60 members (*see* Box 6.1) including broad, thematic, professional and industry. (Interestingly, the Commission has included the pharmaceutical industry, but excluded the tobacco and food industries from this lobbying opportunity.)

Box 6.1 Organisational members of the European Health Forum

Advocacy for the Prevention of Alcohol Related Harm in Europe (EURO-CARE)
Association of European Cancer Leagues (ECL)
Association of European Regions (AER)
Association Internationale de la Mutualité (AIM)
Association of Schools of Public Health in the European Region (ASPHER)
Bureau Européen des Unions de Consommateurs (BEUC)
Coalition of HIV and AIDS Non-Governmental Organisations in Europe (CHANGE)
European AIDS Treatment Group (EATG)
European Alliance of Patients Support Groups for Genetics Services (EAGS)
European Association of Speciality Pharmaceuticals
European Blind Union (EBU)
European Breast Cancer Coalition (EUROPA DONNA)
European Committee for Homeopathy (ECH)
European Disability Forum (EDF)
European Federation of Allergy and Airways Disease Patients (EFA)
European Federation of Pharmaceutical Industries and Associations (EFPIA)
European Federation of Public Service Unions (EPSU)
European Generic Medicines Association (EGA)
European Health Management Association (EHMA)

European Health Telematics Association (EHTEL)
European Heart Network (EHN)
European Medical Technology Industry Association (EUCOMED)
European Midwives Organisation (EMA)
European Network for Smoking Prevention (ENSP)
European Network of Health Promotion Agencies (ENHPA)
European Network Parenthood Federation (IPPFEN)
European Older People's Platform (AGE)
European Organisation for Rare Disorders (EURORDIS)
European Public Health Alliance (EPHA)
European Public Health Association (EUPHA)
European Social Insurance Partners Association (ESIP)
European Society for Mental Health and Deafness (ESMHD)
European Union of Medical Specialists (UEMS)
Global Alliance of Mental Illness Advocacy Networks (GAMIAN-EUROPE)
Groupement International de la Répartition Pharmaceutique (GIRP)
Health Action International (HAI)
Hospitals of Europe (HOPE)
International Alliance of Patients' Organisations (IAPO)
International Union for Health Promotion and Education (IUHPE)
Mental Health Europe (MHE)
Pharmaceutical Group of the European Union (PGEU)
Red Cross
Standing Committee of European Doctors (CPME)
Standing Committee of Nurses (PCN)
Union Européenne de l'Hospitalisation Privée (UEHP/CEHP)
Youth Forum Jeunesse

EU health policy

The emphasis on 'health protection' rather than health services in the Treaty of Maastricht gave a primary direction towards public health for the Commission's health programme. However, because health was seen as a national social issue, controlled within countries, rather than as trade across borders, the activities initially supported by the Commission were about exchange of information rather than engaging in direct public health policy. Even though Commissioner Byrne identified smoking control as his major concern, politics at European level meant that progress was slow. Indeed, when the Health Directorate first achieved consensus for a ban on cigarette advertising, the tobacco industry successfully challenged the directive in the European courts on grounds that it was not covered by the European treaties. (The second directive was successful.)

In 2001, the Health Directorate published a 6-year programme with funding of 50 million euro per year. It has three broad fields: health information, health protection and determinants of health (*see* Box 6.2). The funding supports conferences, databanks, networks, exchanges, training and evaluation. Annual calls to this programme have met with a strong response from health agencies across Europe, and about 50 projects are selected each year.

Box 6.2 European Commission Public Health Work Programme, 2005

1 Information:

- developing and coordinating the health information and knowledge system
- operating the health information and knowledge system
- mechanisms for reporting and analysis of health issues
- eHealth
- supporting the exchange of information and experiences on good practice
- health impact assessment
- cooperation on health systems between member states.

2 Responding to health threats:

- surveillance
- exchanging information on vaccination and immunisation strategies
- health security and preparedness
- safety of blood, tissues and cells, organs
- antimicrobial resistance
- supporting the networking of laboratories.

3 Health determinants:

- community strategies on addictive substances: tobacco, alcohol, drugs
- lifestyles: sexual and reproductive health, HIV/AIDS, mental health
- wider determinants of health
- disease prevention, and prevention of injuries
- genetic determinants for health.

Source: http://europa.eu.int/comm/health/ph_programme/howtoapply/proposal_docs/workplan2005_en.pdf.

In 2005, with enlargement of the EU by ten member states and under Commissioner Kyprianou, an enlarged health programme was proposed. This responded to the increasing interest by EU ministers of health in sharing knowledge on health services as well as on health protection, and improving Europeans' experiences when travelling between countries. Three new programme themes are:

- preventing diseases and injuries (including mental illness, cancer, cardiovascular diseases, rare diseases and accidents)
- improving co-operation between health systems (including patient safety, transnational specialist centres and cross-border care)
- developing structures for emergency preparedness and threats.

Another set of issues for healthcare is the possibility of a Directive on Services of General Interest. This seeks to take forward the EU commitment to markets to include not just capital, labour and goods, but also services. But member states are jealous to retain their national regulations. While markets for services such as insurance, transportation or energy may deregulate slowly, concern is expressed by patients and professionals about creating markets in healthcare. At present, these matters are being treated cautiously, and European Parliamentarians appear to wish to exclude health from a future directive. However, the impetus of the European treaties is to open markets rather than retain national protectionism, and the European Commission is likely to push towards including healthcare in the future.

Environment and health

The area of environment and health has brought the European WHO office and the European Union together – but also shows the differences in approach between them.

WHO initiated a programme on environment and health in the 1980s. The main structure has been joint meetings at international level between ministers of health and ministers of environment. These started in Frankfurt in 1989, and followed at 5-yearly intervals in Helsinki (1994), London (1999) and Prague (2004); the next will be in Rome in 2009. Activities have included reporting on the state of environment and health in Europe, promoting national environment and health action plans, supporting dissemination of local good practice and developing instruments for multi-country collaboration. National environment and health action plans appeared to be a sensible approach to identifying national issues and policies to meet them. But in practice few countries undertook the necessary work, and those that completed the plans did not necessarily implement the action proposed – especially when legislation or finance was needed.

Two approaches have been used for multi-country collaboration. WHO estimate that 120 million people have inadequate access to pure drinking water and adequate sanitation. The Protocol on Water and Health is legally binding for the ratifying countries, and sets standards that countries must meet. It is supported by a broader programme for water development and sanitation improvement.

A second international treaty agreed in London in 1999 was the Charter on Transport and Health. The UK Minister for Transport formally signed the Charter on behalf of all WHO regional countries. But a charter is not a binding legal agreement; and, even though the burden of disease from transport, particularly air pollution and road injuries, is high, European governments have shown less concern for pollution from transport than for industrial pollution. A complicating factor is that transport policy is not usually under control of either the Minister for Health or the Minister for Environment. However, the European work has contributed to raising the issue of environment and health globally for WHO, and in 2004 World Health Day was focused on road traffic injuries (www.who.int/world-health-day/2004/en/).

The European Commission's environment programme for 2004–2010 puts health as one of its four main areas of concern. This meant a change from environmental determinants (e.g. air, noise) towards disease impacts (e.g. respiratory diseases, congenital defects). The work programme also supported development of indicators and research (the latter in coordination with the European Commission's Research Directorate). The Commission has funds for project work at regional and local level (often working through national ministries and matching national funding), which may be particularly relevant in places with chronic pollution problems and in creating a general shift towards cleaner environments.

Health research

The proposals for the 2007–2013 European Union budget include a substantial increase in funding for research, including health research. European health research has traditionally meant laboratory-based research. The 2002–2006 (sixth) EU health research programme was dominated by genomics, with the support of the pharmaceutical industry, while public health research received little funding and attention.

Yet the variations between European countries, both in disease patterns and health systems, both commend further investigation and provide opportunities for new knowledge from comparisons. There have been successful European international epidemiological and comparative studies on heart disease, diabetes, stroke, cancer and neurological disorders, although these studies have been more concerned with aetiology than intervention. Proposals for the seventh EU health research programme (2007–2013) include specific sections on research on disease determinants and health systems.

There are several European health research organisations representing different academic interests, including sociology, economics, health psychology and epidemiology. These different disciplines meet within the European Public Health Association (EUPHA), which publishes the *European Journal of Public Health* and organises a larger research conference each November. The national public health associations which make up EUPHA also have their own conferences, and journals, and there is a challenge to exchange knowledge about health promotion and disease control between practitioners as well as researchers.

Engaging with Europe

How can public health practitioners engage with European public health? They can join local activities that are linked across Europe; they can join projects that link nationally, or link through national associations; or they can work directly with or for international agencies.

Healthy Cities is an excellent example of local collaboration across Europe (www.euro.who.int/healthy-cities). Started in 1985 by the WHO European Regional Office, and following the principles of the 1984 Ottawa Declaration, *Healthy Cities* has become an international activity which allows people to develop health promotion locally. *Healthy Cities* supports intersectoral work and a focus on inequalities. It is usually led by the municipality, where different sectors (e.g. education, planning and regeneration, leisure, social services) can be encouraged to work better with the health sector – and the health sector can be encouraged to see health in a broad perspective rather than just the provision of healthcare.

Yet the *Healthy Cities* model remains underused across Europe; even in countries such as the UK, with long experience and some leadership role, implementation is difficult. Among the issues are the need for continuity of political support, the varying views of professionals, the lack of an evidence base for effectiveness and the absence of a clear budget or cadre of workers: coordination of partners in different organisations towards multiple, shared ends is much more difficult than managing a clearly budgeted programme towards a specific end.

National organisations are increasingly active in linking across Europe. The major professional organisations such as the medical and nursing associations support permanent staff in offices in Brussels, and national associations usually have European committees with member participation. Similarly, both healthcare organisations are coordinated to work at European level, through structures such as the Hospitals Committee for Europe, and there are both patient organisations (e.g. heart disease and cancer and also children's rare diseases), and health behaviour organisations (e.g. against smoking, alcohol). Specific leadership for public health is given by the European Public Health Alliance (www.epha.org), which connects NGOs, and the European Public Health Association (www.eupha.org), which connects public health professional and research associations.

Work directly at European level is more limited. There are not many staff at the WHO Regional Office, and European Commission health offices are divided between Brussels and Luxembourg. While English is nowadays the main language for international discussion, French remains important internally within the European institutions, and Russian and German remain official languages for WHO EURO. People who choose an international career will normally work outside their own country for long periods, which has implications for family life, and the remuneration may be different from their own country. An intermediate possibility is to work in a Brussels office – for example, for professional organisations, health NGOs or regional representatives – for a period, and return home to work afterwards. Experience gained in this way can be particularly valuable for understanding structures and developing contacts that help continuing international work.

A visit to Brussels, for individuals or a group, can usually be organised through European representative offices. The visitors can meet Members of the European Parliament (when in session in Brussels: for 1 week in 4, rather surprisingly, Parliament sits in Strasbourg in France). They can visit appropriate European Commission staff and meet with national representatives, both the national civil servants who prepare for, and attend, the Councils of Ministers, and the regional offices which represent regional and local authorities. And they can meet with representatives of other European industrial, technical and professional organisations.

What is striking, in discussions at European level, is the variety of structures and policies that exist to meet apparently similar problems. A desk officer in a particular field of work at the WHO European Regional Office will know about their field across all the European countries, while most people working nationally are ignorant of even neighbouring countries. They may not have access to comparative information, or a network of colleagues to share knowledge. They may have attended European international meetings, but this is a limited way to build up international knowledge in comparison with visiting people and places. Moreover, as their career develops and responsibilities change, their knowledge needs also change. They will need to read across their field, including free magazines such as *Eurohealth* (www.lse.ac.uk/collections/LSEHealthAndSocialCare/documents/eurohealth.htm) and newspapers such as the *European Voice* (www.european-voice.com).

Probably the most important task of European agencies is to build knowledge and networks between people practising on the ground, and to increase access to comparative information. Thus, EU-funded projects usually encourage participation across countries, and support information sharing and description. Although this may seem relatively 'low-level' activity, it is the necessary precondition for effective joint work.

Future

Health policy at European level is influenced by WHO and the European Union; but, in contrast to the United States of America, European member states hold primary control for the laws governing public health and health systems, and the funds to support them. European Union directives can require member states to introduce legislation, but there have been few examples directly within the health field. Instead, there has been collaboration – in such areas as tobacco and air-pollution control – supported by legal frameworks. In parts of Europe where there are common cultural and language patterns, both patients and service providers are already pushing for open access across borders, and in the future international healthcare providers will increasingly seek markets and regulation at European level. Health policy will probably remain under the control of national governments, but NGOs and industrial groups will seek to influence national policies. There will be more influence of European perspectives on national public health: and anticipating and participating in international policy development is the best insurance to unexpected shocks.

Chapter 7

International public health

Martin McKee

There can be few politicians who remain unaware of how international issues can affect the health of their populations. An obvious example is the way that governments are responding with a sense of urgency to the threat of a pandemic of avian influenza, reflecting their experience of the economic damage that resulted from the emergence of SARS in 2003 (Fan 2003).

The ease with which micro-organisms cross borders has meant that infectious disease has long been the driving force behind efforts to coordinate action on health internationally. It is, however, increasingly apparent that there are many other threats to health that cross borders (McNeill 1976). The spread of tobacco around the world has also been described as an epidemic (Jha 1999). In this case the vector is not the mosquito or the rat flea but the international tobacco industry, often with the support of governments in those countries in the developed world where the tobacco companies are based. The global spread of weapons provides an analogous example of the potential harm arising from some forms of trade, often with repercussions for the exporting countries as many of these firearms reappear in the hands of criminals in the developed world (Holdstock 2001).

The international dimension to health is also apparent through our television screens, as a global communications system can allow us to watch in real time the death of a child from hunger or violence thousands of miles away. This imagery has the power to develop a sense of shared global community, manifest in the outpouring of donations in response to campaigns such as Comic Relief or Red Nose Day. Equally, our improved understanding of the world in which we live is making us more aware of the threats that humans collectively pose to our environment (McMichael 2001); all but a few sceptics (Lomborg 2001) are now convinced of the adverse consequences of climate change for human health.

Less apparent are the many ways in which, in a globally interlinked economy, decisions made in one part of the world impact on health in another (Klein 2001). The closure of a factory in a deprived post-industrial area, decided by a management board in a different continent, may improve a company's bottom line but it may be devastating for that community, propelling it into a downward cycle of hopelessness, fuelled by alcoholism and drug use. The decision to drill for oil in an environmentally sensitive region may equally damage the livelihoods of indigenous peoples (Human Rights Watch 1999).

None of these challenges can be addressed by a single government acting in isolation; they can only be tackled when governments come together to confront shared problems. The countries that emerged from the horrors of the Second World War recognised that new ways of working were required to avoid the failures of the 1920s and 1930s. Their major achievement was the creation of the United Nations, an organisation that has celebrated 50 years of existence. With its specialised agencies, such as the World Health Organization, it provides a mechanism to tackle shared concerns.

The system is far from perfect. Its core budget, provided by its member governments, has never matched the demands placed upon it. It works almost entirely with the consent of national governments, even when those governments engage in the most appalling violations of human rights of their populations. In the areas where it could take more robust action, through the Security Council, there has almost always been at least one of the five permanent members willing to exert their veto. Yet despite all these limitations, it has managed to achieve a great deal.

One of the ways that it can act is by facilitating agreement on international treaties. The 1987 Montreal Protocol began the process of phasing out the use of chlorofluorocarbons. Although it will be several decades before the benefits are fully apparent, this has at least arrested the process of damage to the earth's ozone layer. Fifty years after the end of the conflict, Second World War landmines continue to maim and kill people in North Africa and South-East Asia. Consequently, the benefits that will arise from agreement on a Landmine Treaty will also take decades to have their full effect but at least it will prevent the situation in many parts of the world from getting worse. Most recently, governments came together within the World Health Organization to agree the Framework Convention on Tobacco Control, the first ever treaty where the primary aim was the improvement of health. It requires governments to enact a package of measures that include imposition of restrictions on tobacco advertising, sponsorship and promotion, strengthening health warnings, reducing exposure to second-hand smoke, and clamping down on tobacco smuggling (www.fctc.org/). In these ways it will, over time, save millions of lives.

International treaties are based on the consent of governments to limit their individual freedom to act on the basis that, in the long term, this will benefit both their own population and humanity as a whole. Indeed, the establishment of the United Nations was a clear statement by the international community that the sovereignty of individual governments was constrained by international law. That view has, on many occasions, been challenged. In some cases, the international community has acted, as in the imposition of sanctions against apartheid-era South Africa or the former Yugoslavia during the Balkan wars of the 1990s, as well as through its many peacekeeping operations (Shawcross 2001). In other cases it has not. However, while recognising its limitations, most of which are imposed upon it by its member states, there has at least been a consensus that the United Nations system is a force for good.

The world has, however, changed from the time when the United Nations was created. At that time there was still a balance of power, albeit with different actors from those that had shaped the world in the 19th century, when Germany and Austria–Hungary were still centre-stage. The USA and USSR (Union of Soviet Socialist Republics) emerged from the Second World War as superpowers. The United Kingdom and France had yet to shed their empires and, while clearly in the second division, both had a global reach that, like the USA and USSR, was backed up by nuclear weapons.

At the beginning of the 21st century, the United Kingdom and France are no longer world powers. The USSR is no more and its natural successor, the Russian

Federation, is preoccupied with internal problems. China is becoming stronger, militarily and economically. However, the USA now stands clearly apart from the other four members of the Security Council as the only global superpower, accounting for 40% of the world's defence spending and with a network of military bases that spans the globe. What is the role of multilateral organisations such as the United Nations in this new world order?

One answer was provided for us in 1997 by an American neoconservative policy group, the Project for the New American Century (www.newamericancentury.org/). Its statement of principles was signed by individuals who have since become household names across the world. They include Dick Cheney, Donald Rumsfeld, Paul Wolfowitz and Jeb Bush. Their key message was that America had to assume a global leadership role. This would be based on a substantial increase in defence expenditure, strengthening of ties to America's allies linked to challenges to regimes that are hostile to American interests, and an endorsement of '*America's unique role in preserving and extending an international order friendly to our security, our prosperity, and our principles*'. Three years later, when President George W Bush entered the White House, many of these individuals followed him, achieving senior positions within the Republican administration. The Project for the New American Century became a blueprint for US government policy.

Under this new policy, international agencies are of value only as far as they acquiesce with American interests. In President Bush's first term this meant ignoring or obstructing them. It would have been convenient if the Security Council had agreed to support military action against Iraq but its unwillingness to do so was not seen as an impediment to taking military action. The US government has worked hard to prevent other countries from supporting the creation of the International Criminal Court and has enacted legislation that authorises the use of armed force to rescue any American citizen brought before the court. In one area after another, the USA was signifying its rejection of international treaties as a way of working. Thus, it refused to endorse the treaty on landmines (because it wanted to be able to use them on the Korean peninsula) or the Kyoto Protocol (because it would have harmed its oil and automobile industries). At the same time, senior members of the administration made clear their view that treaties that had already been signed had no legal force (Bolton 1997), exemplified by the argument that one of the longest established elements of international law, the Geneva Conventions, did not apply to those captured in the 'war against terror'. Instead, it worked through 'coalitions of the willing', even trying to set up a new partnership outside the United Nations system to respond to the urgent needs of those affected by the Asian tsunami. The exceptions are those international treaties, such as those protecting intellectual property, that serve its own corporate interests. The USA also sought to constrain the actions of non-governmental organisations working in the international arena, adopting what is formally known as the Mexico City policy, although more often it is referred to as the Global Gag Rule (http://64.224.182.238/globalgagrule/). This denies US government funding to any organisation that provides counselling or referral for abortion, or even lobbies for the legalisation of abortion, anywhere in the world. These developments have been taking place against a backdrop of vilification of the United Nations and, in particular, its Secretary General, Kofi Annan, in right-wing elements of the American media.

The situation has changed in President Bush's second term. At a time when anti-American feeling has reached unprecedented levels worldwide (Berman 2004), the US administration has realised that it needs international organisations. Now the challenge is to ensure that they fall into line with the neoconservative ideology that has taken hold in Washington. This argument has been expressed concisely by John Bolton, President Bush's nominee for ambassador to the United Nations, who has argued that the Security Council should have only one permanent member, the USA (*New York Times* 2005). The new policy is being given effect by the appointment of a series of administration officials to senior positions in the international organisations. Thus, Paul Wolfowitz, until recently Bush's Deputy Defence Secretary and a driving force behind the invasion of Iraq, has been appointed to head the World Bank. Ann Veneman, the incoming head of UNICEF (United Nations Children's Fund), was Bush's first agriculture secretary. The People's Health Movement has chronicled how, in that role, she put the interests of agribusiness above those of the poor, including children of agricultural workers (www.saveunicef.org/).

These individuals can be expected to pursue the neoconservative agenda set out in the Project for a New American Century. It is an agenda in which not only institutions but also scientific knowledge are employed in its own interests, a situation exposed by a series of reports by American scientists (Union of Concerned Scientists 2004) and politicians (US House of Representatives 2003) that have revealed how, in the first Bush administration, there was an unprecedented degree of political interference in science. This interference advanced the interests of two important constituencies, the religious right and corporate America. It involved the suppression of reports of research, the packing of advisory committees by ideologues, many of whom had little if any scientific credibility, and a refusal to support research that risked giving unhelpful answers (McKee and Novotny 2003).

Step by step, the USA is emerging as a 21st-century imperial power, explicitly promoting a policy of *Pax Americana* in which it seeks to mould the world in its own image. For example, one former US ambassador has proposed a campaign to remove the world's remaining dictators by 2025 (Palmer 2003). This is a great responsibility, but even if it was to pursue policies that would make the world a better place, could it deliver? Niall Ferguson is a British academic who has called for the USA to play a greater world role, arguing that '*The world needs an effective liberal empire and the United States is the best candidate for the job*' (Ferguson 2004). Yet he doubts whether it can fulfil this role, arguing that it faces three fundamental deficits. The first is a deficit of money. President Bush has presided over the transformation of a federal budgetary surplus into a record deficit of $412 billion. Wide-ranging tax cuts, disproportionately benefiting the very rich, have taken place at the same time as government expenditure has risen rapidly. Looking ahead, it is far from clear how the USA will pay for the social security and Medicare bills for the generation of baby-boomers, greatly constraining its efforts to project its power globally.

The second is a deficit of people. It is struggling to maintain its military presence in Iraq, dependent on reserve forces, increasingly reluctant allies, and recruitment of people from other countries who are lured by the offer of eventual American citizenship (http://notinourname.net/resources_links/green-card-troops-1sep03.htm).

Ferguson argues that these deficits can be overcome, highlighting, for example, the potential to draw on the two million Americans currently in prison (1 in 142 American residents). It is, however, the third deficit that is most intractable. This is a deficit of attention. Recalling the lack of commitment to Puccini's Madame Butterfly by Lieutenant Pinkerton, he shows how the USA has consistently been unwilling to recognise the long time that it takes to bring about change and to invest the non-military resources that this process requires, a situation exemplified by the failure to rebuild post-conflict Iraq and Afghanistan.

These developments have profound implications for global health. In an increasingly integrated world, where the actions of one government can easily impact on the health of people living far beyond its borders, it is essential to have a means to tackle common challenges that is based on evidence rather than ideology. Instead, the international institutional architecture is being reconfigured in support of vested interests in a single country. Ferguson's analysis suggests that it is unlikely to achieve its own objectives and, even if it did, given the lessons from previous neoliberal policies that are now being pursued with renewed vigour, it would be likely to make things worse (Stiglitz 2002).

There is a widespread consensus that the structures that allow governments across the world to debate shared problems are in need of reform, but much less agreement as to how this should happen. The crucial issue that must be resolved is the position of the USA in relation to the rest of the world. Here views differ, even among those who share a concern about American power. Jacques Chirac has long called for a multi-polar world, with Europe acting as a counterbalance to American power (Chirac 1978). After all, the economy of the enlarged European Union is now larger than that of the USA. However, there seems little enthusiasm in Europe for the massive shift from social to military expenditure that would be required for this to become a reality (German Marshall Fund 2003). Timothy Garton Ash has argued for a renewed engagement between Europe and the USA, based on an explicit recognition of where they agree and disagree (Garton Ash 2004). Joseph Stiglitz has argued for a much stronger voice for the developing world.

These debates may seem to have little to do with public health. Yet without a solution that is based on the values of public health, such as solidarity and sustainability, then the prospects for collective action to confront the increasing numbers of shared threats to health will become even more elusive. The global public health community must not remain silent in the face of the threat posed by the neoconservatives in Washington to international law and the institutions that are charged with upholding it. Unless things change, it will be much more difficult to make the world a safer and healthier place. Some 150 years on, Rudolph Virchow's observation that '*Medicine is a social science and politics is nothing but medicine writ large*' (Rather 1985) remains as true as ever.

References

Berman RA (2004) *Anti-Americanism in Europe: a cultural problem*. Stanford, CA: Hoover Institution Press.

Bolton JR (1997) US isn't legally obligated to pay the UN. *Wall Street Journal*. 17 November.

Chirac J (1978) *La Lueur de l'Espérance: réflexion du soir pour le matin*. Paris: Editions La Table Ronde.

Fan EX (2003) *SARS: economic impacts and implications.* Asian Development Bank. ERD Policy Brief No. 15. Manila: Asian Development Bank.

Ferguson N (2004) *Colossus. The rise and fall of the American empire.* London: Allen Lane.

Garton Ash T (2004) *Free World. Why a crisis of the west reveals the opportunity of our time.* London: Allen Lane.

German Marshall Fund (2003) *Transatlantic Trends.* Washington DC: German Marshall Fund.

Holdstock D (2001) War: from humanitarian relief to prevention. In: M McKee, P Garner and R Stott (eds) *International Co-operation in Health.* Oxford: Oxford University Press, pp.109–26.

Human Rights Watch (1999) *The Price of Oil: corporate responsibility and human rights violations in Nigeria's oil producing communities.* New York: Human Rights Watch.

Jha P (ed.) (1999) *Curbing the Epidemic: governments and the economics of tobacco control.* Washington DC: World Bank.

Klein N (2001) *No Logo.* London: Flamingo.

Lomborg B (2001) *The Skeptical Environmentalist. Measuring the real state of the world.* Cambridge: Cambridge University Press.

McKee M and Novotny TE (2003) Political interference in American science: why Europe should be concerned about the actions of the Bush administration. *Eur J Public Health.* **13**: 289–91.

McMichael T (2001) *Human Frontiers, Environments and Disease: past patterns, uncertain futures.* Cambridge: Cambridge University Press, 2001.

McNeill WH (1976) *Plagues and Peoples.* Harmondsworth: Penguin.

New York Times (2005) The world according to Bolton. Editorial. 9 March.

Palmer M (2003) Breaking the real axis of evil: how to oust the world's last dictators by 2025. Lanham: Rowman and Littlefield.

Rather LJ (ed.) (1985) *Rudolf Virchow: collected essays on public health and epidemiology,* 2 vols. Canton, MA: Science History Publications.

Shawcross W (2001) *Deliver Us from Evil: warlords and peacekeepers in a world of endless conflict.* London: Bloomsbury.

Stiglitz J (2002) *Globalization and its Discontents.* London: Allen Lane.

Union of Concerned Scientists (2004) *Scientific Integrity in Policy Making: an investigation into the Bush administration's abuse of science.* Cambridge MA: Union of Concerned Scientists.

United States House of Representatives (2003) *Politics and Science in the Bush Administration.* Committee on Government Reform – Minority Staff Special Investigations Division. Report prepared for Rep. Henry A Waxman, August. Washington DC: US House of Representatives.

Part 2

Key issues in public health policy

Introduction

A number of key issues forms the basis of this section – the balance between individual freedom and state intervention in people's lives; the importance of inspection and regulation and its application to public health in addition to healthcare; the roles of regional agencies and local authorities in contributing to improved health; how communities can be fully engaged with their health; and the link between sustainability and public health in an attempt to redefine the nature of the public realm at a time when the focus on individual choice and market-style incentives are challenging traditional models of public health and notions of healthy public policy.

At the time of the Labour government's first public health white paper, *Saving Lives: our healthier nation*, published in 1999, there was an explicit recognition of the important role government had in shaping the public's health. By the time of the second white paper, *Choosing Health*, published in 2004, the thinking (certainly in England but perhaps not elsewhere in the UK) had shifted to an emphasis on individual choice and the desire to extend choice to everyone rather than regard it as the preserve of the middle classes. The government was anxious not to encroach on individual liberty and be accused of ushering in the 'nanny' state. These issues, and the balance to be struck between freedom of the individual on the one hand and notions of civic-ness and collective action on the other, are dealt with in Paul Corrigan's chapter. He asserts that doing things to people is no longer an option – rather, individuals and communities have a strong role in improving their own health. Indeed, unpalatable though it may be for public health professionals, the public's health will only improve if people so decide.

The role of government is changing, too, in response to these shifts. There is less emphasis on direct provision and an attempt to limit the role of government to setting the strategic direction and then leaving it up to regulation and inspection to ensure that policy objectives are met. Replacing the Commission for Health Improvement, the Healthcare Commission is one of the new bodies charged with responsibility for ensuring that health organisations perform well. Expectations are high because for the first time, as Jude Williams explains, public health is one of the domains to be inspected. Much of this work can only be undertaken collaboratively with other inspectorates, such as the Audit Commission, since responsibility for improving health goes far beyond the NHS. Hence the importance of joint reviews embracing the NHS and other bodies.

But if central government is looking afresh at its role and responsibilities, so are regional government agencies. When considering the role of government in improving health, the issue goes well beyond central government. Regional government offices and local authorities have important public health responsibilities and these are only now beginning to be fully appreciated. In England, the attempt to establish elected regional assemblies foundered in the North East when, in a referendum conducted in late 2004, the public overwhelmingly rejected what was on offer. However, as Paul Johnstone demonstrates, the public health opportunities at the regional level are considerable and for the most part remain to be realised. The risks are also considerable since working to improve public health requires exceptional leadership and an ability to work across complex boundaries. Johnstone illustrates his arguments drawing on the range of initiatives and activities underway in one English region.

Local government is no stranger to health improvement and yet has often been reluctant to assert a leadership role despite the view of many that it is the 'natural leader' in public health. Tony Elson offers one reason for the reticence. For him, unless we move beyond the rational and scientific to the human and moral arguments around a social justice agenda then the social movement, or tipping point, needed to effect lasting change will not occur. The evidence base is only one side of the argument and will not, in itself, drive change. For that, we need to engage people at the emotional level. Local authorities are well placed to take the lead here building on their experience of engaging with communities.

Chris Drinkwater considers the tricky challenge of getting local communities fully engaged. If the Wanless agenda for public engagement, reaffirmed in the English white paper *Choosing Health*, is to be achieved then new approaches to community involvement are required. Or perhaps they are not so new given the efforts of community development back in the 1960s and the high profile it enjoyed for a time. Perhaps what is lacking is the political will and commitment to embed such an approach on a sustainable basis. Despite the evidence from local projects, we remain some way off achieving the fully engaged scenario set out by Wanless in 2002 and accepted by the government.

In the final chapter in this section, Anna Coote looks at the link between health and sustainable development, focusing on the corporate role of the NHS. The links between public health and sustainable development are critical and yet often overlooked. Poor health is a product of environmental degradation and of social injustice in respect of employment, economic insecurity, and a sense of powerlessness. Unless we tackle these concerns then a focus on public health narrowly conceived will achieve little. The NHS could give a lead through its employment and procurement practices among other things. The issue of good corporate citizenship in the NHS is being promoted by the Sustainable Development Commission and Department of Health. But, as in so many other areas of public health policy, progress will be determined by the presence of political will and sound leadership.

Chapter 8

New social democratic politics of public health in England today

Paul Corrigan

Introduction: the right has a politics of public health too

Most of the self-conscious debate about the politics of public health is the politics of the left. Therefore most of the political disagreements about the politics of public health are framed by those wider politics.

Since the extent of state intervention is one of the main themes of the politics of the left, it is not surprising that the bulk of the discussion within this chapter, and indeed the whole book, is framed by the different ways in which the state should intervene to work with people to improve their health.

But, like too much of the politics of the left, the politics of public health deludes itself into believing that just because the left is the only voice that it hears, that is the only politics that has any effect on the world. In fact, within the public and the wider political arena there is a strong politics of public health which stresses, to the exclusion of all else, the sole importance of personal responsibility. In the 2005 UK general election, the major opposition party gained parliamentary seats on a manifesto which expressed this very clearly:

> *Conservatives believe that people are responsible for their health. We do not believe that food producers are to blame if people eat unhealthily, or that pubs are to blame if people drink or smoke. Therefore we seek voluntary not statutory solutions to public health problems.* (Conservative Party 2005)

Most people within public health fail to notice the strength of this position and assume that all politics of public health concerns different state interventions. We are wrong to do that since the growth of personal responsibility is one of the hallmarks of contemporary societies across the world. If it is only the politics of the right that talks to this personal responsibility then, as I will argue in this chapter, the politics of public health will lose touch with the lives of ordinary people.

My argument rests upon the historical development of 'the public' in English society. If it is true that 'the public' has changed, then anything that depends on a relationship to the public – such as either public health or politics – has to change as well. Those who want to influence the behaviour of the public would be most effective if they recognised these changes. The public and its nature is the determinant in the relationship with public health, and any failure to notice, any belief that public health can tell the public what to do, drastically reduces its efficacy.

In Britain the post-Second World War welfare state settlement saw a 'public' that was primarily male, in full-time employment and lived their lives within a unified culture. This unified view of the public meant that services, such as the NHS, could meet 'the needs of the public' by seeing that public not as a set of individuals with gender, ethnic, age and cultural differences, but as a block. Politics could therefore talk to the public by talking to the large blocks of people whose views were determined by historical forces.

The left failed to notice that over the 50 years since the Second World War, the public changed. Over that period the public not only became much more differentiated one from another, but they wanted that differentiation to take place. People enjoyed being different and wanted, for example, to own their own homes rather than be treated the same as everyone else in council-owned housing.

Over the 10 years from 1984 to 1994, centre-left politics in England slowly understood that the 'public' had developed and changed. By the mid-1990s it recognised that if you want to work with people, then crucially the people had to want to work with you. Under those circumstances you have not only to understand their lives, but also recognise that they do not like being taken for granted and that they have their own hopes and aspirations. And those hopes and aspirations reflect a broad array of differences within British society, not a single public. Equally, given the different aspirations of different people, telling them what to do and how to live their lives did not work as a political appeal at all. People walked away.

What was true about the changing public is also true about the changing health of the public. Like other public services, public health aims to change people's behaviour. It wants people to live healthier lives. If it really wants to achieve this goal it crudely has two ways of going about it. It can follow a particular strand of authoritarian left politics and believe that the best way of changing people's behaviour is by telling them what to do. Or it can follow a different strand of left political activity and, by understanding their current hopes and aspirations, find ways of helping them to change themselves.

My argument is that in the 1990s the centre left in Britain discovered that if you wanted to work with people politically, then you had to find out what the public aspired to and work with them. Telling them what to do would not work.

For public health to have any success in the modern world, its social theory and practice needs to move to work with the public's aspirations.

In the current world of England few public health determinants actually 'determine'

One important example of the way in which an authoritarian politics of the left dominates the politics of public health is the language used. This book is full of examples of public health professionals talking about 'determinants' of health. Most working-class people in Britain in the 21st century do not like to think of their lives as 'determined' by external forces. Of course they recognise that there are big historical structures in society – for example, globalisation, economic change and different sources of power. These have very important impacts on their lives. But if you suggest that their lives are 'determined' by them, people would find that odd. They want to think that they can struggle to have some real say over their lives. In fact many would point to the improvement in their families' lives as coming from the struggle to help shape their own world.

It is interesting that those middle-class people who refer to working-class people as 'determined' by structural forces themselves live lives full of self-determination.

They have higher education qualifications, own houses and look forward to lives with even more self-determination for their children. This struggle for control is one of the main historical themes of an alternative left politics. It stands against the belief that disadvantaged people are determined, and argues that they want to and should be able to control more of their own, their families' and their communities' lives.

This recognition is why the political stance of the government white paper, *Choosing Health* (Secretary of State for Health 2004), is so relevant to the contemporary politics of public health in advanced capitalist societies. Up until recently, most of those involved in the politics of public health have been able to pose politics as a simple bifurcated choice. If you didn't agree with the politics of telling people how to live their lives then, the argument went, you must believe in a simple *laissez-faire* model of society which denies structures exist at all, and leaves everything to individuals.

This simple opposition allowed the politics of 'structural determination' to colonise nearly all of the politics of public health and to claim that this approach is hegemonic. Indeed, as attacks on the *Choosing Health* white paper showed, if you disagree with that politics then, by definition, you must be a neoconservative who does not believe in structures at all.

This approach characterised the UK Public Health Association's response to the white paper (UKPHA 2005). It attacked the idea that members of the public can choose to improve their health with a revealingly absurd analogy.

> *What does choice mean in public health? Public health is principally about organising society for the good of the population's health; at this level of concern, it is no more a matter of individual choice than the weather.*

This is a good clear definition, and one that places 'public health' at odds with most post-enlightenment human endeavour of the last 250 years. One of the lessons that mankind has learnt over that period is that we have the capacity to struggle to gain more control of our environment. But for 'public health' that environment is as out of our control as the weather. We should just give up and look to public health professionals to act as meteorologists to tell us when the rain is coming.

Unlike public health, the politics of many other areas of public service practice has been forced to move on – so that the language of determination in the politics of education has moved on to a much more dialectical approach. Here, the agency of disadvantaged parents and pupils works against the structures that impact upon their lives. In schooling, there has been a strong recognition that educational improvement depends in part on the very hard work of parents and pupils as well as educational policy. It is this hard work, together with the extra resources that the community has put into education, which will improve attainment. The same goes for health.

Over the next few years, public health professionals could engage with an increasingly active public to develop a more dialectical approach. This would stress the relationship between human agency and structures. This will see changes in such structures as poverty and educational attainment coming through that dialectic between individual endeavour and community support. And when public health professionals work with this struggle for self-determination, it will have a considerable impact on the health of the public.

So how did we get here? The problem of 'determinants' of human behaviour

In the past, a public health theory and practice that concentrated on the determinants of health has improved health considerably. If it was correct then, why is it not correct now? Don't theory and practice in health remain the same over time?

It is here that the core of the intellectual problem begins. A part of the theory of public health springs from the theory of medicine and health. This science likes to think of itself – erroneously – as a science of truths that build on themselves in a series of knowledge building blocks. The theory goes that learning about blood, bacteria and genetics is all building on the same corpus of knowledge.

Therefore, if the public's health was determined in the mid-19th century by such issues as water supply and sewage, and if millions of lives were saved by interventions in those determinants, then the same epistemology will work today. Find the determinants, intervene in them and people will have better health. The theory goes that today's determinants, like low levels of educational qualification and low income, work the same way as determinants in the past. Intervene in them and you improve health.

The problem is that the other vital intellectual aspect of public health, the part that differentiates it from most of the rest of the theory of medicine, is essentially social. The social theory and practice of how people and society work in advanced capitalist society has changed radically since the same society started developing mass clean water and sewage.

Some microbes may have stayed the same through history. But over that same history, people have changed a lot.

Only a very few people in political and social science think that social beings are *determined* by structures. Most now understand the way in which social relationships emerge from the interaction of structure and self-activity. They recognise the role of self-activity. In the same way, few people talk of self-development without recognition of social structure.

A determinant means one thing in the intellectual discourse of medicine and another in social and political relationships. The moment you say that, for example, people with lower educational qualifications will have worse health because of those qualifications the very next sentence is forced to say that there will be other factors involved. When it impacts on reality, every 'determinant' is qualified in such a way as to undermine its ability to determine.

Why this matters politically

This is more than semantics. A form of political intervention is 'read off' from this theory of determination. It believes that if people are determined then 'real' political interventions in public health must be big state interventions to counteract these big determinants. People themselves can achieve little or nothing – it is up to the state.

This is made clear in the UKPHA's clarification of who can change the world:

> There should be a refocusing on addressing underlying health determinants, with stronger measures put forward to lift people out of poverty.

It is telling in this quote who is active and who is passive here. Something abstract called *society* has to do the 'lifting' (out of poverty). Something passive called *people* have to be lifted out of that condition. In the real world of poverty it is the poor people themselves who do the heavy lifting.

As I have said, this is only one politics of the left. There is another which stresses that poor people themselves have the aspiration to change their lives. If they do nothing not a lot happens.

Therefore, within the politics of public health a competition between world views is taking place. Classical 'public health' thinks of the world in one way. The government in *Choosing Health* and other white papers thinks of it in another.

For classical 'public health' if a government *cared*, if we *really cared*, and *understood proper public health*, then we would recognise that only *interventions in determinants* will make a difference. So, their argument goes, since government will not carry out these authoritarian structural interventions, government does not really care about health improvement.

But they are wrong. There is a debate, a dispute, a disagreement about politics and philosophy here. *Choosing Health* takes up that debate. It is not that the white paper does not care; it is not that it does not understand. It is that it disagrees with the politics that has flowed from the past.

Lessons from the real politics of the left

The left has always contained twin political drivers for change, and its success has come when they have been brought together, not when they have been separated. The left has always understood that the big structures of society, economy, living conditions, education must be improved for the mass of the population and this calls for intervention at a government level – individuals cannot 'make the world' on their own.

In addition, it has also understood that individuals, especially those from disadvantaged backgrounds, play an active role in improving their own situation and that it cannot be done for them.

Real left-wing movements from the centre to the far left have been peopled by extraordinary women and men who have worked very hard, both in their education and at work, to be able to become a part of a political movement. There is no history of successful progress for the left without powerful aspiration for self-improvement, and without self-improvement the collective improvement does not take place. If disadvantaged people do not do things to move history forward, very little happens.

It just so happens that it was Marx who put this best of all. *'Men (and women) make history but not under conditions of their own choosing.'* The elegance of this sentence is anti-determinist. It points out that conditions do not make the history; rather, men and women do. However, it also points out that our will, our activity, our hopes and possibilities are not unrestrained, but are affected by those conditions. So effective politics needs both.

Why this set of politics matters in an advanced capitalist society such as Britain and how it relates to the health of the public

In politics as in health: if people don't do things very little happens.

Nearly everyone on the British left is engaged in democratic policies. It therefore recognises that there is limited progress to be made without the involvement of large numbers of people. My thesis is that this is also true of improving the health of the public – limited progress is to be made without the involvement of large numbers of people in their own health improvement.

As capitalism has advanced, the prospect of being able to do very much at all without involving people has lessened and lessened. So my thesis is that 'the people' under advanced capitalism are different from 'the people' under an earlier capitalist experience. If the public changes, then surely public health should change too.

The experience of history has changed people for three reasons. First, working people have worked hard together to improve their society through, for instance, educational opportunity, through the National Health Service, through government.

Second, working people have worked hard individually to improve their conditions through their work and by studying at school. People have worked hard to improve their own life chances.

Third, capitalism has interacted with both of these movements and has expanded its opportunities and influences into a very wide set of public life experiences.

Not all the outcomes of this are 'good'. However, for very nearly everyone in our society the possibilities in their lives have improved. In addition, most people do not believe that some abstract like 'capitalism' or 'government' has done this for them. They feel they have done this for themselves either individually or collectively.

More people are more active over more aspects of their lives than ever before. The expectation is that this will grow. Most social and economic policies are developed in order to increase people's capacity for self-activity. Most people grab those opportunities for improvement.

It is very true that for some people the 'conditions' that they live within are very much easier than others. Those easier conditions mean that some people are more active and make much more of their own history than others. People's conditions are not the same and nor are their aspirations. Moreover, these differences must be a theme of all our health-improvement interventions.

Self-activity and its possibilities has become the hallmark of our society. Indeed, one of the main aspects of social inclusion is the right to play an active part in economic and social relationships. Therefore, if we look at the politics of disadvantaged groups, we find groups that struggle for their right to be active.

The hallmark of the politics of all of these groups is their clamour for the right to be active in their own lives. They are right and a decent society supports them in developing that activity.

Given that people want to be more active then anything that starts its discourse with the public around the fact that the public are determined is doomed. The people themselves will drown that discourse out with the clamour for their own right to their own action.

Therefore, in our society both the politics of politics and the politics of public health demand that people should be given the opportunity to be more and more active in determining their own lives.

And what is interesting is that most of us with a bit of extra income and some educational qualifications feel that our lives are better precisely because we do have some more say over them.

So what does this mean for health and how does it influence the white paper, *Choosing Health*?

The white paper is not liked by some sections of the public health community because it does not talk about structure in a way that the public health community recognises. It does very clearly talk about social and economic structures but not as forces that determine human behaviour. It argues that the engine of change is not an abstract, not 'society', but is concrete, namely the individual and the collective actions of millions of people to improve their health.

In fact, it says something very challenging and simple – that if millions of people do not individually and collectively make more healthy choices then the nation's health does not improve. It demonstrates that the public's health improvement is in the hands of the public.

Therefore, the first object of policy is not an abstract determining structure, but is the concrete lives of communities and individuals. If they can become the subject of their own health, if they can choose health, then their health will improve. If they see themselves as the object of other people determining their health then they will not act to improve their own and their communities' health.

This leads the white paper to look closely at the influences on people to help them make more healthy choices. With smoking it recognises that individuals themselves have to make the difficult decision to keep on 'giving up'. Government can't 'give up' for you, nor can it do more exercise or eat more healthily.

The conditions within which people live and the impact on them of government policy can make those decisions easier or harder. It cannot make the decisions for people, but it can help them and support them in making healthier decisions.

The decision by the government to provide a piece of fruit every day for children in primary schools helps those children to make a healthy choice. If the children make the choice to eat the fruit they are offered at school then they are more likely to ask for fruit in their diets the rest of the week. Parents who live under different social and economic conditions will be in different positions to have fruit at home, and local government will have to assist those localities where there is a 'food desert' in order to help set up food co-ops that provide local cheap fruit for poorer families.

Governments can help but the people's choice is the determinant.

Conclusion

The government white paper on health improvement contains a politics of health improvement that demonstrates how individuals and communities have a strong role in improving their own health. It does not see people's health as determined. It does however believe that individuals and communities need to be assisted by government at local and national levels to intervene in the structures that militate against healthy choices and to help people make more choices that will improve their own health.

References

Conservative Party (2005) *Action on Health*. 10 February. London: Conservative Party.

Secretary of State for Health (2004) *Choosing Health: making healthy choices easier*. Cm 6374. London: The Stationery Office.

UK Public Health Association (UKPHA) (2005) *Choosing or Losing Health?* London: UKPHA.

Chapter 9

Inspecting, informing, improving: public health within the Healthcare Commission

Jude Williams

The Health and Social Care (Community Health and Standards) Act (2003) made it clear that the Healthcare Commission had responsibility to consider the extent to which healthcare organisations protect and improve the health of the public and to assess the quality of the delivery of relevant public health systems. Reinforcement for the role comes from the statutory requirement for the Healthcare Commission to take account of the Department of Health's *Standards for Better Health* (Department of Health 2004a), which includes public health issues throughout.

With a clearer central policy framework for improving health and public health that explicitly includes a role for the Healthcare Commission there is an unprecedented opportunity for us to spur on others to make improvements in their activities to improve and protect health. Developing this new agenda has taught us many valuable lessons. This chapter covers the progress made and some of the challenges experienced.

Our new legal duties and assessment framework in relation to public health

The importance of public health is captured in the *Assessment for Improvement: the annual health check*, the document produced by the Healthcare Commission in March 2005 that describes the framework for assessing each healthcare organisation in England through an annual review and rating (Healthcare Commission 2005). Most of the elements of this framework have a significant public health component. The framework includes assessing whether NHS healthcare organisations are meeting the basics on the core standards (one of the seven domains specifically addresses public health and it features within others), value for money and delivering against the existing targets set by government. It also includes assessing what improvement is being made by healthcare organisations by considering the new national targets (many of which relate to population health) and improvement reviews. Local target setting and assessment of progress towards the developmental standards will come on stream in subsequent years. Currently work is taking place to develop an assessment framework for the developmental standard for public health following a positive response from an earlier consultation on proposed criteria.

Systems that deliver improvements in public health include work across organisations, through local and national systems, as well as within individual organisations. Assessment and study tools therefore also need to take a broader, systems view than one that just considers individual organisations. A legal tool which enables us to conduct studies on economy, efficiency and effectiveness is important in this regard, as is our duty to coordinate healthcare inspection enabling us to bring a range of inspectorates together to consider public health.

Other instruments and functions at our disposal include: the annual patient and staff surveys which include public health issues; complaints that we handle when they are unresolved locally; serious investigations which can have direct or indirect implications for the health and safety of the public; and informing the public and patients in a variety of ways on our findings including reporting on the state of healthcare annually. We also have the role of inspecting and regulating private and voluntary sector providers who are delivering healthcare and in the future our work will align with that of the Commission for Social Care Inspection (CSCI). For public health this variety of instruments has resulted in considerable coverage of activity within the first year.

One of our early tasks was to define and scope public health in its relationship to the Commission's roles. As a discipline, public health is concerned with the health of populations and seeks to reduce the overall prevalence and incidence of disease, injury and preventable death with a particular focus on reducing health inequalities. Within the health sector, public health includes all clinical, managerial and administrative activity that contributes to this agenda. Therefore, the extent to which population health profiling and health needs assessment influence commissioning and provision of *all* healthcare is an outcome by which a healthcare organisation ought to be judged. Similarly, the systematic application of evidence about the effectiveness of clinical and other interventions is another useful indicator of high-quality practice.

However, Wanless (2002) clearly illustrated that in order to achieve significant health improvement, effective disease prevention and health promotion delivered in a way that engages the population needed to become critical areas of healthcare activity. Assessment of healthcare organisations on this agenda would ideally involve their direct or commissioned provision; their activities as good corporate citizens; and their role within local strategic and operational partnerships by supporting and leading whole-system change. This latter role recognises the extremely important contribution of local government and other partners to this agenda. Programmes of work at local level draw together comprehensive actions to address complex problems that include the contributions of each partner.

The Healthcare Commission established a range of public health programmes of work during its first year of operations. These are briefly outlined in Box 9.1. Further information can be found on the website: www.healthcarecommission.org.uk

---

Box 9.1 Public health programme within the Healthcare Commission

1 **Core standards based assessment:** The seventh domain contains three core standards that cover health protection, health improvement and tackling health inequalities through partnerships and public health plans and programmes. The criteria developed ensure close alignment with *Choosing Health* (Secretary of State for Health 2004) priorities and

healthcare organisations' systematic delivery of public health work. The model developed takes a planning cycle approach and asks organisations initially to assure themselves against these standards. The Healthcare Commission uses a variety of mechanisms – including nationally available public health indicators and views from Patient and Public Involvement Forums – to determine whether organisations' judgements tally with the data (to roll out in 2006).

2 **Developmental standards based assessment:** Public health was selected as one of the areas to develop a suitable methodology for ongoing assessment of improvement against the developmental standards, to be tested in 2005–06. This will build on the draft public health criteria developed for 'D13' (the developmental standard for public health), which received positive responses during consultation (November 2004–February 2005).

3 **Public health targets: existing commitments 2005/06 and national targets 2006/07.**

4 **Improvement reviews and national briefings:**

- **Tobacco control:** Following piloting on seven sites, the review rolled out to all PCTs (reporting due summer 2006).
- **Sexual health:** Piloting with PCTs was carried out on sexual health (national briefing in summer 2006).
- **Local area study for public health:** A joint study is underway with the Audit Commission. This study will focus on how healthcare organisations, local government and other partners are working in a geographical area to improve health and reduce health inequalities. It is intended that we will cover up to nine areas and will, in part, focus on accidental injury in 0 to 5 year olds. A national report was produced in the summer of 2006 aiming to drive improvement in local delivery of accident prevention programmes and inform national policy makers. The study contributes to our learning about how a joint approach between inspectorates can provide a rounded view of the quality of public health work across organisations.
- **Under-11 obesity public service agreement (PSA):** A joint delivery chain analysis on the under-11 obesity PSA target – undertaken with the National Audit Office and the Audit Commission (published February 2006 and available on the Healthcare Commission website, www.healthcarecommission.org.uk).

5 **Incorporation of public health within other reviews:** All future improvement reviews will be systematically checked for their impact on health and health inequalities. Work has already taken place to integrate public health into the improvement reviews for children (joint area reviews), adult community mental health and substance misuse.

6 **Health inequalities:** Ensuring health equality is fundamental to our public health work. Health inequality work is being embedded into all Healthcare Commission activity. Assessing how elements of system reform impact on health inequalities is an important brief and one which we will focus on while health inequalities are widening. Work is

being undertaken to align our health inequalities work with work on equity and human rights to strengthen both agendas.

7 **Sharing and aligning with other inspectorates and the parallel agencies in Wales:** In addition to the work with the Audit Commission, the National Audit Office and Ofsted (Office for Standards in Education), discussions on public health have been held with CSCI. We are working closely with relevant agencies in Wales to share learning.

Core and developmental standard criteria

The development of the criteria for core and developmental standards involved input from a range of stakeholders and public health practitioners, and they were consulted on widely. The developmental criteria were seen – wherever possible – as a progression or higher level of the core criteria. A simple planning cycle model was used for some of the core and developmental standards to identify the elements each organisation needs to deliver. This approach was assessed as helpful during the Healthcare Commission's consultation period and in pilots of the public health improvement reviews. Figure 9.1 illustrates this approach.

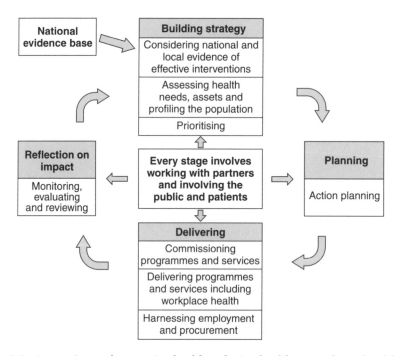

Figure 9.1 Improving and protecting health/reducing health inequalities: local-level cycle.

The importance of a more comprehensive health needs assessment and health profiling having a real impact on prioritisation, planning and commissioning of health improvement and healthcare services fits well with the recently stated roles of PCTs within *Commissioning a Patient-led NHS* (Department of Health 2005).

Improvement reviews

The broad term 'improvement review' covers a variety of ways of measuring progress within specific areas. These can look in depth at a particular condition (such as diabetes), a section of the population (such as older people, people with disabilities), a service (such as drug services) or a certain risk factor (such as tobacco use or obesity). The form the review takes reflects the issues being addressed and its potential to impact on improved outcomes. Some information collected as part of specific improvement reviews will have long-term impact as the information and information systems can be used in the future. This ongoing monitoring will feed into the future annual assessment on the developmental standard.

Healthcare Commission assessments include an initial stage of 'screening' nationally available data and, in the case of improvement reviews, easily collectable and readily available local information. This allows identification of a small proportion of trusts whose performance has been assessed as having the greatest potential for improvement. This 'risk-based' approach means that Healthcare Commission resources can extend farther, to carry out regular core and developmental standard reviews across all healthcare organisations. The breadth of coverage of assessment is supported by in-depth reviews in particular thematic areas.

Our aim is to ensure that inspection in public health has the greatest impact, and supports strategies to improve health of local populations. Driving the selection of tools is the principle of reducing the burden of inspection for local organisations while having maximum impact on health improvement.

Data matters

The Healthcare Commission is working on two strands of activity with regards to data and public health; ensuring it has access to the right information to assess local progress on improving the health of the population while staying 'light touch' and assessing healthcare organisations on their ability to collect, analyse and act on public health information.

These are data-rich times. Technology offers unprecedented opportunities to collect, store and analyse data, making them 'intelligent' for public health strategy and practice. Sources of data vary and there remain challenges in ensuring they are of a quality which enables systematic use of them at all levels. National and local players have a role to play in improving their quality, and ensuring timeliness of provision. National bodies are developing the breadth of their data interests and addressing current shortfalls (for example, the Audit Commission's work in developing local area profiles). In addition, local partners have strong incentives to develop intelligence systems to understand their communities and measure the impact of public health actions.

Developing innovation in data collection is key. Populations are diverse and mobile, and a good understanding of the issues they face is crucial in informing the delivery of public health. Although complex, the relationships between health and socio-economic status, place, health service use, and other factors such as housing, education, and employment are important and demand constant analysis. Linking these in a creative way to other public health data such as the incidence and prevalence of communicable and non-communicable diseases, population ill health and deaths will yield significant results. Clever use of sound data will transform delivery.

Improving understanding about the impact of interventions will add to the confidence of measuring output or process measures. For example, the correlation between partnership working or public health capacity and health outcomes is not yet fully clear. Work with the newly established Centre for Public Health Excellence in the National Institute for Health and Clinical Effectiveness (NICE) will contribute to greater clarity on these issues over time. The Healthcare Commission seeks to play a role in using available and emerging evidence and also to contributing to that evidence base.

Assessing partners and partnership work

The Department of Health (DH) standards have set PCTs the challenge to achieve health protection and health improvement for their local population through, in part, the activities of partner organisations. They can undertake this indirect role through commissioning and also through their support to, and influence on, a range of partners. How much a PCT can be held to account for a poorly functioning local authority, or take credit for a highly performing one, is an issue that needs to be reconciled. We are learning from current pilots and studies how this can be done.

Joint approaches across inspectorates are needed to establish a rounded view of the quality and impact of partnership working, the way in which the larger public health system is operating and the contribution made by each organisation within the system. The Healthcare Commission and the Audit Commission submitted a joint response to the Secretary of State's consultation paper on public health, *Choosing Health* (Secretary of State for Health 2004), which outlined both Commissions' strong commitment to population health improvement and highlighted the potential for aligning their work. Approaches have included exploring how to work together on the assessment of public health capacity in a local area as well as analysing whole-system delivery chains to deliver public health. Another example of an integrated approach is the joint area reviews for children (JARs), which provides excellent opportunities for the Healthcare Commission to incorporate public health issues into a broad programme, involving several inspectorates.

Learning from our work while developing a methodology

One of the challenges for the Healthcare Commission in relation to public health is to be bold in the development and adaptation of methods to explore how we might maximise our impact on this untested area of responsibility for healthcare inspection in this country. Consultation revealed that the inclusion of the few public health elements in the star ratings – though limited – resulted in public health becoming more central to PCT agendas. There is potential to build on this progress and use inspection to drive improvement widely. The particular challenge is to ensure that our systems and methods can adapt quickly, as we learn from our work, our partner inspectorates, and work being undertaken in other national systems.

In addition to our small core team, the Healthcare Commission has contact with a range of individuals with diverse public health expertise to ensure that development and learning is grounded in the realities of day-to-day delivery.

We appointed 26 public health advisers to support our review work. They are public health practitioners, many of whom have review experience, who take time from their 'day jobs' to support our reviews. The Healthcare Commission has also established a Public Health Expert Reference Group to provide high-level support and advice to the evolving programmes.

We have had solid support from colleagues engaged elsewhere in the public health endeavour, for which we are grateful. The Healthcare Commission is only one part of the system that contributes to health protection and improvement and efforts to reduce health inequalities and it is by this involvement from people at all levels in the system that we will ensure that our work encourages continuous improvements in delivery. There are now opportunities to build a convincing account of how local agencies are performing and appropriate assessment systems can help us all make the case for investment in public health. However, this will only be achieved if local strategists and practitioners see inspection as a crucial part of the whole system rather than just external control. Collaboration, of the kind we have started, will contribute to building a system that is more fit for purpose to drive improvement.

References and further reading

Barker DJP, Coggon D and Rose G (2003) *Epidemiology for the Uninitiated*. London: BMJ Books.

Department of Health (2004a) *Standards for Better Health*. London: Department of Health.

Department of Health (2004b) *National Standards, Local Action: Health and Social Care Standards and Planning Framework 2005/06–2007/08*. London: Department of Health.

Department of Health (2005) *Commissioning a Patient-led NHS*. London: Department of Health.

Healthcare Commission (2005) *Assessment for Improvement: the annual health check*. London: Healthcare Commission.

Secretary of State for Health (2004) *Choosing Health: making healthy choices easier*. London: Department of Health.

Wanless D (2002) *Securing Our Future Health: taking a long term view*. London: HM Treasury.

Chapter 10

Public health in the English regions

Paul Johnstone

Introduction

Tackling inequalities calls for a multi-disciplinary, multi-agency strategy operating at all levels – international, national, regional, local and individual.

In the first edition of *Perspectives in Public Health*, David Hunter made this powerful case arguing that multidisciplinary and multi-agency action to tackle inequalities was needed at every level. The 1999 edition concentrated on all these levels – except the regional level. This was because there was little or patchy action on public health at the regional level, particularly on wider determinants of health such as education, transport and economic and social regeneration in a consistent way. Regional public health was part of the outposts of the Department of Health (called regional offices) and largely focused on the NHS and clinical services. Yet Douglas Black (1980) and Donald Acheson (1998) in their landmark reports, and many others including Holland (1999), called for greater action at this regional level of governance.

All this began to change from 2000, with political devolution to Scotland and Wales, including devolved responsibilities for public health, and in England, with the emergence of Government Offices (GOs) of the Regions as a regional tier of central government, including the co-location of Regional Directors of Public Health in 2002. Also in 2000, the Local Government Act gave local authorities statutory responsibility for the wellbeing of their populations. Further developments continued following the publication of Derek Wanless's review of public health and the 2004 public health white paper for England, *Choosing Health* (Secretary of State for Health 2004), which states that public health is everybody's business – including every government department and every sector (Department of Health 2002; Office of the Deputy Prime Minister 2003). We are therefore at the beginning of a new effort to deliver public health action, not just through the health service, but through cross-government action on the wider determinants of health and inequalities, nationally, locally and regionally.

This chapter will focus on the progress made in the last 5 years on public health action in the regions of England, as two stories. The first, to provide context, will be on the evolution of the English regions, which now has the 'footprint' of over 80 government agencies and many other organisations. The second story will describe the development of regional public health action at this important juncture of government and society. Finally, the last section will outline what further work is required, risks and future opportunities.

English regions in the 1980s and 1990s

During the 1980s, a key part of EEC (European Economic Community) economic policy was to target financial assistance to the most deprived regions of Europe.

Alongside such areas in Southern Spain and Italy, some of Britain's more deprived post-industrial areas – particularly in the North of England and Cornwall and parts of Wales and Scotland – qualified for European development assistance. Brussels preferred dealing directly with the regions rather than national governments for this aid. Therefore, the Thatcher government opened offices in some parts of the UK to receive funds from Europe. New 'development agencies' for Scotland and Wales were set up to foster economic development more locally than managing it from Whitehall. In a step to strengthen a more consistent approach, the Major government established nine Government Offices in England in 1994 (*see* Figure 10.1). These housed three Whitehall departments: the Department for Education and Employment, the Department for Trade and Industry and the Department for Environment, Transport and the Regions. The then Environment Secretary, John Gummer, said that the new offices *'will meet the widespread demand that there should be a single point of contact for local authorities, businesses and local communities'*. English regions had become economic as well as cultural entities.

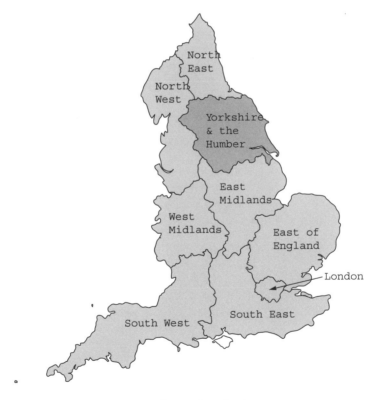

Figure 10.1 The nine Government Offices of England.

Regionalism since 1997

In 1997, the New Labour government shifted UK policy significantly towards devolution and regionalism. Following referenda, political devolution for Scotland and Wales was achieved and each has responsibility for health services and public health. In London, greater powers were handed back to the capital through an elected mayor. At the same time, more Whitehall departments began to look to the regions. By 2002, ten Whitehall departments had a presence in the Government Offices (*see* Box 10.1).

Box 10.1 A table of the ten Whitehall departments in English Government Offices (2002)

- Office of the Deputy Prime Minister
- Department for Trade and Industry
- Department for Education and Skills (DfES)
- Department for Transport
- Department for Environment, Food and Rural Affairs (DEFRA)
- Home Office
- Department for Culture, Media and Sport (DCMS)
- Department of Health (co-located)
- Department for Work and Pensions (DWP)
- Cabinet Office

Government Offices (GOs) continued to establish themselves as the key link between Whitehall and local authorities and played an important role in delivering government policies in the regions. These include neighbourhood renewal, housing, planning, crime, drugs, transport, children and young people's programmes, skills, rural issues, European Structural Funds, voluntary and community sector, resilience and sports, arts and culture.

The Office of the Deputy Prime Minister maintains overall responsibility for GOs. The GOs carry out work on behalf of ten sponsor departments. On behalf of these departments, they are involved in the delivery of over 40 national public service agreements, which cover a huge range of tasks – many of which have both direct and indirect impact on population health and are described in more detail in Chapter 32.

Following the NHS reforms in 2002, *Shifting the Balance of Power* (Department of Health 2002), Regional Directors of Public Health were moved from the Department of Health's eight Regional Offices into the nine Government Offices. This very different arena offered a new opportunity to tackle wider determinants of health, working across Whitehall departments in the Government Offices, the Regional Development Agencies and Assemblies and with over 80 other government agencies that have a footprint at this regional tier.

Other organisations in regions

As Government Offices evolved, a number of other organisations were established at the regional level, two with significant roles – the Regional Development Agencies (RDAs) and Regional Assemblies.

Regional Development Agencies were established by the Treasury and Department of Trade and Industry in 1999. Their main responsibility is to lead 3-year Regional Economic Strategies (or RESs) which set out how the RDA, with local authorities, regional and business partners, plans to regenerate and develop the economies of their regions. They are accountable to Regional Assemblies and Government Offices critically assess their plans. Regional Assemblies, also established in 1999, bring together local authority-elected members, social, economic, voluntary and faith sector partners to provide a 'voice of the region'. They have responsibility for planning in areas such as housing, spatial strategies (including transport) and culture.

The Government Office, Regional Development Agency and Regional Assembly make up what is described at the 'big three' regional organisations. However, there are a host of other organisations, which now have a regional agenda and presence, such as the Countryside Agency, Sport England, a regional cultural organisation, and voluntary sector (*see* Box 10.2). These have significant influence locally, for example in Yorkshire and Humberside, the Voluntary Forum represents 20,000 voluntary organisations in the region with over 450,000 volunteers. As a result, English regions have become important junctures in society, between national government and local communities, and offer important public health opportunities 'through organised efforts of society'.

Box 10.2. Some examples of regional organisations which have a footprint in the regional tier of government and can influence health

- Sport England
- Countryside Agency
- Regional Forum for Voluntary and Community Sectors
- Regional Consortia of Universities
- Regional Cultural Consortium
- Regional Environmental Forum
- Regional Rural Affairs Forum
- Royal College of Nursing
- Care Services Improvement Partnership

While regions in England evolved economic, social and cultural roles, accountability for these actions still rested with Whitehall. Was there an appetite for a political role in the regions? The experience from Scotland, Wales and the mayoral model in London led the government to publish a white paper in 2003 called *Your Region, Your Choice* (Office of the Deputy Prime Minister 2003). It set out a timetable for strengthening all the roles of the three main regional organisations, and, subject to referenda, proposals to develop elected regional assemblies (ERAs). The white paper made the case that ERAs would provide greater clarity of purpose and accountability to regional agencies. The three regions in Northern England were considered as the first wave of interest for ERAs and the first referendum was conducted in the North East region in 2004. However, concerns about extra bureaucracy, a loss of local autonomy and the added value of an ERA led to a no vote in the first referendum, and the government subsequently abandoned this policy. Some argued this decision led to a loss of capacity to deliver regional economic and social agendas – and potentially in public health (Hunter, Wilkinson and Coyle 2005).

With a return of a Labour government in 2005, commitment to develop regionalism over the next few years remains, but not through ERAs. Currently, assemblies retain their statutory roles in planning and they also provide a significant forum for local government. They also continue to provide a collective voice for their region, in England and the European Union (through offices based in Brussels). This was demonstrated in 2004 when the Treasury started basing its 3-year 'Comprehensive Spending Reviews' not just on the relative importance of Whitehall department agendas (such as schools and hospitals nationally) but weighted to evidence-based regional needs through 'Regional Emphasis Documents'. Working with local government at the regional level and making the case for extra resources for regeneration offers important public health opportunities. In the next section, I will describe how we have acted on these opportunities in one regional Government Office.

Public health regional action

It is not difficult to see the public health opportunities of working at the regional level: the potential to tackle the wider determinants of health – working across Whitehall departments in Government Offices, with the RDAs on regeneration and business development, and through Assemblies and others, engaging in organised efforts of society. Regional Directors of Public Health, as part of the Department of Health and co-located in Government Offices, have been in a position to act on such opportunities. In this section, I describe the work we have been leading in the Yorkshire and Humberside Government Office, but acknowledging the development of similar work across all the regions. This tells a story of an evolving new public health agenda, which can be described in four phases:

1 piloting new agendas
2 developing a consistent approach
3 building a coalition for change
4 delivery.

The beginning – piloting new agendas

In setting up the new office, we rapidly assessed the opportunities for action across a wider range of areas. The most obvious place to start was public service agreements (PSAs), which the Department of Health have a responsibility for delivering nationally.

PSAs are a method of delivering cross-cutting policies across all government departments. They are agreed with the settlement for each department in the Comprehensive Spending Review – a 3-year programme of public spending. This policy was developed in order to overcome the short-term annual planning cycle in public service investment and to achieve more coordinated government planning. PSAs have important implications for health improvement. For example, the Department of Health's priority on tackling health inequalities relates to the delivery of 16 other PSAs across eight different departments. Similarly, improving outcomes for people with long-term care conditions is affected, to a greater or lesser degree, by delivery of targets for pensions, safe communities, fuel poverty, social exclusion and transport. Box 10.3 and Table 10.1 summarise PSA topics which have an impact on health with some specific examples for children's wellbeing.

Box 10.3 Summary on cross-government PSAs that have an impact on health

- Tobacco control
- Learning and education inequalities
- Childcare
- Air quality
- Environment
- Adults' skills
- Social exclusion
- Rural areas
- Sustainability
- Employment rates
- Housing
- Fuel poverty
- Pensions
- Access to sports and culture
- Safe communities
- Illicit drugs
- Risks at work

Table 10.1 Specific examples of PSAs having an impact on child health inequalities

Topic	PSA	Government departments
Children	Halt year-on-year rise in obesity in under-11 children by 2010	DH, DfES and DCMS
	Narrow gap in educational achievement between looked-after children and their peers	DfES
Children – Sure Start target	Improve communication, social and emotional development so that by 2008 50% of children reach a good level of development at foundation stage and reduce inequalities between disadvantaged areas and rest of England	DfES and DWP
Young people	Reduce under-18 conception rate by 50% by 2010	DH and DfES
	Increase take-up of sporting activities (minimum of 2 hours a week) to 85% of 5–16 year olds by 2008	DfES and DCMS
Adult skills – the Skills for Life initiative	Improve basic skills levels for employability of 2.25 million adults by 2010, milestone of 1.5 million by 2007	DfES and DWP

Many government departments task their regional presence to lead on delivering PSAs. Boxes 10.4 to 10.7 give some examples of where we made some quick wins based on our work on PSAs and other opportunities working with regional organisations.

Box 10.4 The NHS as an economic regenerator – to tackle poverty and deprivation

Through the RDA's Regional Economic Strategy, we agreed a new approach with NHS organisations to develop their role as economic investors in their communities, as well as providers of healthcare. Local hospitals are often the biggest employers, procurers of local goods and investors in capital development – particularly following the NHS Plan. Many hospitals if floated on the London Stock Exchange would have turnovers equivalent to FTSE 250 businesses. At the regional level, health brings £6.2 billion a year and accounts for 7.2% of all employment in 2004, and over the next decade will experience more growth than any other sector. The RDA subsequently invested £4 million in developing NHS new procurement and employability pilots to forge this new approach. The pilot on employability aimed to establish NHS employment schemes that will create a minimum of 480 learning opportunities with 480 people brought into substantive employment in the NHS. Typical programmes provide pre-employment NHS experience, training – including IT training where relevant – with a prior commitment to ring-fenced posts at the successful end of the training period. The programme seeks to reach those parts of the labour market that do not normally consider work in the NHS or who have difficulty overcoming institutional and other barriers. By the start of 2005 17 separate NHS employers were involved and the scheme was being expanded.

Box 10.5 School Fruit Scheme brings investment to Yorkshire rurally isolated areas

Getting children to develop good eating habits is one of the best ways of promoting their health throughout their lives. It is central to the drive to improve our health and tackle obesity. Following the successful pilot, the School Fruit and Vegetable Scheme was rolled out across England in Autumn 2004. As well as the health benefits, there were clearly potential economic benefits, if local suppliers could be found. Cross-departmental working with DEFRA helped take this on.

It meant the Regional Public Health Team could undertake research with agriculture specialists at the Stocksbridge Technology Centre to scope the potential for local supply and then work with the Purchase and Supply Agency (PASA) to promote the scheme to local growers.

One local family farming business, growing organic carrots, decided to tender to help broaden its customer base beyond the multiple retailers. This was a brave move into a new area and required investment in new processing and packaging equipment. A local primary school was the ideal partner for market research on children's preferences both on shape, size and taste. It also involved persuading the PASA to accept a variation from its specification as the two carrot varieties specified were not suitable for organic growing. Now an estimated 10 tonnes of carrots from 60 acres of fields at Low House Farm, Aldborough, are supplied to schools across the region every week during term time.

The next round of contracts requires an expanded range of produce – including mini cucumbers and strawberries – which offers real opportunities to growers in the region. We are again working with the Stocksbridge Centre, the PASA – and the National Farmers' Union – to identify potential suppliers and practical measures to help them to compete for these large-scale contracts.

Box 10.6 Reducing risks of HIV and hepatitis infections in drugs misusers

Working across Government Office (Home Office, DfES and DH), the police, the National Treatment Agency and strategic health authorities, the group led a crime and health initiative which resulted in the following in Leeds:

- Establishing a 70% return target for needle exchange. The pick-up rate was only 10% – leaving 450,000 needles unaccounted for.
- Improving needle pick-up services and influencing the Drug Action Team to adopt needle pick-up as a priority. The needle clean-up service and hotline are now fully functional and providing rapid services to the public and statutory agencies.
- Agreeing a Rough Sleepers Protocol tying GOYH (Government Office for Yorkshire and the Humber), the police, health, probation, prison, local authority and housing services to reduce the levels of drug-related crime linked to rough sleepers and action to help rough sleepers into housing, education, employment or enforcement. Six months later the number of rough sleepers had dropped from 180 to four.

Box 10.7 Joining up public health intelligence

The public health observatory (PHO) traditionally provided data to the health sector, often generated by the health sector. However, there are many other regional agencies that have 'observatories' and were working in isolation from the health sector. For example, each region has an economic observatory funded by the RDAs, and Regional Sports Boards have developed Sport and Activities observatories. In establishing the work of the PHO, we were able to link its development to work with these other regional observatories and locally with analysts in local government. The outcome has been a more integrated approach to the use of data and better-quality data on the wider determinants.

These early examples opened the way to develop the public health agenda in the region. But in order to encourage deeper understanding and a sustained commitment to this agenda within regional organisations, it was clear that that we needed to draw together, in one place, what is the burden of ill health and show what could be done by regional action, based on learning from these early examples. The next section describes how we did this.

Developing a consistent approach

In 2004, we published the first annual Regional Director of Public Health Report (*see* Figure 10.2) for the Government Office region (Department of Health 2004b) which had the basic message:

- these are the killer facts for people living in Yorkshire and Humberside (*see* Box 10.8)
- here are some regional level actions to support local action
- we believe action requires a new and rigorous partnership.

This type of report was unique as our recommendations were aimed at regional organisations for the first time. The NHS could not deliver health improvements alone, and all regional organisations had important roles, together working with local government and all NHS organisations. The report highlighted 12 health-related themes, underpinned by critical statistics, and suggested 72 possible actions for regional organisations (*see* Box 10.9). A full text of the recommendations and a subsequent framework for action, agreed with 60 organisations, can be found on the website. This created a solid foundation for discussion on which to build a powerful cross-sector coalition of regional and local organisations, committed to working to tackle the causes of poor health and health inequalities in the region.

Box 10.8 Yorkshire and Humber killer facts

- 3,600 extra deaths in Yorkshire and Humberside due to the inequality between this region and the rest of England; 100 of these were babies under 1 year old.
- 10,000 died prematurely from smoking-related diseases.
- 650,000 attend NHS related to alcohol – cost £200 million a year.
- 850 die on roads a year.
- 3,400 more people die in winter months than expected – we have the highest fuel-poverty rates.
- Obesity up from 19% to 26% in last 5 years.

Box 10.9 Themes for regional action identified in *Our Region Our Health*

- Tobacco control
- Food and health
- Alcohol and health

- Physical activity
- Accidental injury
- Mental health and stress
- Teenage pregnancy
- Education, learning and skills
- Housing, homes and health
- Community safety and substance misuse
- Healthy and sustainable communities
- Economic regeneration and NHS role

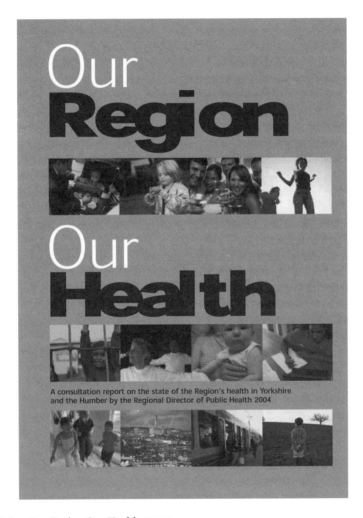

Figure 10.2 *Our Region Our Health* report.

Building a coalition for regional action

The Regional Assembly, as the umbrella organisation for all local authorities and as the 'voice of the region', played a key role in building a coalition for action.

The Assembly endorsed *Our Region Our Health* and backed the development of a Regional Strategic Framework for Health (RSFH) – a plan to implement the actions across a number of regional agencies, as a framework to support local action (Department of Health 2004a). The development of the RSFH engaged over 60 regional organisations including strategic health authorities, the RDA and the Government Office. Rather than develop yet another new set of targets for health, already published in *Choosing Health*, NHS local development plans guidance and local authority community plans, we decided the framework should focus on regional level objectives to support local action on the targets. Therefore, we focused on three overarching objectives:

- to influence all policy development
- to develop effective public health whole systems
- to build public health resources where needed.

The Framework was launched in December 2004, which together with the recently published white paper *Choosing Health* brought together a wider audience of key players for public health action in the region. The six key partners (three strategic health authorities, Government Office, the Assembly and Regional Development Agency) led the signing of a concordat to back the Framework, witnessed by the Local Government Minister (*see* Figure 10.3). The concordat outlined five specific actions that these partners pledged to lead in the first year:

- to realise the benefits of the economic power of the NHS, through the Regional Economic Strategy, as a major employer, investor and economic regenerator in the region, and as a major contributor to the enhancement of sustainable community development
- to implement the Regional Strategic Framework for Health, to improve the public's health – to ensure that regional partners work together to add value to improving people's health and reducing inequalities

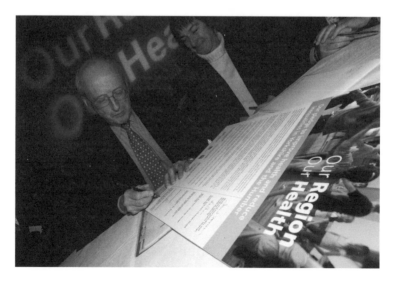

Figure 10.3 Concordat signing with Nick Raynford MP, Local Government Minister.

- to work towards a common approach to assessing performance of health improvement actions, in partnership with local authorities and local strategic partnerships (LSPs)
- to ensure that regional and NHS organisations continue to work together on robust and tested emergency plans as an integral part of local regional resilience
- to provide effective and robust leadership to support delivery in key areas such as supporting the development of smoke-free communities.

Cross-government office plan for health inequalities

At the same time, and integral to developing the Framework with regional partners, we also embarked on a new approach to public health planning across the Government Office. The main driver for this was to align action on jointly shared PSAs, many of which have direct and indirect impacts on population health, described earlier. We particularly focused on areas of high need and high impact, identified in the RDPH report, such as 'excess winter deaths' and 'fuel poverty' accounting for over 3,500 excess deaths in Yorkshire and Humber annually. Details of the action plan can be found at the GOYH website, www.goyh.gov.uk The Government Office subsequently agreed to include 'tackling inequalities' as one of four cross-cutting objectives, alongside economic prosperity, sustainability and the built and natural environment.

Hence with these two approaches, we were able to embed tackling health inequalities and improving the public's health across regional organisations and across Whitehall departments in the Government Office. The next challenge, therefore, was to ensure that these commitments actually delivered health improvements.

Delivering regional action

It is one thing to set up coalitions for action, based on partnerships – quite another to ensure they perform and deliver. This section outlines the approach we have taken and assesses progress so far.

The Concordat and Regional Strategic Framework for Health made specific reference to sharing relevant performance data to support delivery. We also recognised that managing performance required a different cultural approach than say the Department of Health has to strategic health authorities and strategic health authorities to local NHS trusts. While managing performance across the Yorkshire and Humberside partners requires leadership, this recognises that no one organisation is accountable in a hierarchy to any other.

For this reason we developed an intelligence-led performance management system, which we have call 'tracking performance'. This involves pooling data on public health performance from four partners: the NHS via the strategic health authorities, local government, local strategic partnerships and from regional agencies where appropriate. This Framework allowed us to agree on four topics initially to pilot the approach, in tobacco control, sexual health, fuel poverty, and children and obesity. These topics were chosen because effective action can only take place with the commitment from these partners together. The outcome to the first of these topics, tobacco control, can be defined as follows.

While the RSFH provided the leadership and context – 'to achieve smoke-free communities across the region' – we embarked in new areas of work to assess our performance in meeting our commitments in tobacco control across the region. We assessed the contributions needed from the NHS, local authorities and local strategic partnerships and mapped what should be provided to assess our progress (*see* Figure 10.4). This 'map' was also developed for other areas for which we agreed to track performance (childhood obesity, fuel poverty and sexual health) which was published in the RSFH.

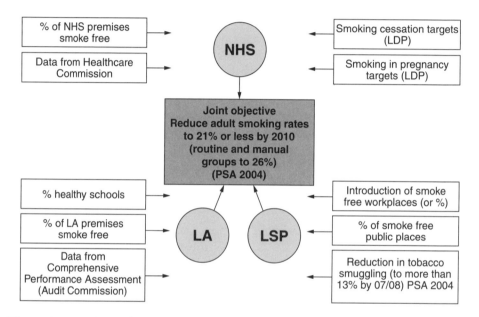

Figure 10.4 Joint performance tracking example in Yorkshire and Humber region.

Subsequently, we were able to combine data from a range of different sources including tobacco-related mortality statistics and number of public sector organisations that had implemented smoke-free policies. By profiling this information, the number of NHS trusts implementing smoke-free policies went up from 1 to 10, and local authorities from 2 to 16.

Thus the publication of available data on health outcomes and performance provided a powerful local lever for change, and the approach was widely welcome.

Other mechanisms to assure performance

Performance on the cross-Government Office plan for tackling inequalities has been incorporated into the Government Office performance-management system. Hence all government departments in the GO report on progress quarterly, and this is presented to the GO Corporate Management Board, which has two non-executive directors. Progress on the Regional Strategic Framework for Health will also be reported to the Assembly through its Overview and Scrutiny Committee, although at the time of writing this function of the Assembly is being reviewed.

Local area agreements

Another important opportunity for implementing the RSFH and *Choosing Health* white paper was developed in 2005 – the local area agreement (LAA). Central government funds about 60 different programmes to local government and individual central departments manage these independently with separate accountabilities and reporting mechanisms. On close inspection, many of these programmes have an impact on health improvement and Box 10.10 shows some examples of these. However, most of these programmes operate separately to the mainstream work of local health agencies.

Box 10.10 Some examples of area-based initiatives that have an influence on health of populations

- **Neighbourhood Renewal Scheme** aims to enable the 88 most deprived local authorities to improve services and narrow the gap between deprived areas and the rest of England.
- **Neighbourhood Nurseries** provide affordable, accessible, high-quality childcare in the most disadvantaged areas.
- **New Deal for Communities** aims to tackle multiple deprivation in the poorest areas.
- **Space for Sport and Arts** aims to build links between schools and communities to encourage social inclusion in areas of deprivation through improving facilities in sports and arts in primary schools.
- **Liveability Fund – based on Sustainable Communities** – building for the future (ODPM 2003). This is a fund to support local authority projects to improve green spaces.
- **Local Network Fund for Children and Young People.** (May 2001) – this provides small grants to local projects for 0–19 year olds in deprived areas.
- **Market Renewal Pathfinders** – funding to support housing schemes in low demand/abandonment areas – targeted to support most socially excluded in Midlands and North of England.
- **Sport Action Zones** – to improve access to sports facilities in deprived areas.
- **Sure Start** – the cornerstone of the government's drive to tackle child poverty and social exclusion. It works with parents-to-be, parents and children to improve their physical, intellectual and social development from 0–4 years, targeted to deprived areas.

LAA pilots sought to streamline bureaucracy to deliver these programmes in ways which are more locally responsive and accountable. Local agreements were negotiated with each central department through the Government Offices, where targets, funding and performance management arrangements were agreed. The effect of this basic approach revolutionised the relationship between local and central government – with a new role for Government Offices. The first wave of LAA negotiations was divided into three blocks: 'Children and Young

People', 'Safer Stronger Communities' and 'Healthy Communities and Older People'. In 2005, the second wave of LAAs included a fourth block on 'Local Enterprise and Economic Development'.

LAAs are a significant opportunity to tackle the wider determinants of health, implementing *Choosing Health* local actions and forging a new role for local authorities in public health. Experience from the first wave also points to the need to refine the process and allow more national programmes to be placed in the pool for local negotiations to continue to reduce bureaucracy and develop streamlined performance systems. Yet, despite these early teething problems, there is strong support from local authorities, and many if not all local authorities will have LAAs by 2007.

Local authorities have drawn on their connections and expertise of local community development to engage with stakeholders, including PCTs. While most effort has been focused on the Healthy Communities block, it is widely recognised that health opportunities exist in working with all four blocks. While only a handful of programme budgets have been devolved so far, local interest has focused on how better to organise PCTs, LAs and LSPs to be fitter for purpose to improve health.

Therefore, a number of performance-assessment opportunities currently exists and I have demonstrated four adopted so far: intelligence-led performance tracking, GO performance-management systems, local and regional Overview and Scrutiny Committees, and the LAA process. Like many regional public health initiatives, these are new areas of work and are likely to adapt and evolve still further. As in any new initiative, threats and opportunities exist. The last section of this chapter looks at these and explores future roles for regional action on public health.

Opportunities, risks and the future for regional public health

I have described two stories in this chapter. The first, to provide context, is the story of regionalism in England, not just organisational developments of Government Offices as the regional tier of government, but the economic, cultural and social roles of over 80 government agencies and many other non-government organisations which have a footprint on the English region. The second is a story of opportunistic development by public health practitioners working with these agencies to improve public health and tackle the wider determinants of health. Most of this work is to align and join up to support local action, and I have described one region's approach to deliver this through a Framework for Health. Other regions have also developed similar approaches. I have also referred to the new roles for local government, with their new responsibilities for 'wellbeing' and the evolution of the local area agreement, all requiring regional support and action to complement population health improvement.

So what will the future hold? Labour's third term is likely to see more in this direction of travel – tackling the wider determinants of health and health inequalities. There will be more emphasis on empowering local government still further, to shift power to local communities and 'places', promoting choice of public services and enabling deprived communities in particular. The regional tier of government will play a role supporting this. LAA pilots will be rolled out to many if not all local authorities over the next 2–3 years and are expected to deepen and broaden in what they can do. This represents a significant public health opportunity both locally and regionally.

There are risks, however. Agendas for health improvement do require effective partnership at any level – and this is equally relevant for the English regions. Partnership working requires clarity of purpose, visibility and leadership. We need to be clear about what regional organisations 'do' and what they support. Performance management will need exceptional leadership – particularly in setting strategy and assessing performance across different organisations. The task of performance managing actions across a complex set of determinants to improve health, and across several regional and local organisations, each with different cultures, requires a quite different approach to performance managing a waiting list target in one organisation. There will be a risk if the NHS remains a separated player both locally and regionally. However (at the time of writing), the NHS is planning to work more closely with regional organisations, through larger strategic health authorities working more closely with regional organisations, as will PCTs with local authorities. Finally, there will be risks, as in any middle tier of any organisation, about changing expectations from both above (the government) and below (local organisations), particularly as central government tends to want more or less power over time. Most important will be the need to add value to the agenda, so that Government Offices really do join up government and local area agreements really do reduce bureaucracy and lead to improvement of health and public services.

However, despite these risks, the development of the Department of Health presence in the regions, working *for* health and the NHS, has been an important step forward.

Acknowledgements

I would like to thank Diane Bell for comments on earlier drafts and my regional public health team for an exciting and innovative 3 years!

References

Acheson D (1998) *Independent Inquiry into Inequalities in Health (The Acheson Report).* London: Department of Health.

Department of Health (2002) *Shifting the Balance of Power*. London: Department of Health.

Department of Health (2004a) *A Regional Strategic Framework for Health*. Leeds: Department of Health.

Department of Health (2004b) *Our Region Our Health. A consultative report from the Regional Director of Public Health*. Leeds: Department of Health.

Holland W (1999) In: S Griffiths and D Hunter (eds) *Perspectives in Public Health*. Oxford: Radcliffe Medical Press.

Hunter DJ, Wilkinson J and Coyle E (2005) Would regional government have been good for your health? BMJ. **330**: 159–60.

Office of the Deputy Prime Minister (ODPM) (2003) *Your Region, Your Choice*. London: The Stationery Office.

Secretary of State for Health (2004) *Choosing Health: making healthy choices easier*. Cm 6374. London: The Stationery Office.

Townsend P and Davidson N (1982) *Inequalities in Health. The Black Report*. London: Penguin.

Chapter 11

Local government and the health improvement agenda

Tony Elson

One morning, early in 2004, I was sat having a conversation over a cup of coffee with a councillor who had for many years represented a ward in the West Yorkshire Council where I was working as Chief Executive. I had just been explaining that I was involved in co-chairing the Delivery Task Group as part of the national consultation in preparation for the white paper on public health, and that I was intent on ensuring that the role of local government in improving health was fully recognised.

The response from my political colleague took me by surprise. It was passionate and to the point. She told me that she had just finished reading the local Director of Public Health's annual report, and she was truly shocked by the level of health inequalities that it revealed in the area she represented. In what was closer to an evangelical witness than a calm statement of political objectives, she told me that if she achieved nothing else as a Councillor she would be satisfied if she could help to improve this situation. She was looking to me as Chief Executive to help her gain the support of the Council to make this a key priority for us.

I was completely taken aback by the strength and emotion expressed in her response. It was not breaking news that infant mortality in parts of her ward were among the worst in the country, and that preventable deaths from heart disease were far higher than the national average. I knew that because I had taken reports to Council committees and shared this information widely among members on many occasions in the past.

Health was also already high on my Council's agenda, with significant investment in health programmes and many policy commitments recorded in planning documents. They had been very happy to give me time to serve on the government's Cross-Cutting Spending Review on Health Inequalities in 2002, and had seconded me a year later for 1 day a week to work with the Health Inequalities Unit to advise on local government's role in delivering health improvement.

Nor was this a new topic of conversation between the two of us. On many occasions she and I had talked about the way that Council services can have an impact on health, and the need to address health as an important step to progress other local authority priority agendas. If I had to name ten councillors who were well briefed on the topic she would have been at the top of the list.

So why was I so surprised by her response? It was simple. In spite of all the information that I had given her over recent years and the arguments that I had put to her and her colleagues to persuade them to invest in a health programme, for her the shocking statistics on health inequalities in the area she represented had come as news.

Overnight the intellectual knowledge that we had imparted with such care was overtaken by an emotional understanding of what this meant to real people's lives. It was personalising the debate about health inequalities, and for this Councillor it had become very real and personal. She could relate the arguments to the experiences of people she knew. Suddenly for the first time this had become her responsibility as a community leader and advocate for her area in a much more direct way than before.

For me that conversation was one of those milestones that we experience in life, one of those events that give you a sense of the movement that we have to achieve as we seek to engage everyone in activity for health improvement. The debate has to move beyond the rational and the scientific to the human and the moral arguments that will really lead to the social movement that we need to embed health improvement at the centre of public policy and private endeavour.

It serves as an essential reminder of the true challenge we face in embedding the change that local government is expected to make in delivering health improvement. It is easy to do the analysis and repeat the usual truisms about the importance of the wider determinants of health, and to relate this to the new responsibilities that Councils have for co-delivery of the white paper.

It takes no effort to agree that we need to improve the evidence base and understand better how to intervene to have greater impact on health. We can use familiar words – partnership, community engagement, improved access. However, none of this will lead to the significant changes we aspire to achieve until we can break through the intellectual arguments and engage people at the emotional level.

It shouldn't come as any surprise that this takes us back to the foundations of the white paper. The principles on which it is based spell out the need to reach outside traditional institutional and professional territory, to find new ways of helping people make their own choices to improve their lifestyles and through those changes improve their health and wellbeing. The challenge of changing behaviour applies to individuals, communities and to organisations and professions, and while rational argument plays an important part in responding to that challenge we need to understand far more about the way that people change their opinions.

Choosing Health (Secretary of State for Health 2004) recognised that the influences on people's lives rest as much in their engagement with their neighbours, and with the wide range of social, community and commercial interests that make up society. The idea that any single part of the public sector can act on its own to persuade people to change is at best naïve – at worst it is arrogant.

As we enter the early delivery phases of the white paper we go through a very sensitive period of development. In the next few months we can rely on traditional institutional approaches that embed a number of discrete activities in our normal bureaucratic processes, or we can add to this new and creative approaches that challenge the traditional and deliver a far wider social movement for health. It will be easy to underestimate the conservative forces that will look for comfortable, familiar solutions, particularly when the drive to demonstrate early progress on national public service agreements dominates parts of the debate.

The strong messages about the shared responsibility on local government and PCT's to co-deliver the objectives in the white paper are a welcome recognition of the need for a shared approach to this agenda between these two organisations, but it must not lead to the role of other players being undervalued as we move forward.

Messages that stress the sharing of leadership responsibility must not create confusion or uncertainty about who leads on individual programmes. PCTs and local authorities have distinctive but complementary roles. The former have access to much of the specialist information and advice that is necessary for progress to be made locally. PCTs will form views on what interventions are most likely to lead to health improvement given local circumstances and the evidence base that exists at present, and will bring this to public attention and will provide advice to their partners.

Local authorities' leadership responsibilities are more focused on ensuring that the partnership infrastructure exists locally and that health improvement is fully recognised in sustainable community planning processes. Local authorities also have a responsibility to build on their experience of engaging with communities to ensure that the dialogue about health, lifestyles and health inequalities takes place on the street corner as well as in the Council Chamber and round the table at local strategic partnership meetings.

The nature of this wider role within communities, and their democratic base, gives them a perspective of where ordinary people are in their thinking. Given a change agenda that depends upon people choosing to adopt the lifestyle changes that public health colleagues advocate, we need to use this intelligence to help plan approaches that are going to be accepted by local people. The best evidence-based knowledge is of little value if people will not act on it.

In local government the health agenda is increasingly seen as part of the wider wellbeing agenda, and this is helping to move it from a separate silo to the centre of thinking about economic regeneration, skill development, educational performance and community cohesion. The power to promote the wellbeing of local people may have been introduced in the Local Government Act 2000, but it has only been in the last couple of years that its significance has begun to be recognised more widely within the local government sector.

The importance of community engagement in shaping and responding to public opinion also reflects a wider debate about the future of local government. The challenge from central government to the local government sector has been to demonstrate that all their activity is geared to delivery of change within local communities.

The Comprehensive Performance Assessment (CPA) regime placed an emphasis on 'impact' from the beginning, challenging councils to show how people's lives had been improved rather than relying on measurement of activity, or even on recorded outcomes. That challenge rather uncomfortably tested the extent to which local government even knew whether its services met the needs and aspirations of the people that they are designed to serve.

The approach will be strengthened in the next round of CPA and is increasingly influential in other areas of audit and inspection work within local government. It is precisely the style of assessment that is required as we strive to implement public health reforms. We cannot simply measure success by the number of health trainers employed by PCTs or the number of new initiatives that have been funded. What matters is the impact that these developments have on people's lives. Do people who have used these services or this support make life-improving decisions which they sustain for years to come?

Much of the earlier debate about the balance of responsibility between the NHS and local government for the public health agenda has tended to focus on the services that each provide and the probability of these being given priority within mainstream budget processes. Often health improvement through local government was almost a by-product of action to achieve other objectives such as improved educational performance, lower levels of fuel poverty or increased involvement in leisure activities. It was welcomed, but not seen as part of the core agenda.

That attitude has been changing. Where as recently as 2 years ago it was difficult to get councils to volunteer to take part in nationally sponsored health programmes, more recent experience demonstrates a far higher level of interest and commitment. This significantly is also increasingly led from the top – it is less likely to be the result of individual enthusiasts in middle-ranking positions in their organisations.

It isn't too hard to see why this is the emerging position. In 2003 individual councils could choose whether they signed up to the Shared Priority pledge on health improvement negotiated between the Local Government Association and central government. That has been overtaken by the requirement to demonstrate progress on health improvement as part of the performance-management framework for local government.

Inspectorates will measure council contributions to health improvement as part of the new round of CPA and the joint area reviews of children's services, and they will not just look at what initiatives have been taken; they will be seeking evidence that the community has noticed the difference.

This agenda is also centrally placed in the framework that underpins the new local area agreement (LAA) approach. LAAs are an important development, although they are still very much in their infancy. There are dangers that they may become too bureaucratic and stifle some of their original purpose of stimulating a more focused approach to local planning and delivery. This said, there is a clear commitment from central government to build on the initial pilot programme, with an intention to roll LAAs out to all upper-tier council areas by the spring of 2007.

The local government sector has displayed enthusiasm for the approach, as demonstrated by the high level of applications to be considered for the first two rounds of the LAA process. Early indications are that there will be significant gains from the direct focus on health improvement as one of the main themes, coupled with the less direct health dimensions found in the other areas for the agreement around children and young people, safer and stronger communities, and economic development and enterprise.

For the first time local authorities, on behalf of their local strategic partnerships, are signing commitments to deliver health improvements over the next 3 years. Even though some of the targets selected in the first pilots may be a little questionable, they will focus the attention and raise the priority given to health and wellbeing within local government.

The programme is also raising complex challenges about the working relationships between County and Shire District Councils, and between regional public health teams and the National Health Service. Both of these areas of tension have been with us for some time, but there is the prospect that the difficulties that do exist in some of the working relationships will be brought to a head by the LAA process, and will lead to action that will resolve long-standing difficulties.

So what conclusions do I take from the thoughts in this chapter? It is always dangerous to make predictions about the way that public services will develop, not least because we never seem to be operating in a steady state. Colleagues in the NHS are looking nervously at a further period of structural change, and display an increasing unease about the financial stability of present funding arrangements. Local government colleagues are speculating about structural change for two-tier local government, and will certainly be going through a period of significant change in children's and adult services. They also face the uncertainties of a new CPA round, and are experiencing significant financial pressures.

All of this can distract attention from a new health improvement agenda, but the drivers of change on the local government side of co-delivery are sufficiently robust to ensure that progress will take place. It remains to be seen how well the NHS can rise to the challenge. If the commitment is there from the top, what has been a marginal interest can very rapidly become everyone's interest given the management culture of the organisation. There are promising signs in some regions – the next 12 months will determine whether we are on track for rapid progress or a slower pace of change.

Reference

Secretary of State for Health (2004) *Choosing Health: making healthy choices easier*. Cm 6374. London: The Stationery Office.

Chapter 12

Getting fully engaged with local communities

Chris Drinkwater

Introduction

There is a growing recognition both nationally and internationally that the modern public health challenges of obesity, mental illness, sexual health and long-term conditions require new approaches. During the last two centuries public health and epidemiology made a significant contribution to understanding and controlling infectious diseases. This success has not been replicated in the control of behaviourally determined diseases. We know a great deal about the determinants of such diseases but as a number of commentators, including Derek Wanless, have pointed out there is a dearth of evidence about effective interventions (Wanless 2004). This lack of rigorous evidence is at the same time challenged by an increasingly powerful body of opinion that argues that the best way of improving the health of the population is by building social capital and social cohesion and not by specific health interventions. This argument has been put very cogently by Cottam and Leadbeater (2005), who suggest that:

> in the 20th century, big gains came from formalising the provision of professional knowledge through systems of training and provision of institutionalised, mass service provision. In the 21st century the big gains will come from professionals mobilising a far larger body of lay knowledge among users. Organisations that can mobilise the intelligence, investment and imagination of their users will reap huge gains in cost, productivity and innovation.

This challenge has been reinforced by the second Wanless report which argues that the inexorable rise of healthcare costs can only be effectively contained if the public are fully engaged in relation to behavioural change to improve health. This economic debate has occurred in parallel with increasing investment across the developed and developing world in involving local people in regeneration, renewal and development of their communities.

Much of this investment has been almost intuitive, driven by the evidence that the most disadvantaged communities have the poorest health, the highest levels of crime and the lowest levels of civic engagement, as measured for instance by voter turnout at elections. This has resulted in a political drive to rebuild civic engagement at a local level and reflects renewed debates about the balance between central control and universality of provision versus local autonomy and diversity.

This chapter tries to take stock of the current state of play in respect of community engagement and health with particular reference to the UK. It looks at the overall strategic framework and more importantly at the opportunities provided by the renewal of interest in public health. Using examples of good practice it also makes recommendations about the way forward.

Community engagement and health

Over the last 20 years there has been a gradual shift from 'doing to' communities to 'doing with' communities. This is probably best exemplified by a shift in both the nature and the spending pattern of urban regeneration programmes. Early programmes, such as City Challenge in England, spent most of their money on physical capital; the underlying assumption was that investment in new buildings would drive regeneration and that this would bring in new businesses and run-down areas would be revitalised. What generally happened however was that some new businesses were created but in the main any new jobs went to people from outside the local area who had the required skills. Similarly public sector housing was upgraded but, because the local area was still not seen as a place where you would want to live, populations continued to decline with those who could moving out, leaving increasing numbers of vacant properties and a residual population with high levels of need (Robinson 1997). The result was that only a few years later local authorities ended up demolishing vacant properties that had only recently been renovated. The clear message was that investment in people, social capital, is as important as investment in buildings.

Cognitive therapy is an illustrative analogy. This is a successful psychological therapy that has been developed to address the negative thought patterns and the low self-esteem characteristic of depression. In the same way there are depressed communities that have negative images. Perhaps not surprisingly, these communities also have a much higher than average prevalence of mental health problems. This links to the increasing strong evidence that psycho-social factors are key determinants of negative health behaviours that ultimately determine health outcomes (Marmot 2004; Wilkinson 1996). Investing in buildings without trying to change underlying behaviours is akin to our current obsession with treating the symptoms of depression with expensive antidepressants without dealing with the causes of depression and the context in which it is more likely to develop.

The evidence from spending patterns in current regeneration programmes such as New Deal for Communities and the Neighbourhood Renewal Fund is that the lessons have been learnt and that greater amounts are now invested in revenue projects to improve the life and circumstances of local people. The best example of this is the lengthy document on *Creating Healthier Communities: a resource pack for local partnerships* published by the Neighbourhood Renewal Unit (2005). This document clearly illustrates the change in direction with improvements in health and partnership with local communities seen as key elements of regeneration. This gradual change has run in parallel with a renewed public health interest in the importance of neighbourhoods and communities for the health of individuals.

Neighbourhoods and public health

In England, the Chief Medical Officer's *Project to Strengthen the Public Health Function* that started in 1997 identified sustained community development and public involvement as one of the five major themes essential for a successful public health function. The final report of the project published in 2001 (Chief Medical Officer 2001) produced five key recommendations about community development:

1 Rebuild sustainable community capacity to improve local health and wellbeing through the involvement of individuals and community groups.
2 Local agencies need to take a strategic approach to community development, including a review of capabilities and availability of skills in each locality, with an action plan as necessary.
3 Professionals need more understanding of appropriate models and techniques of community development.
4 Short-term, marginal projects are rarely a cost-effective investment and lead to disillusionment in communities as well as workers.
5 The involvement of those that are hard to reach because of social exclusion or poor health should be actively sought in local programmes to raise awareness of public health issues and action.

These recommendations have been further strengthened by *Choosing Health: making healthy choices easier* (Department of Health 2004), which devoted a whole chapter to 'Local communities leading for health'. This document explicitly states that *the environment we live in, our social networks, our sense of security, socio-economic circumstances, facilities and resources in our local neighbourhood can affect individual health.* It identifies unacceptable differences in people's experience of health between different areas and between different groups of people within the same area and highlights the need to empower and support communities to take action to improve local health. These unacceptable differences are explicitly linked to the concept of social capital and to the increasing evidence that shows a clear link between low status, low self-esteem, poor mental health and adverse health outcomes.

Neighbourhoods and health: the evidence

A comprehensive review of all of the evidence is contained in *Neighbourhoods and Health*, edited by Kawachi and Berkman (2003). The brief summary is that in studies that have controlled for a range of individual socio-economic and other characteristics, there remains a statistically significant association between neighbourhood environments and health. How this effect is mediated is more problematic and their review goes on to explore some of the complexities that include the different weight to be given to issues such as the influence of social selection versus social causation (do healthy people selectively leave poor neighbourhoods leaving unhealthy people behind and is this the cause of the disparity rather than any direct effect of the neighbourhood?), psychosocial versus material explanations (is it poverty *per se* or is it low self-esteem and lack of autonomy that impacts on health outcomes?) and is it geographically bounded neighbourhoods or other forms of community such as workplace, race or religious affiliation that determine outcomes? These issues are important for policy makers and practitioners involved in urban and rural regeneration who have to make decisions on the basis of partial evidence and they go to the heart of the debate about what sort of society we want to live in. Do we want to live in an increasingly segregated society where the rich increasingly live separately from the poor and where older people with good pensions live in secure gated communities, or do we want to equalise incomes, welcome diversity and move towards a society in which quality of life and sustainable development are as important as economic growth?

The evidence from the work of researchers such as Marmot (2004) and Wilkinson (1996) clearly demonstrates that perceived status and rank in hierarchies has an effect on individual health outcomes. This applies both to the workplace, as the longitudinal study of civil servants in Whitehall (Marmot and Shipley 1996) has demonstrated, and to the wider society. There is also evidence that the countries with the greatest income differential also have the greatest inequalities in health (Wilkinson 1996). Sadly, unlike antibiotics for infectious diseases, there is no simple intervention to address these issues. Community-based interventions are complex and require political leadership and long-term investment which often sits uneasily with the increasing need to demonstrate value for money and measurable short-term gains.

Building community engagement

There is a parallel between building engagement in communities and building engagement in frontline staff. Smithies identified clear connections between management theory and community development theory (Smithies 1991) and the NHS implicitly accepted this analogy in the policy document *Shifting the Balance of Power* (Department of Health 2001), which talked about the need for a cultural shift in the scale and quality of staff, patient and community involvement. A potential model for delivering this cultural change is illustrated in Figure 12.1.

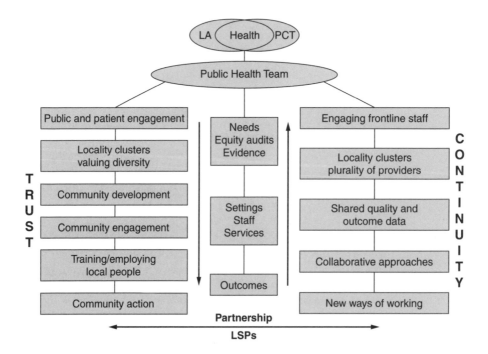

Figure 12.1 Staff, patient and community engagement.

There are a number of prerequisites for this model to work effectively.

1 There needs to be effective partnership between the local authority and the PCT and there needs to be a shared public health team with the commitment and leadership skills to drive this forward.
2 The public health team needs the skills and competencies not only to deliver the central, specialist core of this model – which is about needs, equity audits, evidence, and making best use of resources to deliver outcomes – but also the ability to build staff, patient and community engagement.
3 Building relationships, trust and continuity over time is essential for effective sustainable delivery. Disadvantaged areas have often been subjected to a succession of initiatives without any obvious change on the ground. In the same way frontline staff have often seen a succession of different managers and they themselves are also more likely to move than has been the case in the past.

What works

Coote and colleagues, in a review of complex community-based initiatives (Coote *et al.* 2004), highlighted the fact that where you have a highly specific and relatively straightforward health risk, such as falls in the elderly, it is possible to combine community development and capacity building with a rigorous approach to evidence. Where, however, you are addressing a more complex problem, such as lack of social cohesion, this is much more difficult partly because of lack of evidence but also because people's views of what should be done are likely to be more divergent. It therefore seems appropriate to end this chapter by looking at two practical examples that illustrate the two extremes of this spectrum.

Healthy Communities Collaborative Falls Prevention Initiative

The Falls Collaborative (National Primary Care Development Team 2005) was established in 2002 with the aim of reducing falls by engaging older people in developing new and innovative approaches to prevention. They developed a systematic approach to engaging older people and to getting them involved in partnership with health professionals in three different geographical areas of England. As part of this process they used the Plan–Do–Study–Act (PDSA) model for improvement in local learning workshops in order to tap into new ideas and to develop strategies for improvement. This generated a range of initiatives that included physical activity, footwear and footcare, better lighting, accident prevention and medication reviews. This is a much broader range of initiatives than would have been generated by a medical approach and there was also good evidence of significant community involvement. The outcome of all of this work was a 32% reduction of falls across the three geographical areas.

A healthy living network in Newcastle

HealthWORKS Newcastle, a healthy living network run by the West End Health Resource Centre (Drinkwater 2001) and funded by the New Opportunities Fund, rather than taking a focused approach to one condition has developed an approach that involves three key elements:

1 an experienced team of community development workers
2 training and employment of local people in disadvantaged communities as health link workers
3 an Activities Development Fund which is locally controlled and which allocates funds against agreed criteria.

Because the project aims to engage as many local people as possible, it has supported the development of community-led initiatives covering a range of areas that include:

* accident prevention
* working with black and ethnic minority communities
* diet and nutrition
* education
* homelessness and housing
* physical activity
* substance misuse
* sexual health
* supporting vulnerable communities.

The outcome of this approach has been high levels of community engagement with as many as one in ten of the local community involved and with a clear focus on those most likely to be excluded. The downside has been that it is more difficult to demonstrate clear outcomes and, although local people see it as a joined-up approach, it can sometimes be seen as a confusing medley of unconnected projects that are unsustainable. It does however go to the heart of the dilemma about community engagement. Is it about setting up systems in which local people control the agenda, however diverse it might be, or is it about looking at ways in which local people can be successfully engaged to meet nationally set targets?

References

Chief Medical Officer (2001) *Report of the Chief Medical Officer's Project to Strengthen the Public Health Function*. London: Department of Health.

Coote A, Allen J and Woodhead D (2004) *Finding Out What Works: building knowledge about complex community-based initiatives*. London: King's Fund.

Cottam H and Leadbeater C (2005) *Red Paper 01. Health: co-creating services*. London: Design Council. www.designcouncil.org.uk

Department of Health (2001) *Shifting the Balance of Power Within the NHS: securing delivery*. London: Department of Health.

Department of Health (2004) *Choosing Health: making healthy choices easier*. London: Department of Health.

Drinkwater C (2001) A primary care perspective: reflections from the West End Health Resource Centre. *Local Governance*. **27**(4).

Kawachi I and Berkman L (2003) *Neighbourhoods and Health*. Oxford: Oxford University Press.

Marmot M (2004) *Status Syndrome: how your social standing directly affects your health and life expectancy*. London: Bloomsbury.

Marmot M and Shipley M (1996) Do socioeconomic differences in mortality persist after retirement? 25 year follow-up of civil servants from the first Whitehall study. *British Medical Journal.* **313**: 1177–80.

National Primary Care Development Team (2005) Healthy Communities Collaborative to reduce falls in older people. www.npdt.org

Neighbourhood Renewal Unit (2005) *Creating Healthier Communities: a resource pack for local partnerships.* London: Office of Deputy Prime Minister.

Robinson F (1997) *The City Challenge Experience: a review of the development and implementation of Newcastle City Challenge.* Durham: University of Durham.

Smithies J (1991) *Management Development Theory and Community Development Theory – making the connections in roots and branches: papers from the OU/HEA 1990 Winter School of Community Development and Health.* Milton Keynes: The Open University.

Wanless D (2004) *Securing Good Health for the Whole Population.* London: HM Treasury.

Wilkinson RG (1996) *Unhealthy Societies: the afflictions of inequality.* London: Routledge.

Chapter 13

Health and sustainable development

Anna Coote

In this chapter I explore the connections between health and sustainable development and the implications for public policy, focusing on public health and on the corporate activities of the National Health Service.

The Sustainable Development Commission

First, a word about the Sustainable Development Commission. It is a non-departmental public body, set up in 2000 under the chairmanship of Jonathon Porritt, reporting directly to the Prime Minister. It consists of 19 Commissioners drawn from different areas of expertise, and a small secretariat. Its UK-wide remit is to promote sustainable development, to monitor progress and to advise government. For the Commission's purposes, sustainable development is seen as having three main dimensions, which are interrelated: social, economic and environmental. A fourth, linking theme is democratic engagement, on the premise that sustainable development can only be achieved if individuals and communities can freely and actively participate in decision making at all levels.

From the start, an important strand of the Commission's work has been concerned with health-related matters – demonstrating the benefits to health of sustainable practices and ways in which the pursuit of health and sustainable development can be mutually reinforcing. Other key issues with which the Commission is concerned – such as climate change, energy, sustainable consumption and production, transport, housing and education – all have important implications for population health. The Commission has established a 'Healthy Futures' programme, with support from the Department of Health, which is dedicated to making these connections – working with NHS trusts, health departments and other stakeholders to identify and spread good practice (Sustainable Development Commission 2005b).

Public health

It is now widely acknowledged that social isolation, poor education, fear of crime, disrupted family life and unhappiness are bad for health: new research suggests that people who have a positive attitude live on average 7 years longer than unhappy people (Lyubomirsky *et al.* 2005). Likewise, poverty, joblessness, powerlessness and economic insecurity are bad for human health. These are the social and economic dimensions of sustainable development. And environmental damage is bad for health – air pollution, contaminated water, poor food supplies, heavy road traffic, dislocated neighbourhoods, poorly designed buildings. Climate change brings extremes of heat and cold, flooding, storms, drought and threatens the very essentials of human life (DH 1998; King's Fund 2002).

What's more, these health risks tend to pile up in the lives of poor and dispossessed people in ways that are vividly reflected in health statistics. Poor people get ill more often and die much younger than people who are well off.

The UK government produced its public health white paper *Choosing Health* in 2004 (DH 2004). This followed two reports to the Treasury by Derek Wanless. The first showed that failure to prevent illness would cost the taxpayer some £30 billion extra a year by 2020 (HM Treasury 2002). The second pointed to ways of achieving what Wanless called a 'fully engaged scenario', in which individuals were willing and able, and appropriately supported by government, to make choices that prevented illness and preserved good health (HM Treasury 2004b).

Choosing Health acknowledges that '*the environment we live in, our social networks, our sense of security, socio-economic circumstances, facilities and resources in our local neighbourhood can affect individual health*'. It also calls for a '*strong role for Government in promoting social justice and tackling the wider causes of ill-health and inequality in health*'.

The new sustainable development strategy for the UK, *Securing the Future* (HM Government 2005), published a year later, includes indicators that measure progress towards sustainable development in health terms – the same as those used by the Department of Health to measure progress in public health: inequalities in infant mortality, adult life expectancy, healthy life expectancy, premature death rates from cancer and heart disease, and trends in smoking, diet and childhood obesity.

So there is strong evidence, backed up by major new public policy initiatives, that the pursuit of sustainable development can profoundly influence population health, and the pursuit of preventive public health measures can help attain the goals of sustainable development. This should, in theory at least, be a winning combination – helping to channel the energies and enthusiasms, resources and actions that are required to bring about change.

The corporate activities of the NHS

Now let's look at the NHS. Consider all the things it does routinely to enable it to provide health services – employment, procurement, management of energy, waste and transport, landholding and commissioning new buildings and refurbishments. This is the largest single organisation in the UK and one of the largest and most powerful in the world. Its annual budget is more than £60 billion a year. It employs more than a million people. It spends more than £11 billion a year on goods and services (King's Fund 2002).

Seen from this angle, the NHS has huge potential to do good – or harm – to the health of the nation and to the cause of sustainable development.

Take employment, for example. The NHS suffers continuously from staffing shortages. It cannot find enough doctors and nurses, so recruits instead from the developing world, leaving many poor countries perilously short of trained clinicians. Yet many NHS trusts in the UK are located in neighbourhoods where there is high unemployment, and where conditions are such that people get ill because they are jobless, insecure, poor and unable to take control over their own lives. If the NHS invests some of its billions in basic training for local people, to prepare them to take the first steps into employment, they will get a chance to come into hospitals and health centres as workers rather than as patients. Getting jobs makes them less vulnerable to illness; the fact that they live locally provides the NHS with a reliable, committed workforce. It doesn't work straight away; it doesn't work for everyone. But in the longer term it can create a virtuous circle – helping to improve health in the community, reducing preventable disease, lessening the burden on the NHS and freeing it up to provide better services for those with unavoidable ill health.

This potential is already being harnessed in some parts of the country. In the North East, for example, a group dedicated to 'Widening Participation in Health and Social Care' is working with the NHS to improve recruitment and retention of local staff in the region. The group focuses on lifelong learning and coordinates training networks, funding sources and job opportunities in areas of deprivation or high unemployment. Their schemes have been successful in putting unemployed people in touch with NHS jobs and providing training and support in preparation for employment (Sustainable Development Commission 2005c).

One of the scandals of the NHS is that some patients leave hospital suffering from malnutrition. The food is poor, they don't like it, or can't eat it and, even if they do eat, it doesn't do their health any good. This slows down patient recovery rates and makes them vulnerable to further ill health. This is the same point that Jamie Oliver (Channel 4 2005) has made about school food – children do better at school if they eat well; patients do better in hospital if they eat well. If the NHS uses its resources more carefully – arranging its purchasing and catering policies so that it provides nutritious food in ways that encourage people to eat and enjoy – it could do marvels not only for patients' health, but for the health of staff and visitors too. It could also use its power, as one of the largest food purchasers in the country, to encourage local and sustainable food production, to strengthen local economies, to reduce the environmental damage caused by shipping foods across vast distances, and to promote organic and other environmentally sound agricultural practices. Here again is a virtuous circle, where buying and serving food in ways that promote health and sustainable development can help to safeguard the effectiveness and long-term viability of the NHS.

In Cornwall, five NHS trusts are doing just this, working together to purchase high-quality food from local suppliers and to develop more jobs locally. The Cornwall Food Programme, hosted by the Cornwall Partnership Trust, has been developed within the Royal Cornwall Hospital Trust. It aims to secure contracts with local businesses for sandwiches, fruit and vegetables, dairy products, eggs and fish. At present, 30% of total food expenditure is from local sources and this figure is expected to grow. Experience is showing not only that the local community, economy and environment benefit, but also that patients, visitors and staff prefer the local produce, so that more food is eaten and less wasted (Sustainable Development Commission 2005a).

The NHS is currently engaged in the largest capital development programme of its lifetime. Hospitals and primary care premises are being built or refurbished on a vast scale, right across the country, involving huge sums of public and private money. A good building can provide a healthy environment to work in, reducing absenteeism and improving staff performance. It can provide a good environment to receive treatment and care in – increasing patient recovery rates. Building design can affect the ease with which infections such as MRSA (methicillin-resistant *Staphylococcus aureus*) can be isolated, or spread. A building can be constructed using sustainable materials and local labour. It can make maximum use of natural heating and ventilation, reducing energy consumption and carbon emissions. It can be located and designed to facilitate water conservation, minimise waste and encourage walking, cycling and public transport rather than private car use. It can be situated on a brownfield site, helping to preserve green spaces.

The challenge is to make optimal use of the contracts that are currently being let under PFI (private finance initiative) and LIFT (local improvement finance trust) schemes, to insist that new buildings and refurbishments are undertaken according to the principles of sustainable development. If the government is serious about wanting to promote a healthier nation and a sustainable future, it should make this obligatory.

Some NHS organisations are managing to incorporate a range of sustainable practices into their building projects. The Norfolk and Norwich University Hospital, for example, is a PFI project designed to be energy efficient with a combined heat and power plant that reduces carbon emissions and produces lower cost energy for the hospital. The Burnley Central LIFT redevelopment aims to reduce the amount of travel it generates by combining clinical facilities with a leisure centre, café and crèche on a site that is accessible by public transport, walking and cycling. And the Whipps Cross University Hospital NHS Trust PFI redevelopment aims to reduce the amount of waste going to landfill sites by up to 30% by identifying markets for materials from the old hospital buildings, and by using at least 10% recycled materials in construction (Sustainable Development Commission 2005b).

The Department of Health has recognised the importance of what it calls 'Good Corporate Citizenship', which signals the deployment of NHS resources in matters such as employment, procurement and buildings, to promote health and sustainable development – creating virtuous circles that minimise risks to health and help to ensure the long-term viability of the NHS. This approach has been endorsed by the *Choosing Health* white paper, which commits the Department of Health to working with the Sustainable Development Commission to develop the capacity of NHS organisations to use their resources more wisely. It also commits the government to sponsoring a debate on corporate citizenship right across the public sector, leading to *'firm recommendations for action for all public and private sector employers to demonstrate how they can organise their activities in ways that improve the health of employees and the wider community'*. And the UK Sustainable Development Strategy commits the government to 'lead by examples', with every department having to produce an action plan, setting out practical steps to promote social, economic and environmental sustainability.

The Sustainable Development Commission is currently working with the Department of Health to develop a self-assessment model aimed at helping NHS organisations to judge how far they are contributing to good corporate citizenship and to develop their capacity to act as good corporate citizens. This means looking closely at how they contribute to strong local economies, community cohesion and a healthy environment, through their daily corporate activities. It is a voluntary model, aimed at chief executives, board members and operations managers, for use within performance-management processes, and it focuses on employment, procurement, community engagement, facilities management, buildings and transport. It encapsulates and builds on existing work, providing ideas about good practice with examples from exemplary trusts, and points the way to relevant guidance and resources, and was launched in March 2006 (www.corporatecitizen.nhs.uk).

Like the public health agenda, the drive to promote 'good corporate citizenship' points to a potentially powerful, mutually reinforcing connection between health and sustainable development. But on both fronts – public health and NHS corporate activity – there are some seriously inhibiting factors.

The first and perhaps most obvious is that health policy is developed by the Department of Health while most factors that seriously affect health come under the auspices of other departments – work and pensions (DWP), education (DfES), trade and industry (DTI) and environment, food and rural affairs (DEFRA). The challenge is not simply to get other departments to sign up to their role in preventing illness (although that can be hard enough), but to drive through implementation, when every department and every ministerial team has its own priorities on which it wants to be judged.

The second inhibiting factor is that most health professionals don't have a driving interest in preventing illness. They derive their income, status and job satisfaction from making people better after they have become ill. The professional groups that are most powerful in the field of health policy tend to be more interested in policies that improve the health services they provide than in policies that aim to prevent people needing their services in the first place. The point is not that doctors conspire to make people ill – of course they don't – but that it is treatment and cure rather than prevention that gives them a sense of urgency and full-on commitment.

A third problem arises from the 'choice' agenda. This is the 'big idea' in the *Choosing Health* white paper, which is mainly devoted not to tackling the social, economic and environmental causes of illness, but to encouraging individuals to 'choose' healthy lifestyles through behaviours related to smoking, diet, exercise, alcohol and sex. Yet health policies that focus on choice – whether it is choosing health services or healthy behaviour – usually favour the better off. They don't have the same effect on people who are poor, disadvantaged, socially excluded – the very people whose health is most at risk. Choice may be highly desirable in theory. But individual choice as a policy driver, unless firmly rooted in policies to promote shared responsibility and equal capacity to choose, is likely to widen health inequalities and so undermine the goals of public health and sustainable development (House of Commons Public Administration Select Committee 2005).

Another inhibiting factor is the government's drive for 'efficiency', led by the Gershon review (HM Treasury 2004a), which implicitly encourages purchasing decisions that go for economies of scale rather than longer-term value. There is still important work to be done to redefine 'efficiency' in sustainable terms and to embed that in the work of regulatory bodies such as the Audit Commission and the Healthcare Commission. The need to develop whole-life costing and accounting is acknowledged in the UK sustainable development strategy, but the message has yet to get through to those who spend public money out in the field.

A final problem relates to priorities and incentives. The prevention of illness and the pursuit of good corporate citizenship are endorsed in policy, but they are not the sort of thing that ambitious health professionals and managers build their careers upon.

As the saying goes, 'vision without action is hallucination'. What counts in the end is whether there is sufficient energy, enthusiasm, political will, leadership and power to drive through the actions that must be taken and to keep the action going over very considerable periods of time. The point is to make, manage and sustain change, not simply to draft policies or legislation (Hunter and Marks 2005).

To sum up, it is possible to achieve better health outcomes by pursuing sustainable development, and to achieve more sustainable outcomes by preventing illness, reducing health inequalities and using NHS corporate resources strategically. Put together, health and sustainable development should be a winning combination.

To make this happen, it will be important to get a lot better at cross-departmental policy making and practice, to address traditional interests and power relations within the health sector, to take a far more thoughtful and critical approach to the 'choice agenda', to redefine efficiency and to change incentive structures in the health sector, providing strong, unequivocal and sustained leadership, not just within the Department of Health and the NHS, but right across government.

The price of failure is vast – in terms of wasted resources and wasted lives. The prize of success is worth a lot more effort than it is getting at the moment.

References

Channel 4 (2005) *Jamie's School Dinners*: www.channel4.com/life/microsites/J/jamies_school_dinners

Department of Health (DH) (1998) *Independent Inquiry into Inequalities in Health: The Acheson Report*. London: The Stationery Office.

Department of Health (DH) (2004) *Choosing Health: making healthy choices easier*. London: The Stationery Office.

HM Government (2005) *Securing the Future: delivering UK sustainable development strategy*. London: The Stationery Office.

HM Treasury (2002) *Securing our Future Health: taking a long-term view*. London: HM Treasury.

HM Treasury (2004a) *Releasing Resources to the Front Line: independent review of public sector efficiency*. London: The Stationery Office.

HM Treasury (2004b) *Securing Good Health for the Whole Population*. London: HM Treasury.

House of Commons Public Administration Select Committee (2005) *Choice, Voice and Public Services; fourth report of session 2004–05, Volume 1*. London: The Stationery Office.

Hunter DJ and Marks LM (2005) *Managing for Health: what incentives exist for NHS managers to focus on wider health issues?* London: King's Fund.

King's Fund (2002) *Claiming the Health Dividend: unlocking the benefits of NHS spending*. London: King's Fund. www.kingsfund.org.uk/resources/publications/claiming_the_1.html

Lyubomirsky S, King L and Diener E (2005) The benefits of positive affects: does happiness lead to success? *Psychological Bulletin*. **131**(6): 803–55.

Sustainable Development Commission (2005a) *Cornwall's NHS Food Project*. www.sd-commission.org.uk/publications/downloads/Cornwall-NHS-Food-Project.pdf

Sustainable Development Commission (2005b) *Healthy Futures: buildings and sustainable development*. www.sd-commission.org.uk/publications/downloads/HF3-final.pdf Launched June 2005.

Sustainable Development Commission (2005c) Widening Participation in Health and Social Care Group. www.sd-commission.org.uk/publications.php?id=187

Part 3

Priorities for health

Introduction

The public health agenda is potentially huge, covering extensive tracts of public policy and human activity. It is easy to become overwhelmed by the complex nature of the task and range of issues to be tackled. Establishing priorities is therefore essential. Not surprisingly, these include tobacco, obesity, child health, sexual health, mental health, alcohol, transport, health in the workplace and the role of genetics. The chapters in this section deal with all of these.

Andrew Hayes reviews current policy initiatives in the area of tobacco control in the context of the issue posed in the last section, namely the balance to be achieved between personal choice and public concern. The issue was a particularly vexed one in England where the government appeared reluctant to invade personal liberty and be accused of acting as the nanny state. While elsewhere in the UK the devolved administrations were impressed by and sought to emulate the progress made in Ireland and the largely favourable public response to a total ban on smoking in public places, within England central government prevaricated. Local authorities and regional bodies made the running by seeking to control smoking within their communities, representing the growing role of sub-national govern-ments in promoting health that was described in the last section. Eventually, in the face of mounting political pressure, a free vote was allowed and an English ban on smoking in public places will be introduced in 2007.

Obesity, like smoking, is another health issue which excites passions. Often more heat is generated than light in arguments about obesity and how it can best be tackled. It is, as Tim Lang points out, a 'complex policy terrain'. The answer he believes lies in injecting more realism and responsibility into supply-chain pol-icy, something which public health practitioners may support but may feel ill equipped to progress. Lang believes the evidence base for such an approach already exists so, once again, it is not lack of evidence which is a barrier to action. The challenge also links to the issue of sustainability covered in Chapter 13 since at issue should be not the volume of production but its quality, impact on diet, and sustainability in the long run.

Healthy childhood is seen as vital if issues like smoking, obesity and sexual health are to be tackled successfully. Paul Lincoln reviews the issues, noting that only recently has a comprehensive national policy emerged on child health. He claims that this deficit was partly the result of an assumption that children have been perceived as healthy and disease free. But through the development of life-course epidemiology, public health practitioners now recognise the importance of childhood and early intervention in preventing chronic diseases and establishing healthy behaviour and wellbeing. Health inequalities in children are well docu-mented and affect not just the health state of children but also their educational attainment, susceptibility to child abuse and so on. Reducing low income among poor families in combination with interventions in early life, like Sure Start, are the key instruments to tackle poverty, as is the development of health-promoting schools. These help equip children with the knowledge and skills essential for life although these have tended to be marginalised by the school curriculum and pre-occupation with exam subjects, not to mention the growing commercialisation of childhood more generally.

Sexually transmitted infections (STIs) are on the increase in the UK at an alarming rate. There are links between STIs and the effects of alcohol and patterns of drinking, especially the phenomenon of binge drinking. As Anne Weyman and Caroline Davey note, sexual health is a central element of the public health agenda. Yet this centrality does not appear to be fully appreciated by government if judged by the poor state of sexual health services. It is a state of affairs Weyman and Davey believe can be linked directly to a widespread reticence in the UK to address sexual health openly and honestly. Although progress is being made, there remains a long way to go.

Mental health is another forgotten area of public health and subject to taboos about what can, and cannot, be discussed openly and honestly. As Lionel Joyce states, millions of lives are destroyed by mental health problems and the stigma these attract. The social consequences are significant. It is an issue which, once again, the different countries making up the UK are tackling in different ways. Promoting good mental health is as important as promoting physical health and is a priority of the English white paper, *Choosing Health*, although for many it is still regarded as a Cinderella service. It is a situation only likely to be redressed by tackling the stigma and discrimination associated with mental health. Mental health policy in England is guided by the National Service Framework for Mental Health and supported by the National Institute for Mental Health in England. In Scotland, there is a National Programme for Improving Mental Health and Wellbeing informed by four aims: raising awareness and promoting mental health and wellbeing, eliminating stigma and discrimination, preventing suicide, and promoting and supporting recovery. People with poor mental health tend to experience poorer physical health than the rest of the population. Yet, the evidence shows that a healthier lifestyle improves mental health and wellbeing. Regular physical activity reduces the risk of depression and has positive benefits for mental health. It is also likely to help prevent suicide and reduce the chance of developing dementia. The public health contribution to mental health is therefore considerable but possibly insufficiently appreciated.

Alcohol has attracted considerable public and media attention as governments wrestle with a desire to allow responsible drinking at any time without undue restriction on the one hand while confronting evidence from the police and others on the likely effects of such a policy on the drinking patterns of young people and a drinking culture (and drinks industry) that promotes excessive drinking and associated antisocial behaviour on the other hand. Against such a context, Geof Rayner claims that public policy towards alcohol has been fragmented, public health considerations marginalised, and interventions introduced with limited effect. The powerful drinks industry appears to hold sway over policy and to point the finger of blame at irresponsible individuals and their antisocial drinking habits. Rayner believes this is to duck the issue and that government has a responsibility to tackle the 'problem' with alcohol in a more open and honest way. As in other areas, it seems that England lags behind policy developments elsewhere in the UK.

Transport has always been a difficult issue for governments to tackle, especially in an integrated way. The dominance of the car culture shows no sign of waning even when the evidence on climate change shows the significant contribution car use makes to the situation. Harry Rutter reviews the policy initiatives needed, although to achieve success would seem to be something of an uphill struggle. Efforts to encourage healthier modes of transport have not had significant success and government seems to have all but given up on any hope of significantly reducing car usage and getting people to adopt other forms of transport which might also contribute to healthier lifestyles through, for example, walking and cycling. Again, it is an area where public health practitioners perhaps need to become more forceful advocates for change.

Work and health has for long been recognised as vital if only because a healthier workforce is likely to be a more productive and happier one. It was an area acknowledged by Derek Wanless as important although somewhat neglected. The NHS as a major employer could be leading by example since, as Kit Harling shows, the workplace is an ideal setting for promoting health. The relationship between work and health is one where more evidence is needed.

Still on the theme of work and health, Lord Hunt sets out the government's thinking and policies. These are aimed at getting people back into work and then staying in work. He sees this strategy as important in reducing health inequalities. The government is also intent on more effective joined-up working between the Department of Work and Pensions and the Department of Health in order to improve the health of working-age people.

Public health and genetics attracted considerable interest some years ago in the context of the human genome project. As Mark Kroese, Ron Zimmern and Simon Sanderson observe, the impact of genetics on human health will not happen suddenly but incrementally over time. The impact on population health could be considerable and a new field of public health has been created to explore the implications called public health genetics or genomics. Genetic factors play an important role in influencing the risk of disease but they interact with other factors in complex ways. It is these interactions which determine whether disease will develop. For public health genetics to achieve the impact it could requires the support and engagement of the public. Both the public and public health practitioners will require education and training in order to appreciate the implications of genetic science.

Chapter 14

Tobacco: current issues

Andrew Hayes

Introduction

In October 1604, James I of England showed remarkable public health prescience in his *Counterblaste to Tobacco*, describing '*A custom loathsome to the eye, harmful to the brain, dangerous to the lungs*' (James I 1604). It was not until the mid-20th century that the real import of his intuition became clear. Tobacco is not only 'loathsome to the eye': it kills its consumers at an astonishing rate. Every other regular smoker dies as a direct consequence of his or her nicotine addiction, losing on average 10 years of life (Doll *et al.* 2004).

Tobacco is an accident of history. It is a product that would never be allowed onto the market today, given present knowledge of its impact on personal and public health. Even the tobacco industry, which had long denied any link between tobacco and ill health, now acknowledges the risks involved:

> *Cigarette smoking causes lung cancer, heart disease, emphysema and other serious diseases in smokers. Smokers are far more likely than non-smokers to develop diseases such as lung cancer. There is no such thing as a 'safe' cigarette.* (www.philipmorrisinternational.com/PMINTL/pages/eng/smoking/ S_and_H.asp)

The scale of the problem

But a 50:50 prospect of dying from tobacco-related disease is not a 'risk'. It is a dead certainty for half of all smokers. The consequence, for the community as a whole, is devastating: 114,000 deaths each year in the UK alone (Peterson and Peto 2004), around 650,000 in the European Community (Peto *et al.* 2004), and nearly five million worldwide (Peterson and Peto 2004).

According to the findings of the 2003 General Household Survey (www.statistics.gov.uk/ghs), 26% of adults aged 16 or over in Great Britain smoke cigarettes. This average figure masks considerable variation between age groups and, to a lesser extent, between men and women (*see* Table 14.1).

Table 14.1 Estimated current smoking prevalence

| | *Estimated current smoking prevalence %* | | |
Age	*Males*	*Females*	*All*
16–24	36	36	36
25–34	38	35	36
35–44	34	30	32
45–54	30	28	29

Table 14.1 (Continued)

| Age | Estimated current smoking prevalence % | | |
	Males	Females	All
55–64	24	23	23
65–74	18	18	18
75+	10	10	10

Source: Twigg, Moon and Walker 2004.

Sadly, tobacco kills not only those who smoke but also bystanders who breath in their smoke – variously described as side- or slip-stream smoke, second-hand or environmental tobacco smoke (SHS or ETS), or as passive smoking. SHS comprises smoke that comes from the tip of a lit cigarette and also smoke exhaled by the smoker. Of the 4,000 or so chemicals contained in tobacco smoke, 60 are known or suspected carcinogens (www.ash.org.uk/html/factsheets/html/basic01.html).

The health effects of SHS have been reviewed twice by the Scientific Committee on Tobacco and Health (SCOTH), in 1998 and 2004 – confirming that exposure to SHS risks lung cancer and ischaemic heart disease and has a strong link to adverse effects in children (Scientific Committee on Tobacco and Health 1998, 2004). A more recent estimate of deaths attributable to SHS in the UK calculated a likely annual total of more than 11,000. Most of these relate to exposure at home, but passive smoking at work could account for 600 deaths a year including more than 50 employed in the hospitality industry (Jamrozik 2005).

Dying for a fag: personal choice or public concern?

Tobacco presents the public health case study par excellence: how to tackle a totally preventable epidemic, unnecessary morbidity and avoidable premature mortality. But it is a case study with a difference. The vector in this case is not human-to-human infection. It is not the mosquito. It is not malnutrition. It is not impure water or inadequate sewage disposal. Rather, it is the tobacco industry, and the many vested interests that the industry's activities have spawned over the years. These have exerted, and continue to exert, significant influence over the development and implementation of public policy.

There is one concern that tobacco does share with some other threats to public health: namely, the 'lifestyle' issue. The debate around personal choice and responsibility, as against governmental interest in the public good, is relevant to tobacco, alcohol, obesity and sexual health (and probably much more besides). 'Give them the facts, explain the risks and let them choose' is the mantra of the free market. But how does this *laissez-faire* approach square with any government's responsibility to protect the health of its citizens?

Current policy initiatives

The health consequences of tobacco have been researched and documented since the middle of the last century. Despite this, successive governments, and the health community generally, took very little coordinated action against smoking. The climate began to change in the early 1990s, partly as a consequence of the *Europe Against Cancer* programme – which initiated EU-wide legislation on maximum tar levels, health warnings and tobacco advertising. These proposals proved controversial. The consequent policy debate stimulated public interest and awareness, encouraging health professionals and the voluntary sector to become more focused on seeking political support for effective action. The publication of the white paper *Smoking Kills* (Department of Health 1998) in 1998 suggested that tobacco had finally become recognised, politically as well as professionally, as a substantial health threat in the UK: one that warranted serious policy and programme initiatives at national level and throughout the NHS. Monies were earmarked to establish tobacco control alliances at local level and to fund NHS provision of local Stop Smoking Services.

No single tobacco control measure will work in isolation (Jamrozik 2005). Various parallel steps have to be put in place – and sustained over time – to have any prospect of lasting impact. The benefits of this approach can be quite substantial. New York City Health Department, for instance, claims an 11% drop in smoking prevalence between 2002–2003 as a result of intensive and broadly based tobacco control programmes (Frieden 2005).

In England, current DH initiatives are structured around a six-strand strategy, ranging from product regulation (e.g. health warnings, advertising restrictions, no sale to minors, etc.), price controls (through tax policy) and media campaigns, to support for would-be quitters – service provision and availability of nicotine replacement therapy (NRT), etc. On the basis of published research, both national and international, the DH has calculated the benefit of each measure in terms of potential reduced prevalence – i.e. the percentage figure next to each of the bullet points.

- Greater awareness: information and education campaigns – 2%.
- Regional and local action, including effective Stop Smoking Services – 1%.
- No tobacco promotion (e.g. banning advertising) – 2.5%.
- Rigorous regulation of tobacco products (e.g. labelling requirements) – 0.5%.
- Reducing supply (especially illicit sales) and availability: 1% price increase = 0.3% prevalence reduction.
- Reducing exposure to second-hand smoke – up to 4%.

The white paper *Choosing Health* (Secretary of State for Health 2004) and the subsequent Delivery Plan (Department of Health 2005) restate the multi-pronged approach and outline a variety of commitments to promote smoking cessation, to reduce exposure to second-hand smoke, and to reduce smoking prevalence. Suggested action includes:

- offering stop smoking (SS) advice as part of surgical care
- establishing an 'effectiveness and efficiency' SS task force
- identifying and disseminating good SS practice
- providing free products (NRT rebate scheme) to PCTs to help target 'hard to reach' groups
- extending the national awareness campaign
- shifting the balance in favour of smoke-free environments
- introducing smoke-free work and public places
- supporting nurses' smoke-free role
- introducing graphic warnings on tobacco products
- enforcing 'point of sale' regulations and ban on underage sales
- ending brand-sharing and internet advertising
- tackling illicit sales.

Much of this echoes the title of a 1999 report published by the Health Education Authority, *Been There, Done That: revisiting tobacco control policies in the NHS* (Health Education Authority 1999). But the white paper goes far beyond the NHS alone. It implicates the community as a whole and, in its smoke-free commitments, proposes policy innovation that can only be effected through legislation.

The white paper proposals on 'going smoke-free' have provoked controversy on all sides. The tobacco industry and some parts of the hospitality trade are dismayed at the prospect of restrictions that cover all workplaces, with limited exceptions for pubs that don't serve food (so-called 'wet pubs') and for membership clubs. The health community, on the other hand, cannot discern any logic or consistency in banning exposure to second-hand smoke on health and safety grounds – but then allowing it in certain circumstances. If SHS is a health risk in one setting, it is a health risk in any setting and should be treated accordingly. This is especially so, given the type of variable policy on offer – one that will effectively add to the disadvantage of existing disadvantaged groups. Most 'wet pubs' are located in communities already adversely affected by health inequalities (British Medical Association 2005).[1]

It is not only the health community that regards this approach as inimical. Some leading pub chains have also called for a comprehensive policy: in their case, in order to secure a 'level playing field' (http://news.bbc.co.uk/1/hi/business/4201053.stm). And many employees in the hospitality trade – those whose health is most at risk (British Medical Association 2005) – would prefer to work in a smoke-free atmosphere: 87% according to a recent survey by Caterer-online (www.caterersearch.com).

Tobacco's footprint: local and international

Tobacco is a product that permeates and impacts society at every level. People start to smoke for many different reasons. They then continue to smoke because they have become addicted to nicotine and find the addiction hard to break. But the most basic and straightforward reason for starting is that 'it is there': people couldn't smoke if there were no tobacco to be had. The pathway to consumption and addiction, with the inevitable ill health and early death suffered by so many smokers, starts with tobacco seeds and tobacco farmers. Planting, harvesting and processing of the tobacco leaf; manufacture, distribution and marketing of tobacco products; promotion and sale in local retail outlets: all are recognisable features of any normal supply chain. So are governmental interests in terms of tax policy. Less recognisable, but seemingly inevitable, are the side effects of the tobacco trade (which is dominated by a few multinationals operating in a globalised economy). Among these are child labour (www.christian-aid.org.uk/indepth/0201bat/batresp.htm); deforestation and soil erosion; illicit sales and tax evasion – smuggling and counterfeiting (World Bank 1999); and tobacco litter (Register 2000), with its environmental degradation and waste disposal consequences. All of these side effects impact on the health of local communities.

---

[1] The Health Bill is still under consideration. The House of Commons voted overwhelmingly in favour of smoke-free legislation without exemptions in February 2006.

It is not surprising, then, that leading international agencies have become involved in the struggle against the tobacco epidemic. In particular, the World Bank has done much to document the economic costs of tobacco, and to refute the industry's claim that tobacco control damages local economies. The World Bank argues strongly in favour of comprehensive tobacco control measures as sound fiscal policy (World Bank 1999).

In May 1999, the World Health Assembly adopted a resolution paving the way towards negotiations for the world's first international health treaty – to combat the world's biggest health threat, namely tobacco. The negotiating process took 4 years, culminating in a treaty signed (as at May 2005) by 168 countries and ratified by 66 countries. The UK ratified the Framework Convention on Tobacco Control (FCTC) on 16 December 2004 (www.fctc.org/treaty/index.php). The Treaty itself came into effect on 27 February 2005, having been ratified by the necessary 40 countries. Countries ratifying the FCTC commit themselves to a range of measures (*see* Box 14.1).

Box 14.1 Key requirements of FCTC

- Ban tobacco advertising, sponsorship and promotion.
- Ensure health warnings covering at least 30% of pack.
- Protect people from second-hand smoke in public places.
- Draw up strategies to combat smuggling.
- Adopt tax policies which discourage smoking.

So far, so good?

The past 15 years have seen significant progress towards more effective tobacco control locally, nationally, regionally (e.g. EU) and now worldwide. There is a broadly based tobacco control community that is increasingly well-informed, articulate, media savvy and battle hardened. This derives in part from the explosion in new communications technologies. Online data exchange and instant networking have become the tools of trade for tobacco activists – wherever they are based, whatever their perspective – whether they are clinicians, public health specialists, smoking cessation advisers, health promoters, government officials or politicians (www.globalink.org/).

There has been a common agenda behind all these efforts: to dissuade non-smokers (especially young people) from starting, and to persuade smokers to stop. This amounts to a process of 'de-normalising' tobacco use – i.e. non-smoking is presented as the norm and smoking as socially unacceptable. The intention is to reduce tobacco consumption, and thus the prevalence of tobacco-related morbidity and mortality. This overall, if unspoken, objective appears to have been embraced by the health community as a whole. Any disagreement – or healthy debate – has concerned emphasis or means, but not the general 'direction of travel'. However, today's implicit harmony may soon be sorely challenged.

In England, the issue of smoking cessation targets – how they are set, how they are measured and whether they are meaningful – has already provoked debate (West 2004). The Department of Health set a target of 800,000 successful quitters for the 3-year funding cycle 2003–2006. This overall target was then attributed to all PCTs on a 'per head' population basis. Individual PCTs chose whether to divide their local target equally over each of the 3 years, or whether to stagger them (e.g. to reflect potential service growth). Outcome is measured according to the number of clients who self-report successful quits (2 weeks' abstinence) 4 weeks after setting a quit date.

The advantage of this approach, which is linked to PCT star ratings, lies in the senior management interest engendered at local level: every PCT chief executive is keen to ensure good results. There are very real concerns, however, as to how valid an average population target is (when it fails to reflect local demography and tobacco consumption patterns in different communities); how the numbers are being counted; whether they are strictly comparable from one PCT to another; whether individual quitters receive sufficient long-term support to sustain their abstinence; and whether any meaningful public health gain is being achieved – e.g., in terms of reduced prevalence. The Healthcare Commission has included tobacco control among the first of its public health 'improvement reviews', to assess whether Stop Smoking Services effectively target groups most at risk (www.healthcarecommission.org.uk).

The controversy over quit targets concerns practice rather than principle. It should be resolved, over the next few years, once the new review mechanism has taken effect and on the basis of those old trusties: trial and error, and the 'sharing of good practice'. More controversial, and less easy to resolve, are various concerns that are more a matter of principle.

Prohibition

In December 2003, *The Lancet* called for an outright ban on tobacco – a suggestion promptly ridiculed by the tobacco industry, but also greeted with very little enthusiasm by most tobacco control advocates. There is only one country in the world that has banned tobacco *per se*: Bhutan (November 2004) (http://news.bbc.co.uk/1/hi/world/south asia/4305715.stm). While both developments have been largely ignored, they create more of an immediate challenge for the tobacco control community than for the tobacco industry. They effectively pose the question: what is the end game? What are we trying to achieve in tobacco control? Continued reductions in tobacco-related harm? Or no tobacco at all?

Harm reduction

From time to time, the tobacco industry has considered developing and marketing a 'less harmful' product. The concept has failed to take off for various reasons, including the following.

- Internal legal advice: tobacco industry lawyers advised that the notion of harm reduction implicitly acknowledged 'normal' products as harmful, and could render the companies vulnerable to successful litigation.
- The fear that 'less harmful' products would be perceived as less macho products, and therefore prove impossible to market.
- The reality that there is no such thing as a safe cigarette, that 'harm reduction' offers no tangible health benefit and that the whole notion is therefore meaningless.

However, there is one product on the market in some Nordic countries for which less health harm is claimed. This is snus, a form of oral tobacco, manufactured by Swedish Match. On entry to the EU in the mid-1990s, Sweden negotiated a derogation from the ban on oral tobacco that applies to all other member states. When the EU Tobacco Products Directive was recently recast, Swedish Match campaigned for the ban to be lifted – arguing, *inter alia*, that snus causes less health harm than smoked tobacco products.

This claim is supported by many tobacco control experts in Europe, who have made the case for market liberalisation on the basis that it is illogical to allow the sale of tobacco known to be a major health risk, but not a form of tobacco that causes less health harm – i.e. that priority should be focused on reducing the risk exposure of those addicted to nicotine. Others suggest that the health arguments are not proven, and that it ill becomes the health community to advocate legalisation of the one form of tobacco that is currently banned in much of Europe (Yach *et al.* 2005).

The controversy is set to run. For it posits a fundamental dichotomy: is tobacco control about reducing consumption by tackling nicotine addiction? Or is it about eliminating death and disease caused by tobacco?

Product regulation

No regulatory authority would approve tobacco as a new consumer product, if today's 'health and safety' requirements had to be taken into account. Tobacco, which causes nothing but harm, is subject to next to no control compared to other products – such as pharmaceuticals – which are meant to do us good. This anomaly is particularly poignant when one considers NRT, which is subject to the full rigours of medicines' approval regimes.

The EU Tobacco Products Directive outlines several future steps towards more rigorous regulation: these include disclosure of ingredients and additives, justification for additives, and the introduction of graphic health warnings (www.eu.int/scadplus/leg/en/cha/c11567.htm). Tobacco activists have also suggested generic packaging.

The EU and member states will have to consider whether to introduce some form of Tobacco Regulatory Authority. Even this is controversial, for it implies an element of cohabitation with the tobacco industry. It could also be seen to let the industry off the hook: approval of their products by an official authority (whether EU or member state) would surely diminish the scope for liability litigation.

Lessons for the wider health community?

Tobacco is a product quite unlike any other. It kills about half of all regular smokers, when used exactly as intended by the manufacturer.

Apologists representing a free-market view of the world try to suggest that any restrictions on tobacco manufacture or marketing are the 'thin end of the wedge'; that a ban on tobacco advertising, for instance, will inevitably lead to a ban on advertising alcohol or cars – for they both cause death and destruction. This claim is easily refuted, for neither alcohol nor cars necessarily cause damage in 'normal' use. In their case, it is abuse of the product that carries risks. With tobacco, it is everyday use. So there is no comparison.

There is, however, a comparison between advocacy for tobacco control and advocacy for health generally. The process, the tasks, the skills: all are similar and transferable. The content and the contacts may be different, but the lessons can all be used in the wider public health context.

References

British Medical Association (2005) *Booze, Fags and Food*. Published online: www.bma.org.uk/ap.nsf/Content/boozefagsandfood.

Department of Health (1998) *Smoking Kills: a white paper on tobacco*. London: The Stationery Office.

Department of Health (2005) *Delivering Choosing Health: making healthier choices easier*. London: Department of Health.

Doll R, Peto R, Boreham J *et al.* (2004) Mortality in relation to smoking: 50 years' observations on male British doctors. *BMJ*. **328**: 1519.

Frieden T (2005) *Adult Tobacco Use Levels After Intensive Tobacco Control Measures: New York City, 2002–2003*. New York: New York City Department of Health and Mental Hygiene.

Health Education Authority (1999) *Been There, Done That: revisiting tobacco control policies in the NHS – policy monitoring tool*. London: Health Education Authority.

James I (1604) *A Counterblaste to Tobacco*. London: R Barker.

Jamrozik K (2004) Population strategies to prevent smoking. *BMJ*. **328**: 759–62.

Jamrozik K (2005) Estimate of deaths attributable to passive smoking among UK adults: database analysis. *BMJ*. **330**: 812–16.

Peterson S and Peto V (2004) *Smoking Statistics*. London: British Heart Foundation.

Peto R, Lopez AD, Boreham J *et al.* (2004) *Mortality from Smoking in Developed Countries 1950–2010*. Oxford: Oxford University Press.

Register K (2000) Cigarette butts as litter – toxic as well as ugly. *Underwater Naturalist*. **25**: 2.

Scientific Committee on Tobacco and Health (1998) *Report of the Scientific Committee on Tobacco and Health*. London: Department of Health.

Scientific Committee on Tobacco and Health (2004) *Secondhand Smoke: review of evidence since 1998. Update of evidence on health effects of secondhand smoke*. London: Department of Health.

Secretary of State for Health (2004) *Choosing Health: making healthier choices easier*. London: The Stationery Office.

Twigg L, Moon G and Walker S (2004) *The Smoking Epidemic in England*. London: Health Development Agency.

West R (2004) *Identifying Key Factors for Success in Delivery: report of the NHS Stop Smoking Services workshop, 30th September 2004*. London: Department of Health.

World Bank (1999) *Curbing the Epidemic. Governments and the economics of tobacco control*. Washington DC: World Bank.

Yach D, McKee M, Lopez A *et al.* (2005) Improving diet and physical activity: 12 lessons from controlling tobacco smoking. *BMJ*. **330**: 898–900.

Chapter 15

Food: time to shift from classical to ecological public health

Tim Lang

Introduction

As the British state labours under rising healthcare costs, attention has returned once more to the role of diet in public health and whether food behaviour should receive deeper intervention. Obesity has sparked this resurgence of interest. This chapter explores the complex policy terrain of diet and health, suggesting some key drivers and lessons in history, as well as some major issues ahead. It proposes that a new ecological public health approach – linking health and environment, and thinking holistically – would refine strategy for getting the supply-chain to take health seriously. The alternative is for health to be left to the whims of the market, where public health spending will always be outclassed by big corporations' spending.

Food and health in Britain: crazy paving or advance?

Food as a public health concern has a chequered past in Great Britain, not least because the four nations that make up the UK have such varied cultures and histories as well as systems of food and public health governance. To talk of British food is, even today, a puzzling notion. We are a culture which now deems its national dishes to include pizza and 'curry' (an Anglo-Indian concoction of the imperialist Raj, not of Indian cuisine *per se*) and which created that wonder of modern cuisine the deep-fried Mars bar and whose favourite condiment is merely known as brown sauce.

Alongside these frontiers of food experience and despite massive coalescence of eating styles, driven by mobility, foreign travel and supermarketisation, there is some residual regionality in tastes, far less than, say, Mediterranean or Indian regions but discernible nonetheless. And there is certainly a rebirth of consciousness of local foods, aided by a combination of support from Regional Development Agencies, pursuit of foreign export sales and localism harnessed by indefatigable Women's Institutes on the one hand and the Italian imported Slow Food movement on the other. Generally over the last 30 years, Britain has witnessed a remarkable and strong demand for better quality, more affordable and a greater range of foods. Restaurants and supermarkets, for all their critics and serving of 'globo-food' or 'bistro fusion mock Mediterranean', have fed public consciousness of food. There is divergence alongside convergence (Hawkes 2006). Rising affluence, helped by TV cooking shows, has seen an explosion of cuisine consciousness, far beyond the greyness of post-Second World War days and rationing (Cooper 1967; Driver 1983). Optimists therefore argue, with reason, that food has at last begun to improve in Britain. Realists remind us, however, of our highly processed diet and that there are considerable gaps between the choices of the affluent and the poor. The lower a household's income, the more restricted is its diet, and the worse its health (Dowler, Turner and Dobson 2001; Mackenbach and Bakker 2002). This is a truism of food and health, even in an affluent society like Britain; more so in poorer societies (Commission on the Nutrition Challenges of the 21st Century 2000).

It is against this crazy-paving past and present of British food and culinary culture that food's role in public health has to be inserted and judged. Dietary impact on health has long been known to be very high. It is a key factor in preventing and contributing to major sources of ill health and premature death (WHO 1990; WHO/FAO 2003). Since 1974, the government's own advisory body has made that clear (COMA 1974, 1994). Yet on the one hand the British people are living longer, albeit fractured by social class; and on the other hand there is a strong resistance to improving some behaviour known to be vital for health. We eat far too much fat, salty foods, and far too little fruit and vegetables. We use cars to get to supermarkets rather than walk or bicycle. Targets set to eat five-a-day have not been met. On average, the British stubbornly eat well below half that; Scottish children even less (Caraher and Anderson 2001). Despite setting targets in 2001 to raise consumption of fruit and vegetables to the five-a-day goal, in 2005 the government reported that '*since 2001 there has been no improvement in fruit and vegetable consumption for the most disadvantaged groups and no significant narrowing of the gap*'. Its response was to establish more five-a-day projects in deprived areas (Department of Health 2005). The analysis offered here is that the issue is more deep-rooted into British food culture and its supply chain than can be ameliorated by just targeting the poor. Fruit and vegetables are expensive compared to biscuits, fried and other filling foods.

The troubled place of food in British history

From medieval times, there were attempts to regulate standards of quality and to limit adulteration. Thus if health was not in the driving seat, it at least featured in a political economy otherwise dominated by survival and commerce (Paulus 1974). Until industrialisation, a process that began in England in the late 18th century but accelerated and swept the country in the 19th, the main policy concern at state level was land. The Domesday Book, created in 1086 at the end of William the Conqueror's reign, is testament to the sensitivity of land a thousand years ago (Williams and Martin 2002). The invading French (Norman) rulers needed to know where the best land was, what its worth was, what rents and yields it gave and above all who owned it and whether it could be taxed or tithed (church taxes). For 200 years, as the French ruled, they built, ploughed, introduced crops, exploited agricultural labour. Spencer's magisterial *British Food* argues that these two centuries laid down a pattern of thinking about food which still has echoes today: that food is fractured by social class, ethnicity, family traditions, aspirations, extremes of wealth and poverty; the rule being that the rich eat well, the poor survive (Spencer 2002). But with the demise of the feudal manorial system and rise of tenant farming, there was expansion; tenants looked to clear new ground (Drummond and Wilbraham 1939). Despite the Black Death, villages grew, as did output. In the 17th to 19th centuries, extensive drainage increased productivity (Wade Martins 2004). In Scotland and England, enclosures, forced and voluntary, shaped an approach to food and land alike. A split between the town and the country was enshrined which continues but which has attracted deep concern on health grounds at times. In the 1920s and 1930s, the rural areas were appealed to as wells of health; they ought to give not just food, but breathing space, recreation, resources, peace (Fielding 1923; Stapledon 1935). These themes are again re-emerging in the literature on links between rurality, greenery and health (Pretty *et al.* 2003). It is detectable in the demand for organic, contaminant-free foods (Conford 2001).

But British food, and its health impact, has not been the unmitigated disaster story a certain strand of élitism implied. In the 20th century, some argued that it was only the spread of the French (again) civilised approach to food and wine which brought good food and therefore health to Britain, and enabled a healing process whereby people could see food as pleasure not just needed fuel (Morrah 1987). This version of history denies the culture of good local foods and traditions, some born from necessity, regionalism and experience (Driver 1983; Hartley 1954; Steven 1985). Britain may have had to import its wines – a matter of deep regret to Cobbett who fulminated against tea as well, exhorting the English working people to stick to home-grown beers (Cobbett 1830)! – but its fish and meats were famed across Europe. There has been a steady strand of evidence about good foods and comparatively well-fed people alongside the more troubled tradition of food riots, machine smashing (Luddism) and other hunger marches. Edward Thompson, writing about the resistance of English crowds to the arrival of industrial relations in the late 18th century, remarked on the importance of the shift from the paternalism of the feudal legacy where there was a notion of right to foods, and its replacement under urban industrial capitalism by the 'stand on your own feet' individualism (Thompson 1993).

The history of British food, then, is fissured. The considerable literature of the last two centuries in particular is not just testament to the skill of our historians but to the immense complexity of food mores and behaviour as society went through an astonishing transition. If the greatest post-evolutionary change was the shift from hunter-gathering to settled agriculture – a process widely agreed to be in the human cultural lexicon by around 10,000 years ago (Smith 1995; Tudge 1998) – the next mega-shift was the transition to industrial capitalism around 200 years ago. The former transition occurred in the Fertile Crescent of the Middle East; the latter on this wet northern island. The former gave us at least five key grains; the later pioneered mass white bread! Industrial steam-roller mills enabled systematic separation of flour, giving the urban poor the chance to eat routinely what previously had only been affordable by the rich. Status framed what people ate, even to the detriment, science has taught us, of our health (Cleave 1974). This extraordinary history, coupled with its waves of immigration and emigration, is what makes Britain's food and health history, present and policy so interesting. It also makes its public health challenge particularly poignant.

Food as a challenge to public health

The history of thinking about food and public health in the modern era (the last 200 years) has been summarised elsewhere (Lang 2005; Lang and Heasman 2004). It is a history essentially of conflict over and between interests: the state, civil society, supply chain and natural environment. Within each node of this quartet, health politics divide interests. Food and farming may have dominated state interests for centuries, but at times the need for healthier populations has also surfaced. Being an island, security of supply has been important. After the great experiment of reliance on the colonies to feed it, the British state awoke to the importance of feeding its working people – at least if it needed a decent, healthy army. The Boer war and lousy recruits were a shock to the system. But other determinants of health and health amelioration vied for attention, too. Champions presented evidence about food's role in poverty, squalid town experience, the case for welfare food, continuing worries about food safety and quality, economic inefficiency, market concentration, and environmental impact. These themes have surfaced, submerged and resurfaced for decades. They have suffused, on the one hand, Britain's class politics with its hunger marches (Hannington 1936), and on the other hand its paternalism, with industrialists arguing the case for better feeding (Crawford and Broadley 1938; Rowntree 1921). This has been described as the long struggle between forces trying to control society through food versus the demand to democratise food. Public health proponents have sat and can sit in both camps. Sometimes we want to impose taste and patterns; other times we are more hands-off. Often the division is whom we work for.

The British state has had a chequered involvement with food and health. Britain had, in the early 20th century, the largest directly controlled empire humanity has yet seen – more extensive than the Athenian, Roman, Venetian, Ottoman, Persian, Chinese, Japanese or even the present virtual US empire (Ferguson 2004). But its policy went through constant revision; the state and key industrial interests first built up home agriculture, then let it quietly collapse, then were forced to rebuild it again due to the First World War's constraints, then abandon it again, only to have to rebuild it for the second time in the Second World War, and then put it on a more measured basis for strategic interests, and finally merge productionist interests into the European Union's food and farming policy, the Common Agricultural Policy. All this in 200 years. The track record on public health policy through food is slightly less breathless but sometimes as contorted. Across the same last 200 years, food and health policy has veered through benign neglect, fierce support for markets, welfarism, emphasis on consumer choice and now sits with an uneasy combination of guidance and consumerism.

Consider obesity: it is now recognised as a major public health cost (overweight and obesity cost an estimated £6.6–7.4 billion (Health Committee of the House of Commons 2004), is a precursor to key diseases and is rising rapidly. The Chief Medical Officer rightly issued a stern warning (Donaldson 2003). Yet there is a curiously low-key response across Europe, not just the UK: a mixture of threats, pilot projects, encouragement and policy stick-wagging and consensus-building with big business. But there is relatively little confrontation of the marketing industries or food industries that pour out fat, sugar and highly processed foods whose activities are strongly associated with the supply side of the obesity problem (Lang and Rayner 2005). Privately, many believe that such hands-off, consumerist public health strategies are doomed to failure; hiding behind consumer choice appears democratic but consigns many to ill health. The challenge is to confront culture. A healthy society will need to be not just more equal but to have health-enhancing behaviour rooted in its daily way of living, whether this is eating or exercise or work (Marmot 2004; Marmot and Wilkinson 1999; Wilkinson 2005).

A crisis of policy, vision or institutions?

The tension between food democracy (giving more power to people to decide their diets) and food control (constraining and directing food supplies) has permeated struggles over food and health in modernity. In the 19th century, food prices were driven down to constrain wages but standards were driven up because of public health alarm about adulteration, poisoning and poor health of working-class consumers. Critiques of the exploitation of the public through its food were a feature of the emerging public health movement of the mid-19th century. Chadwick, Hassall, and other mid-19th-century pioneers of what we now term classical public health (Coley 2005), all saw food as central to their vision of re-engineering society to improve health. The Pure Food Laws that were fought for through much of the 19th century are the testament to the alliance of professionals, campaigners, activists and 'ordinary' people who felt that no society is civilised if its people are fed lousy food.

In the 20th century, with the laws now in place and new institutions created to begin to deliver public protection locally (through medical officers, sanitary inspectors, school education, etc.) and nationally (through ministries and boards for health, agriculture, trade, etc.) state attention was drawn to the running sore of inequalities largely by working-class demands for better conditions, together with middle-class support. Even here, in what became a half-century struggle for a decent welfare safety net and threshold of adequacy, food played an important role.

One of the first Acts of the modern welfare state was the Education (Provision of Meals) Act of 1906. This created the school meals service; more in principle than reality, since the Act allowed local authorities to levy a rate, an opportunity that few authorities took up, but which led directly to the collapse of the faltering charity meals system that preceded it. It was only the 1914–1919 war's demand for female labour, and particularly the Second World War, that created the meals service in Britain. Again it was an alliance of campaigners and public health and nutrition specialists which delivered advances. Using Rowntree's work on basic minimum nutritional requirements in his studies of his home chocolate city of York from 1899 (in turn inspired by Atwater's late 19th-century USA work), a coalition of poverty researchers, the medical establishment and welfarists persuaded the wartime Conservative Education Minister to lay down nutritional standards for children and therefore their food at school (Le Gros Clarke and Titmuss 1939; Webster 1997). These were systematically removed under the Thatcher experiment in contracting out of public services in the 1980s, with the 1980 Education Act removing the 1944 Education Act's commitments to nutritious food at school. It took a TV series by Jamie Oliver, a celebrity chef, in 2005 to embarrass government to toughen up 'soft' guidelines that replaced the vacuum. Evidence of the urgent need to alter children's diets now had piled up for years to little avail but much academic frustration (Lang 1997), a reminder perhaps not to over-rely upon reason in pursuit of evidence-based policy!

In fact, for much of the 20th century, the British food supply chain was dominated by the stricture to increase output, rather than for public welfare. But this production-focused policy was itself to some extent a response to evidence of health effects of under-production in the 1930s (Boyd Orr 1936, 1943). Great heroes of food and public health such as Sir John (later Lord) Boyd Orr had championed the need to increase output coupled with social justice in distribution;

a conservative, he became radical. The hallmarks of productionist food and health policy was to tackle yield, price, quantity, efficiency and waste reduction. This new paradigm may be represented as a policy equation (Lang and Heasman 2004):

science + capital + state support (finance + policy) → increased production, which if distributed appropriately → health + wellbeing.

It is this paradigm which is now unable to deal with the complexity outlined and endlessly rehearsed in the literature on food and health. If the food problem was conceived as under-supply, the policy response cannot now deal with the new realities of over-, under- and mal-consumption within and between societies and households. As the evidence mounted from the 1960s to 2000s on diet's role in non-communicable diseases, obesity, childhood eating, price signals, the power of marketing, the dangers of food culture driven by choice and price signals, the productionist policy could only stick to its course. Governmental and industry silence was deafening and at times recoursed to blaming the victim, urging consumers to look after themselves when the need for an entirely different approach to food was increasingly apparent.

But tipping points for change in food and health policy have a habit of emerging from off-field. In the late 1980s, a radical non-interventionist Conservative government was forced to impose tough controls to tackle food safety and try to win back public trust. Again, this happened in 2005 for school meals, known to insiders as the Cinderella service. Might it be possible that in the early 21st century, it will be obesity that breaks the public health logjam? The costs are certainly high and noted, *inter alia*, by Sir Derek Wanless's two reports in 2002 and 2004. Pressure is also building, via the enormous (almost 19th-century style) coalition around the Children's Food Bill coalition (www.sustainweb.org/child_index.asp), to take control over profligate marketing of unwholesome foods at children. Again, the evidence for action has long been known and presented to the state (Hastings *et al.* 2003). Food companies have formidable marketing budgets; McDonald's and Coca-Cola both spend around $1.7 billion a year globally. What health education department can compete with that consciousness moulding, let alone have the manpower to use texting, sponsorship, education materials and other less overt marketing methods? In the UK, Coca-Cola spent £26 million in 2002, compared to the Consumer's Association's (now Which?) £200,000 and the Food Standards Agency's £8 million (much on research) (Lang 2004).

A number of environmental crises faces the infrastructure of food supply and health. Climate change, water shortage, excessive use of oil to transport food to people, animal-born viruses (avian flu H5N1 in particular), all point to the possibility of enforced radical change ahead, to which food culture will have to accommodate. National food security, long provided by EU CAP (Common Agricultural Policy) surpluses, is uncertain; within Whitehall there is once more talk of abandoning agriculture altogether, a re-run of the mid-19th-century Repeal of the Corn Laws. Strategically, this carries major risks. The USA had to be paid to feed the UK in the Second World War under the Lend-Lease programme. In the 21st century, the USA is more interested in feeding China's demand for meat than the UK. Not growing food, when you have the land and climate to do so, is historically unsound and sourcing foods long distance generally makes little sense ecologically; this the government itself recognises (Smith *et al.* 2005). It also conflicts with the Food Industry Sustainability Strategy (or reduces that policy to tokenism).

At the institutional level, although there is much talk about obesity, the truth is that public health action is weak. The enormity of change required meets political resistance. Consumers are exhorted to eat less, but lower prices (celebrated by economists) encourage the reverse; and building exercise into daily life is nigh impossible with transport and home-work distances as they are. There is some policy structural movement however. After years of being accused of 'agency capture' (i.e. favouritism to farming interests), in 2001 the old Ministry of Agriculture, Fisheries and Food was rightly abolished and replaced by the new Department for Environment, Food and Rural Affairs (DEFRA). Although DEFRA has made good steps to link farming and environment, the health connections are still slight, not helped by the Department of Health (DH) going through a major labour-shedding process. Nordic societies offer a different role model, trying to join up food, health and environment thinking, and using policy councils to monitor and advise on food, physical activity and public health. The UK should follow suit (Lang *et al.* 2005).

The UK, led by its Treasury, has tried to reform the EU's CAP. This plays well to Euro-scepticism but is in fact well underway. Subsidies for production are being phased out. The UK might take a more positive role if it emulated Sweden in health auditing CAP (Elinde 2003; Whitehead and Nordgren 1996). CAP's impact on health is its achilles' heel, and ought to be done to meet Amsterdam Treaty commitments (Belcher 1997; Commission of the European Communities 1995). A tougher pro-health line on food and agriculture would not come amiss at the World Trade Organization either, whose goals of pursuing liberalisation can sit at odds with member-state commitments to environmental protection.

Conclusion

Food policy and practice provide salutary reminders of some old public health lessons. Public health is never given, it has to be gained and organised for. Diet is a significant factor – and often most preventable – in the major causes of ill health. Hence the challenge to public health to think ecologically before it is forced on us. How much evidence will it take?

References

Belcher P (1997) Amsterdam 1997: a new dawn for public health. *Eurohealth.* **3**(2): 1–3.

Boyd Orr J (1936) *Food, Health and Income: report on adequacy of diet in relation to income.* London: Macmillan and Co.

Boyd Orr SJ (1943) *Food and the People.* London: Pilot Press.

Caraher M and Anderson A (2001) An apple a day ... *Health Matters.* **46**: 12–14.

Cleave TLS-G (1974) *The Saccharine Disease. Conditions caused by the taking of refined carbohydrates, such as sugar and white flour.* Bristol: John White.

Cobbett W [1830] (1932) *Rural Rides.* London: JM Dent and Sons.

Coley NG (2005). The fight against food adulteration. *Education in Chemistry.* www.rsc.org/Education/EiC/issues/2005Mar/Thefightagainstfoodadulteration.asp (March).

COMA (1974) *Diet and Coronary Heart Disease: report of the Advisory Panel of the Committee on Medical Aspects of Food Policy (COMA).* London: Department of Health and Social Security.

COMA (1994) *Nutritional Aspects of Cardiovascular Disease: report of the Cardiovascular Review Group of the Committee of Medical Aspects of Food Policy.* London: HMSO.

Commission of the European Communities (1995) *On the Integration of Health Requirements in Community Policies. First report. COM(95) 196 final.* Luxembourg: Commission of the European Communities.

Commission on the Nutrition Challenges of the 21st Century (2000) Ending malnutrition by 2020: an agenda for change in the millennium. Final report to the ACC/SCN. *Food and Nutrition Bulletin.* **21**(3 Sup): whole issue.

Conford P (2001) *The Origins of the Organic Movement.* Edinburgh: Floris Books.

Cooper D (1967) *The Bad Food Guide.* London: Routledge and Kegan Paul.

Crawford W and Broadley H (1938) *The People's Food.* London: Heinemann.

Department of Health (2005) *Tackling Health Inequalities: status report on the programme for action. A report by the Scientific Reference Group on Health Inequalities chaired by Prof Sir Michael Marmot.* London: Department of Health.

Donaldson L (2003) *Annual Report of the Chief Medical Officer for England 2002.* London: Department of Health.

Dowler E, Turner SA and Dobson B (2001) *Child Poverty Action Group (Great Britain). Poverty bites: food, health and poor families.* London: Child Poverty Action Group.

Driver C (1983) *The British at Table 1940–1980.* London: Chatto & Windus.

Drummond JC and Wilbraham A (1939) *The Englishman's Food: a history of five centuries of English diet.* London: Jonathan Cape.

Elinde LS (2003) *Public Health Aspects of the EU Common Agricultural Policy.* Stockholm: Statens Folkhalsoinstitut/National Institute of Public Health.

Ferguson N (2004) *Colossus: the price of America's Empire.* New York: Penguin Press.

Fielding SC (1923) *Food.* London: Hurst and Blackett Ltd.

Hannington W [1936] (1977) *Unemployed Struggles 1919–1936.* London: Lawrence and Wishart.

Hartley D (1954) *Food in England.* London: Macdonald.

Hastings G, Stead M, Macdermott L *et al.* (2003) *Does Food Promotion Influence Children? A systematic review of the evidence.* London: Food Standards Agency.

Hawkes C (2006) Uneven dietary development: linking the policies and processes of globalization with the nutrition transition, obesity and diet-related chronic diseases. *Globalization and Health.* **2**(4). www.globalizationandhealth.com/content/2/1/4.

Health Committee of the House of Commons (2004) *Obesity. Third report of session 2003–04, HC 23-1, volume 1.* London: The Stationery Office.

Lang T (1997) Dividing up the cake: food as social exclusion. In: C Walker and A Walker (eds) *Britain Divided: the growth of social exclusion in the 1980s and 1990s.* London: Child Poverty Action Group.

Lang T (2004) *Food and Health Wars: a modern drama of consumer sovereignty.* Economic and Social Research Council and Arts and Humanities Research Board Cultures of Consumption Programme, Cultures of Consumption Working Papers series, no. 14. London: Birkbeck College ESRC Cultures of Consumption programme. www.consume.bbk.ac.uk.

Lang T (2005) What is food and farming for? The (re)emergence of health as a key policy driver. In: F Buttel and P McMichael (eds) *New Directions in the Sociology of Global Development: research in rural sociology and development,* vol. 11. Oxford: Elsevier, pp.123–45.

Lang T and Heasman M (2004) *Food Wars: the global battle for mouths, minds and markets.* London: Earthscan.

Lang T and Rayner G (2005) Obesity: a growing issue for European policy? *Journal of European Social Policy.* **15**(4): 301–27.

Lang T, Rayner G, Rayner M *et al.* (2005) Policy councils on food, nutrition and physical activity: the UK as a case study. *Public Health Nutrition.* **8**(1): 11–19.

Le Gros Clarke F and Titmuss RM (1939) *Our Food Problem and its Relation to Our National Defences.* Harmondsworth: Penguin.

Mackenbach JP and Bakker M (2002) *Reducing Inequalities in Health: a European perspective.* London: Routledge.

Marmot MG (2004) *Status Syndrome: how your social standing directly affects your health and life expectancy.* London: Bloomsbury.

Marmot MG and Wilkinson RG (eds) (1999) *Social Determinants of Health*. Oxford: Oxford University Press.

Morrah P (1987) *André Simon: gourmet and wine lover*. London: Constable.

Paulus I (1974) *The Search for Pure Food*. Oxford: Martin Robertson.

Pretty J, Griffin M, Sellens M *et al.* (2003) *Green Exercise: complementary roles of nature, exercise and diet in physical and emotional well-being and implications for public health policy*. CES Occasional Paper 2003-1. March. Colchester: University of Essex Centre for Environment and Society.

Rowntree BS (1921) *The Human Needs of Labour*. London: Longmans.

Smith A, Watkiss P, Tweddle G *et al.* (2005) *The Validity of Food Miles as an Indicator of Sustainable Development. Report to DEFRA by AEA Technology*. London: Department for the Environment, Food and Rural Affairs.

Smith BD (1995) *The Emergence of Agriculture*. New York: Scientific American Library/WH Freeman.

Spencer C (2002) *British Food*. London: Brub Street.

Stapledon SG (1935) *The Land: now and tomorrow*. London: Faber & Faber.

Steven M (1985) *The Good Scots Diet: what happened to it?* Aberdeen: Aberdeen University Press.

Thompson EP (1993) The moral economy of the English crowd in the eighteenth century and Moral economy reviewed. In EP Thompson (ed.) *Customs in Common*. Harmondsworth: Penguin.

Tudge C (1998) *Neanderthals, Bandits and Farmers: how agriculture really began*. London: Weidenfeld and Nicolson.

Wade Martins S (2004) *Farmers, Landlords and Landscapes: rural Britain, 1720–1870*. Macclesfield: Windgather.

Webster C (1997) Government policy on school meals and welfare foods, 1939–1970. In: DF Smith (ed.) *Nutrition in Britain: science, scientists and politics in the twentieth century*. London: Routledge, pp.190–213.

Whitehead M and Nordgren P (1996) *Health Impact Assessment of the EU Common Agricultural Policy: a policy report*. Stockholm: National Institute for Public Health, Sweden.

World Health Organization (WHO) (1990) *Diet, Nutrition and the Prevention of Chronic Diseases*. Technical Report Series 797. Geneva: World Health Organization.

World Health Organization and Food and Agriculture Organization (WHO/FAO) (2003) *Diet, Nutrition and the Prevention of Chronic Diseases. Report of the joint WHO/FAO expert consultation*. WHO Technical Report Series, No. 916 (TRS 916). Geneva: WHO/FAO.

Wilkinson RG (2005) *The Impact of Inequality: how to make sick societies healthier*. London: Routledge.

Williams A and Martin GH (eds) (2002) *The Domesday Book*. London: Penguin Books.

Chapter 16

Healthy childhood and a life-course approach to public health

Paul Lincoln

Mankind owes to the child the best it has to give. (UN Charter)

Introduction

Until the development of the National Service Framework for children's health in 2004 there had never been a national plan for child health in England. Recent child public health policy developments have been driven first by the exponentially increasing trend in early chronic conditions such as obesity and diabetes and the linked early life adoption of a plethora of unhealthy behaviours, and second by the development of the science of life-course epidemiology and the realisation that early life experiences are key determinants of health and disease prospects, especially avoidable chronic disease.

Control of childhood infections has been a great success with the recent and extraordinary exception of measles, mumps and rubella. The prevention of accidents and avoidable chronic diseases remain key challenges. This chapter focuses on preventing avoidable chronic diseases from an early age through the promotion of positive health behaviours and the development of a supportive health-promoting environment. This chapter identifies some of the key public health challenges in England and the policy implications.

Child public health policy developments

In the second half of the 20th century, adult chronic disease became the main public health problem of industrialised countries, responsible for 86% of deaths in developed economies (Beaglehole 2005; WHO 2002, 2005).

From the beginning of the NHS, national public health policy in the UK has been dominated by adult health priorities. This tradition was continued in the first public health white papers in England – *Health of the Nation* (Department of Health 1993) and *Saving Lives: our healthier nation* (Department of Health 1999). Health policy had been centred around chronic disease-based reduction targets with interventions in adulthood. One consequence of this policy has been a neglect of prenatal and child health policy when the origins of lifelong chronic diseases begin.

Indeed until recently there has not been a comprehensive national policy framework on child health, with the exception of childhood immunisation programmes and some aspects of accident prevention. Not since the Court report (DHSS 1977) which was an expert advisory report has there been any semblance of competent child health policy. This has recently changed with the publication of the white paper *Every Child Matters* (Department for Education and Skills 2003) and the first ever National Service Framework for child health (Department of Health 2004). This was the first ever comprehensive development of national child health standards which addressed the wider aspects of child health, especially chronic diseases such as obesity.

For too long children have been perceived as healthy and disease free and this supports the illusion that chronic disease develops later in life and can be prevented if not treated in later adulthood. Chronic diseases are perceived as an acceptable risk in life's lottery based on the belief that children are resilient and a fatalism that suggests everything will be fine when they grow up. However, public health scientists and practitioners have increasingly emphasised that the origins of disease and health inequalities and the building of health capital and the maximisation of health potential originates from the very beginning of human life.

Biological markers such as obesity and positive (and conversely negative) health behaviours such as physical activity and a healthy diet are very good indicators of a child's health/disease status and future adult health/disease prospects.

Public health scientists and practitioners have now acquired the epidemiological knowledge and sufficient intervention know-how to prevent future epidemics of chronic disease which fortuitously at the same time promote health and wellbeing.

A key public health challenge is to develop a mindset among policy makers that automatically considers the early most influenceable origins of health and disease.

The rest of this chapter explores key policy issues and related challenges for reducing the size and severity of the epidemic of avoidable chronic diseases in future generations. Indeed the policy mission in England could be summarised as follows:

> *Every child born in England today should be able to live to at least the age of 65 free from avoidable chronic diseases.*

Current policy issues and future public health challenges

A life-course approach to public health

The avoidable chronic diseases are cardiovascular diseases, hypertension, obesity, diabetes, respiratory disease and many cancers. These chronic diseases are theoretically largely avoidable and develop through lifelong exposure to the key risk factors – inappropriate diet, tobacco, alcohol and physical inactivity. These often linked chronic diseases manifest themselves later in life depending upon an individual's genetic disposition and individually and environmentally determined exposure to risk factors.

In a recent book on life-course epidemiology Kuh and Ben-Shlomo (2004) stated that:

> *The prevailing aetiological model that predominately emphasised adult lifestyle, such as smoking, diet and lack of physical activity has been successfully challenged, by growing international evidence that impaired early growth and development, childhood infection and poor nutrition, and socioeconomic or psychological disadvantage across the lifecourse, affect chronic disease risk. The study of these exposures and the lifecourse pathways through which they have their effects lies at the heart of lifecourse epidemiology.*

The physiological risk factors for coronary heart disease (high blood pressure, high blood cholesterol) have been shown to have their origins in childhood. Similarly their determinants (poor diet and physical inactivity) are habits that, together with smoking, are often adopted in childhood and carried through to adult life. Research indicates that children and young people's lifestyles are increasingly unhealthy, resulting in a rising prevalence of overweight and obesity among this group, and diagnosis for the first time of type 2 diabetes among teenagers (young@heart 2003).

Most cancers are largely determined by the risks of tobacco consumption and an inappropriate health-damaging diet.

Obesity, a major risk factor for many chronic diseases, is rising in prevalence worldwide. Early-life prevention is important as treatment of established obesity is largely ineffectual. Evidence is growing that factors in the prenatal period through adolescence are important determinants of excess weight gain. These factors range from upstream socially determined environmental to individual lifestyle and genetic factors. There is a vicious cycle of obesity developing between generations.

There are many factors that have adverse health impacts over the rest of the life course. If you smoke by the age of 20 years you will probably continue into adulthood; food preferences are formed between the ages of 2 and 7; the quality of a child's exposure to physical activity will translate into the development of neuromuscular skills and an accompanying enthusiasm and enjoyment for activity later in life; breastfeeding offers many benefits including emotional security, mental health and immunity to infectious diseases; an overweight child has a 50% chance of being an overweight adult; poverty can adversely influence health by affecting access to resources for health such as nutritious food, play, education, housing, etc. (young@heart 2003).

The development of life-course epidemiology is critical to our understanding of the early life origins of health. Life-course epidemiology can help us to understand which developmental periods are irreversible or optimal for intervention. Life-course epidemiology can also improve health and disease modelling and help shape longer-term investment in health and social policies.

The prevention of avoidable chronic diseases is one of the biggest contemporary public health challenges facing society. The stark reality is that the current generations of children and young people and adults are more likely to be affected by the avoidable chronic diseases than previous generations. Indeed there is a very real likelihood that today's children and young people may not live as long as their parents and will suffer more chronic disease morbidity and disability.

The reversibility of ill-health behaviours and the promotion of health

Over the last 30 years there have been significant reductions in death rates from chronic diseases such as coronary heart disease (CHD) in many developed economies. According to Critchley and Capewell (2002) up to 70% of this decline in the countries he studied such as England are as a result of changes in lifestyle risk factors. This is due to a combination of reduction of risk, in particular decreases in smoking prevalence. However, the epidemic of chronic diseases still accounts for most adult mortality, morbidity and disability and these diseases can just as easily increase as decrease. This is of great concern because younger generations, unlike previous ones, are now exposed to a new range of ubiquitous health-damaging risk factors such as highly processed, energy-dense, fatty, sugary and salty foods, an education, home and built environment that encourages low levels of physical activity and high levels of alcohol consumption in ways never experienced by any previous generation accompanied by the continuing threat from the traditional risk factors such as tobacco.

In the last 25 years in England the attributable avoidable chronic disease risk factor profile between generations has significantly changed with the exception of poverty as a determinant!

One key reason for early behavioural intervention is the prospect of being able to reverse unhealthy behaviours. By definition behaviours are less ingrained and more reversible the earlier they are tackled in life. Similarly profoundly influencing lifelong positive and negative health behaviour is more likely in early preschool and primary education years when rules and knowledge are more easily accepted and not prone to post-puberty and early adulthood instinctive counter-reactions.

Public health's primary goal for child health should be to promote health capital and potential from the beginning of life through encouraging positive health behaviour and provide a nurturing and supportive health-promoting environment. This approach has the added benefit of reducing and/or delaying the prospect of chronic disease later on in life. The key influenceable and cost-effective intervention years probably being from the prenatal period to early adolescence.

Below are outlined some of the key health-promoting environmental and life/health skills determinants.

Life conditions – the environment and the intergenerational cycle of health inequalities

There are major health inequalities in the distribution of chronic diseases between social groups. This is due to the differential exposure between social classes to a lifetime's exposure to the major risk factors. Smoking currently accounts for 50% of the excess deaths from CHD between social groups. Fruit and vegetable consumption is very much lower in families of social groups 4 and 5. Obesity is beginning to display a social gradient particularly among women. The levels of childhood poverty in the UK are the highest in the EU countries. In the UK nearly a third of the 11 million children experience poverty. Due to the hazardous built environment that accompanies poverty there is poor access to resources such as play and recreation areas and facilities and families often live in areas often aptly described as food deserts. The environments are from a life-course perspective 'toxic' and thus could variously be described as obesogenic, cardiogenic, carcinogenic and diabetogenic, etc.

Not surprisingly avoidable adverse health outcomes are worst in poorer social groups being associated with undesirable living conditions, stress and poverty. Although mortality and morbidity in childhood has fallen overall, the differential between social groups has widened.

The evidence for health inequalities in children covers infant mortality, low birth weight, low breastfeeding rates, dental disease, iron deficiency, accidents, development and educational attainment, behavioural problems and child abuse (Hall and Elliman 2003).

The public health challenge is to reduce the levels of absolute and relative poverty in low income:low wealth-ownership families through mechanisms such as through minimum income standards like the minimum wage and by ensuring adequate maternity benefits for pregnant women of all ages to assure the level of resources necessary to confer a healthy diet, decent housing, basic needs such as access to play and leisure, etc. This should be in combination with providing targeted welfare services and interventions in early life such as Sure Start which provide direct support to children and parents to ameliorate or compensate for the impact of poverty.

The main public health challenge is to end child poverty in the UK, break the intergenerational cycle of health inequalities and ameliorate its damage where it has left its mark on adults. This can be achieved by a combination of general poverty reduction measures combined with a targeted programme of health and welfare interventions that directly benefit children.

Life skills and the educational culture in the UK

The development of health knowledge, life skills and developing a positive attitude to life forms the basis of the health-promoting schools programme. Equipping young people with health knowledge and skills and positive health values is a vital preparation for life. Knowing what will build and destroy health is essential life-enhancing knowledge. Knowledge is necessary but not sufficient; children and young people need the life skills to acquire health such as being aware of commercial and peer-group pressures and being able to resist them. They also need to understand and clarify their own and others' values. The capability to develop a health decision-making capacity from an early age is vital for a healthy life.

Personal health and social education have been marginalised in the school curriculum by the preoccupation with examination subjects. The bottom line for the education system is focused around the traditional preparatory subjects for universities and employment based on a still-powerful UK tradition of grammar-school subjects and notions of a liberal education. Preparations for other aspects of life take second place. One major victim is physical education. The amount of time allocated to physical education declined dramatically in the 1990s and is still only guided by the government recommendation of a minimum of 2 hours a week. This is in stark contrast to the 1960s. Current education policy is to build sport and physical activity into the school day by extending the school day so that breakfast clubs and after-school activities become part of the school day. Food technology has replaced cooking skills in response to an acceptance of the processed food culture. Young people and many young parents are being deskilled and disadvantaged in health terms compared to previous generations.

One example of the way in which schools could make a major contribution to health beyond the formal curriculum is through the provision of nutritious school meals. School meals are, for children in poverty, often the only cooked meal of the day. The appalling and shameful state of school meals in England was highlighted by the celebrity chef Jamie Oliver who showed how processed food of low nutritional quality was being widely provided and school catering staff had been demoralised and deskilled when kitchen facilities were sold off in the 1980s. From the 1980 Education Act until 2000 schools were no longer obliged to meet statutory school meal standards. In 2000 the government introduced a few food-based standards. Recent OFSTED/FSA reviews of school food show that these standards have not been successful. Unfortunately the government chose not to introduce nutrient-based standards, which are the only reliable means for setting and monitoring the quality of school meals. However, there is every indication that through the public health white paper *Choosing Health* (Secretary of State for Health 2004) the government is reconsidering the position. One further complication is the fact that many local authorities and schools have contracted out to private providers' school meals with low standards for the next 25 years. Over the previous 25 years the school food culture has been one of neglect and cost savings at the expense of children's health. The situation in the UK contrasts badly with many countries in Europe and has been a factor in devaluing the importance of fresh natural and locally produced food which has had wider implications for the UK food culture.

A key public health challenge is to develop the culture of education establishments such as nurseries, schools and colleges so that they take an active responsibility for the health development of children and young people and make themselves integrated community-based health-promoting organisations.

The role of the state and the commercialisation of childhood and effective controls on the processed foods, alcohol and marketing industries

The role of the state in respect of public health has been redefined in the white paper *Choosing Health* (Secretary of State for Health 2004). The white paper legitimises the role of the state as a 'nanny' in respect of nurturing and protecting children. Public health controls are fully justified in relation to protecting children, particularly vulnerable children where their health is at risk and beyond their immediate locus of control such as being recipients of second-hand smoking or being exposed to the ruthless, exploitative, unethical and relentless marketing of foods high in salt, sugar and fats from an early age.

In recent years many public health, religious and other commentators on children's rights including the Department of Health's Children's Czar have raised concerns about the commercialisation of childhood. Obesity has increased in the UK by over 400% in the last 20 years. During this period there have been major changes in the UK's food culture. This is what many Europeans refer to as the Americanisation of our diets – the shift towards our diets being dominated by the consumption of low production cost, highly processed foods which are high in sugar, fats and salt. This is accompanied by a huge investment in their marketing and a rapid decline in cooking skills and changing lifestyles. The trend is to market these health-damaging products to ever-younger cohorts of children.

The role of the state should be a nurturing role to maximise health potential in childhood and in adulthood.

Most worryingly children, including preschool children, have become the focus of a huge investment in direct and indirect marketing for these highly health-damaging foods through ruthless and unethical marketing. These products usually have low production costs and enormous marketing budgets. Research by the Food Standards Agency has demonstrated that this marketing clearly influences children's diets, demands and 'pester power'. Eighty per cent of foods are purchased in the big four UK supermarkets, of which 85% of the food available is now highly processed.

Amazingly in the UK there are no statutory controls or standards on the marketing of fatty, sugary and salty foods to children. The codes that exist are not fit for purpose and any new unhealthy food product can be promoted with immunity from any meaningful and punitive sanctions being applied. The concept of self-regulation for a highly competitive global industry such as food manufacturing which operates on thin margins is totally flawed. Unless controls across the whole marketing promotional mix are introduced, specific codes on TV advertising will be ineffectual as they will result in the expansion of other promotional means and media. The vested food and marketing interests are wealthy and thus very powerful; they have been resistant to any effective controls and prefer to provide the minimum of information to the public and represent the public health case as someone else's concern.

A key public health challenge is to develop a health-promoting economy and ensure effective and comprehensive controls on the tobacco industry, alcohol and processed food industries to prevent the unethical exploitation of children, their childhood and the destruction of their health prospects.

The UN Convention: children's rights and voices

The UN Convention on the Rights of the Child (1989) established the importance of working with and listening to children and young people. Children's rights should be respected and children's and young people's views should be heard when developing services. All too often such mechanisms of participation and involvement do not exist or when they do they are at best tokenistic and thus result in intervention or service failure. The involvement of children in decision making is vital to an appreciation of democracy and citizenship. Such an approach also enables children to appreciate the broader determinants on their lives and health and allows them to develop influencing skills.

Health promotion is defined as *'the process for enabling people to increase control over the determinants of health and thereby improve their health'* (Ottawa Charter, WHO 1986). The four countries of the UK have now developed the office of Children's Commissioners to act as advocates for children and they report directly to Parliament. The *Children's National Service Framework* (Department of Health 2004) rightly warns against treating children in a reductionist way as 'mini adults' and not respecting their rights. Children's rights to a voice and involvement should be recognised as set out in the UN Children's Charter. It is generally accepted that most children develop a more worldly critical consciousness by the age of 8 years old. The development of children's citizenship skills via School Councils and their general empowerment in influencing adult decision making is key to ensuring successful interventions.

A key public health challenge is to develop accepted and effective mechanisms for engaging children and young people to become citizens and shape their health prospects.

Supportive, health-enhancing built environment and radical changes in transport policy

To make the healthy choices the easy choices especially for the poor and vulnerable we need a supportive environment to realise those choices. Inner-city children may not have access to playgrounds locally or in their schools; traffic may be a deterrent for parents; fresh food may not be available or too expensive; the built environment is ugly and soul destroying; there may limited facilities and choices available for young people. In rural areas the pub may be the only place for young people to go.

Many inner-city areas are being regenerated but the built environment lacks the sort of standards needed to promote and protect health and encourages unhealthy lifestyles for young people – a toxic environment for nurturing children and young people, e.g. for enabling physical activity in terms of cycle tracks, pedestrian priority areas, attracting pub ghetto areas and fast-food outlets and more recently gambling establishments. Many new schools are being built or refurbished but not necessarily with provision for sport and physical activity or cooking facilities.

Radical changes are required in transport policy. The car is king – pedestrians take second place. Gridlock is predicted on UK roads in the next 10 years with a doubling of cars expected. Society has become unhealthily dependent upon the car. Short journeys to schools are taken in the new fashionable 'four by fours' which offer increased protection for the occupants but increased risks to the environment for all and pedestrians and other road users. Challenges to these norms face many vested interests. Speed is revered and glamorised. It is often difficult for schools to introduce 20 mph zones. Public transport requires 20-plus years of investment and the development of public interest standards as has been demonstrated in France and Germany. Safe travel routes to schools are being promoted nationwide through the Department of Transport and the Department for Education and Skills (DFES).

Radical and long-term changes in values and practices are needed. A key public health challenge is to establish enforceable standards for health promotion and protection in planning the built environment, especially in poor neighbourhoods, and radical shifts in transport policy.

Social care and pension policy

We need to reduce morbidity and disability in old age as well as decrease mortality. One major implication is to develop policies that compress morbidity to the end of the lifespan and increase healthy life expectancy. This has implications for child health policy and investment in health from an early age. The EU countries are particularly exposed in macroeconomic terms given the current imbalanced demographic ratio of the young to the old. WHO Europe recognises this in its report on public health action for healthier children and populations (2005) where good health is key to social and economic development.

The public health challenge is to invest in child health to sustain the economy and quality of life for young and old alike and the intergenerational contract of mutual dependency necessary at different stages of life.

Final remarks

Life-course science and approaches to public health are only just beginning to inform public policy. Most importantly public health practitioners and policy makers should realise that decisions affecting the future need to be taken now not in the future!

Finally:

> *A child is not a thing to be moulded but a person to be unfolded.* (Quote from the cathedral in Georgetown, Guyana)

References

Beaglehole R (2005) Preventing chronic disease. *Lancet*. October.

Critchley TA and Capewell S (2002) Why model coronary heart disease? *European Heart Journal*. 110–16.

Department for Education and Skills (2003) *Every Child Matters*. London: TSO.

Department of Health (2004) *Children's National Service Framework*. London: Department of Health.

Department of Health (1993) *Health of the Nation*. London: Department of Health.

Department of Health (1999) *Saving Lives: our healthier nation*. London: Department of Health.

Department of Health and Social Security (1977) *Court Committee Report on Child Health Services*. London: DHSS.

Hall MB and Elliman D (2003) *Health for All Children* (4e). Oxford: Oxford University Press.

Kuh D and Ben-Shlomo Y (2004) *Chronic Disease Epidemiology. A lifecourse approach* (2e). Oxford: Oxford University Press.

National Heart Forum (2003) *A Lifecourse Approach to Coronary Heart Disease Prevention. Scientific and policy review*. London: TSO.

Office for National Statistics (2004) *Health Survey for England*. London: Office for National Statistics.

Secretary of State for Health (2004) *Choosing Health: making healthy choices easier*. Cm 6374. London: The Stationery Office.

United Nations (1989) *UNICEF Convention on the Rights of the Child*. New York: UN.

World Health Organization (WHO) (1986) *Ottawa Charter for Health Promotion*. Geneva: WHO.

World Health Organization (WHO) (2002) *World Health Report*. Geneva: WHO.

World Health Organization (WHO) (2005) *Preventing Chronic Disease: a vital investment*. Geneva: WHO.

WHO (Euro) (2005) *Public Health Action for Healthier Children and Populations*. Geneva: WHO.

young@heart (2003) *Towards a Generation Free From Coronary Heart Disease*. London: National Heart Forum and TSO.

Chapter 17

Sexual health: the challenges

Anne Weyman and Caroline Davey

Introduction

Sex is a natural part of life, and should be seen as a positive force which can contribute to creating a happy society. But often we stigmatise sex by associating it with negative experiences and consequences, particularly when talking about sexual health.[1] Sexual health is not just about the absence of ill health; rather it is about enabling people to have fulfilling relationships, which are good for their physical, mental and emotional wellbeing.

In this context, it is vitally important to recognise sexual health as a central element of the public health agenda. As the consultation for the 2004 public health white paper *Choosing Health?* noted, '*sexual health is one of the few health areas that affects the majority of the population and is relevant through the greater part of our lives*' (Department of Health 2004). Good sexual health has an enormously positive impact on people's emotions, relationships and overall health. However, there has long been a reticence in the UK to address sexual health openly and honestly, and this awkwardness has contributed to the sexual health problems that are only now beginning to be addressed. In recent years, national policy on sexual health has transformed it into a key priority, but challenges remain to tackle the more deep-seated fears and concerns around sex and sexual health which are embedded in the population.

Sexual health today

A legacy of unwillingness by successive UK governments to tackle sexual health problems in a comprehensive way has contributed to a situation where we now suffer from poor sexual health in a number of different areas. Over the last decade diagnoses of sexually transmitted infections (STIs) in genitourinary medicine (GUM) clinics have risen sharply: diagnoses of chlamydia, gonorrhoea and infectious syphilis have more than doubled since 1996, and chlamydia is now the most commonly diagnosed STI in GUM clinics (Health Protection Agency 2004). Table 17.1 shows the percentage increases in the number of new diagnoses of selected STIs between 1995 and 2003.

STIs are on the rise across all age groups, and early results from the National Chlamydia Screening Programme in England indicate that as many as one in ten sexually active young people aged 16–24 are infected (LaMontagne *et al.* 2004). There have also been record levels of HIV diagnoses in recent years, with an increase of around 150% since 1996 (Health Protection Agency 2004). In addition,

---

[1] fpa defines sexual health as '*the capacity and freedom to enjoy and express sexuality without exploitation, oppression, physical or emotional harm*'.

the Health Protection Agency estimates that almost a third of people with HIV in the UK have not yet been diagnosed (ibid.).

Table 17.1 Number of new diagnoses of selected STIs: GUM clinics, England, Wales and Northern Ireland (NB: data from Scotland not available)

	% change 1995–2003
Chlamydia	190%
Genital warts	27%
Gonorrhoea	137%
Genital herpes	15%
Syphilis	1062%

Source: Health Protection Agency (2004).

The UK also has the highest rate of teenage pregnancy in western Europe. Despite recent reductions in the rate – figures show that there was a 9.8% reduction in the under-18 conception rate between 1998 and 2003 – this still remains high at 42.3 per 1,000 young women aged 15–17 in 2003 (Office for National Statistics 2005). Although many areas have seen a slow but steady decline in their local teenage pregnancy rates in recent years, there are still a persistent minority of 'hotspots' which have seen their rates rise over the same period of time. Indeed, the most recent statistics show that 50% of all under-18 conceptions occur in the 20% of local authority wards with the highest rates (Teenage Pregnancy Unit 2005).

Contraception has been free for all on the NHS since 1974, and approximately 75% of care is now provided in general practice (fpa 2002). However, many women are still not offered the full range of contraceptive methods, and have particular difficulty in accessing longer-acting methods such as implants, the intrauterine system (IUS) and the intrauterine device (IUD). Many PCTs have cut funding to specialist contraceptive clinics, which in many areas are the only place where women can access the full range of methods and expert advice, and there is also a growing shortage of specialist professionals working in this area. Indeed, the inadequacy of current contraceptive services is indicated by the fact that approximately a quarter of all pregnancies in England and Wales end in abortion, and this figure rises to a third of all pregnancies in London (Office for National Statistics 2001).

Abortion is one of the most common medical procedures, and on average one in three women will have an abortion during her lifetime. In 2003, 181,600 abortions took place in England and Wales: 58% of abortions took place under 10 weeks, the vast majority (87%) took place under 13 weeks, and 80% were paid for by the NHS (Government Statistical Service 2004). However, there is still a huge variation in waiting times and funding across different areas of the country; for example, the proportion of abortions that was funded by the NHS in 2003 varied from 66% in the worst-performing strategic health authority to 94% in the best-performing (ibid.). Women may also find it difficult to access abortions at later gestations, and many areas impose an informal upper time limit far below the legal limit of 24 weeks – this can be anything from 12 weeks upwards, forcing women to travel outside their local area or to pay for an abortion themselves (All-Party Parliamentary Pro-Choice & Sexual Health Group 2004).

Current policy and practice

There has been a significant increase in the priority given to sexual health at a national level over the last 5 years. The first step in this process came in 1999, when the Social Exclusion Unit *Report on Teenage Pregnancy* prompted the launch of the Teenage Pregnancy Strategy in England. This set out a 10-year programme to 2010, with targets for reducing conceptions among under-16s and under-18s, and for increasing the participation of teenage parents in education and work to reduce the risk of social exclusion (Social Exclusion Unit 1999).

In 2000, the Welsh Assembly launched the *Strategic Framework for Promoting Sexual Health in Wales* (National Assembly for Wales 2000). The following year, the government launched the *National Strategy for Sexual Health and HIV* in England, which aimed to improve services across all of sexual health and proposed a comprehensive and holistic model of sexual health, as follows:

> *Sexual health is an important part of physical and mental health. It is a key part of our identity as human beings together with the fundamental human rights to privacy, a family life and living free from discrimination. Essential elements of good sexual health are equitable relationships and sexual fulfilment with access to information and services to avoid the risk of unintended pregnancy, illness or disease.*

The *National Strategy* outlined the main elements of a modern, comprehensive sexual health service as: contraceptive care and abortion; diagnosis and treatment of STIs and HIV; prevention of STIs and HIV; and services that address psychological and sexual problems (Department of Health 2001). In 2002, the *National Strategy* was followed by an *Implementation Action Plan* (Department of Health 2002). In 2004, a sexual health promotion strategy for Northern Ireland was issued for consultation, but to date the final strategy has not yet been launched. Finally, in 2005, the Scottish Executive launched *Respect and Responsibility: a strategy and action plan for improving sexual health* (Scottish Executive 2005). These national strategies have been important landmarks in raising the profile of sexual health and HIV across the UK, but progress on the ground has been frustratingly slow in their first few years.

In 2003, the House of Commons Health Select Committee produced a hard-hitting report on sexual health, which described the situation as a 'crisis' (House of Commons Health Committee 2003). This report served to refocus attention sharply on the need for dramatic improvements in sexual health services. In response to this and other criticisms of the slow progress being made at local level, in November 2004 the government incorporated sexual health as a key theme within the public health white paper *Choosing Health*, a blueprint for improving the public health of the nation as a whole (Department of Health 2004). To support the sexual health proposals contained within the white paper, £300 million was committed to investment in sexual health services over the 3 years 2005 to 2008. *Choosing Health* highlighted a number of key areas for action, which are detailed in Table 17.2.

Nonetheless, despite a strong focus on sexual health at a national policy level, it has been difficult to achieve any prioritisation at a local level. Primary care trusts (PCTs) have been reluctant to prioritise sexual health, particularly as they have so many other competing priorities on which they are more rigorously monitored and performance managed (BHIVA, PACT & Terrence Higgins Trust 2005). It is clear that monitoring and performance management make a huge difference – one area where there has been some improvement has been in the proportion of NHS abortions carried out under 10 weeks, which has been part of the balanced scorecard for PCTs and therefore has been a greater priority. In 2003 52% of all NHS-funded abortions took place under 10 weeks (Government Statistical Service 2004), and many PCTs are taking steps to speed up access to abortion to improve this figure further (All-Party Parliamentary Pro-Choice & Sexual Health Group 2004). However, the urgent need for further improvements is demonstrated by the fact that, in 2002 (the latest year for which we have detailed figures), although the best-performing PCT conducted 79% of NHS abortions under 10 weeks, the worst-performing PCT conducted only 9%, a truly unacceptable variation (Government Statistical Service 2003).

Table 17.2   Key sexual health elements of the white paper *Choosing Health*

Proposal	*Funding allocation*
Upgrading of contraceptive services: audit of contraceptive provision followed by central investment to meet gaps in local services	£40 million
New national awareness and prevention campaign: targeted particularly at young people	£50 million
Accelerated implementation of chlamydia screening programme: to cover the whole of England by March 2007 (brought forward from 2008)	£80 million
Modernisation of GUM clinics: national review of services followed by investment in both services and infrastructure	£130 million

Source: Department of Health (2004).

However, the absence of other strong sexual health indicators within the PCT star ratings system means that it has not been at the top of the agenda for PCT chief executives. *Choosing Health* provides a number of levers to overcome these local barriers – in particular, the requirement that sexual health must now be included in PCT local delivery plans will help to give it higher priority, as will the requirement that strategic health authorities must now performance manage PCTs more strongly in this area. The introduction of a new waiting time target of 48 hours for GUM services, to be achieved by 2008, should also serve to focus attention at a local level. However, although these new levers should help, it remains a problem that the money allocated to sexual health will not be ring-fenced, and therefore could potentially be siphoned off to other areas by PCTs if there is not strong commitment to the prioritisation of sexual health from the PCT's Board.

Key issues

Recent national policy initiatives and investment in the arena of sexual health have been a welcome step forward in tackling this vital area of public health. However, there are a number of key issues which must be addressed now to ensure that maximum benefit is gained from current policy initiatives and investment.

First, it is vital that all policy on sexual health addresses the issue holistically. There is a tendency in some quarters to interpret the term 'sexual health' as only relating to STIs (including HIV). This is an extremely short-sighted and limiting interpretation, which does not take into account the inter-related nature of all aspects of sexual health, including contraception, abortion and sexual wellbeing as well as infections. Specifically, at a funding and commissioning level there must be sufficient focus on contraception and abortion services in order to enable people to manage their fertility, as a crucial element of promoting public health. The legalisation of abortion (in 1967) and the availability of free contraception (since 1974) are two of the most significant public health advances of the 20th century, and it is vital that current policy serves to reinforce the benefits that these two services provide. Consistently high rates of unintended pregnancy indicate that contraceptive services are not currently able to meet people's needs, and there is an urgent need to give greater prioritisation to these services in order to reduce rates of unintended pregnancy over the long term.

The second key issue to address is the balance between the need for short-term improvements in services and the need for longer-term health-promotion programmes to enable people to make informed decisions and healthier choices about their sexual health. Clearly, current high rates of STIs, teenage pregnancy and unintended pregnancy make it vital for STI, contraceptive and abortion services to be improved so that they meet demand. However, at the same time it is necessary to effect improvements in sexual health over the long term. Central to this is establishing an effective programme of information and education on sexual health – including comprehensive sex and relationships education (SRE) in schools from primary school onwards – to enable people to protect their own and their partners' sexual health and to promote sexual wellbeing.

In this context, the third key issue to tackle is the prevailing attitude of embarrassment and fear around sex which is common across much of the media and the population as a whole. Despite an increasing sexualisation and liberalisation within popular culture, the long-standing 'stiff upper lip' approach to sexual health remains among many sections of the population, and it is still very rare for people to talk openly about sexual health issues. This kind of attitude is particularly prevalent when talking about young people and their need for comprehensive SRE and confidential access to services. Evidence clearly shows that these are the most effective means of promoting sexual health, but there is often a knee-jerk resistance to developing such programmes. Over the long term, high-quality, comprehensive SRE must be the cornerstone of public policy to promote sexual health for all, and in order to achieve this there needs to be a clear reassessment of our collective attitudes towards sex.

Challenges for the future

Even with the recent prioritisation of sexual health within the broader public health agenda, there remains a number of barriers to be overcome in planning for a sexually healthy future. A principal challenge is to develop a clear and comprehensive understanding of sexual health, which resonates with the public, policy makers and professionals. Over the longer term, there must be a move towards recognising that a holistic approach towards sex, relationships and sexual health is the optimum way of securing real improvements in this area. In order to do this effectively there will be a need to break down professional barriers and make best use of the skills mix of a range of different professionals, particularly taking into account the recent increase in nurse-led services in this area and the need to integrate sexual health services.

In particular, there is significant scope to improve abortion services by amending the law both to allow suitably trained nurses to perform early surgical and medical abortions, and to make uncomplicated early abortions available at community level. These changes would make a real difference to the delivery of abortion services and would improve access to and availability of abortions, as well as making best use of the contribution that nurses can make in this field (Mawer and McGovern 2003).

In the future, it will be important to focus more attention on developing proactive approaches to health promotion in the field of sexual health, in order to influence people's behaviour *before* they have sex. Successful public health policies work best when they are preventive rather than curative, and this is particularly the case in sexual health where effective interventions can promote positive sexual health and wellbeing while minimising risk. In order to achieve this, there will need to be a cultural shift to a situation where sex and relationships are talked about more openly, services are easily accessible for all, and where young people are encouraged to build up their confidence and self-esteem in order to make the right decisions about sex for them. There must also be a greater focus on interventions – particularly in schools and at an informal community-based level – which work to change attitudes and behaviour at the stage before services are required.

A new and open climate around sex and relationships would be a huge leap forward for the development of positive sexual health for all. Indeed, a more honest and rational atmosphere of debate and discussion would help policy makers and professionals to navigate some of the finer complexities and inconsistencies within sexual health messages. This would help, for example, in balancing the message that condoms are the most effective protection available against STIs, against the fact that condoms are not universally effective protection against *all* STIs. A more open climate would also help in ensuring that the needs of all are catered for in terms of both health promotion and delivery of sexual health services. This would be of particular benefit to communities which are currently marginalised by mainstream messages and services, such as black and ethnic minority communities and gay, lesbian, bisexual and transgender communities.

Finally, there remains a significant challenge to address not only individual and societal attitudes towards sex and relationships, but also the impact of an increasingly vociferous minority. In recent years we have seen a growth of fundamentalist movements which poses a real threat to sexual health and which are standing in the way of improvements in treatment and services. Most notably, this movement has concentrated its efforts on opposing abortion, and is starting to gain ground in pushing for a reduction in the time limits. Other areas which have also come under threat include SRE, particularly with the growth of the abstinence movement, which was born out of Christian fundamentalism in the United States (www.lifeway.com/tlw; www.silverringthing.com/index.html). Those who hold these extreme and conservative views are a tiny but vocal minority, and it is vital that they are actively challenged at all levels to ensure that their influence does not grow further.

Conclusions

We have come a long way in the field of sexual health over the last decade, but there remains a long way to go. Sexual health is now slowly being established as a central feature of the public health agenda at the national level, and there have been significant improvements in the prioritisation of and investment in sexual health services. It has taken a real crisis to prompt this change, but we should not have to wait for a further crisis in order to turn this change into long-lasting improvement.

Recent policy developments have, quite rightly, focused on the short-term needs of sexual health services, and should help to deliver significant service improvements within the next few years. What we now need is a more long-term and strategic approach to the sexual health of the nation as a whole, which recognises the positive benefits that good sexual health can bring as well as the savings to be accrued from preventing sexual ill health. Policy makers and professionals will need to work together to engender a more positive and holistic approach to sex and relationships, which in turn should help to achieve the ultimate goal of a population with the knowledge and skills required to negotiate good sexual health, for life.

References

All-Party Parliamentary Pro-Choice & Sexual Health Group (2004) *NHS Abortion Services: a report on a survey of primary care trusts*. London: TSO.

BHIVA, PACT and Terrence Higgins Trust (2005) *Clinical Trials? The third annual survey of how English HIV and sexual health clinicians and primary care trusts view their services*. London: Terrence Higgins Trust.

Department of Health (2001) *Better Prevention, Better Services, Better Sexual Health: the National Strategy for Sexual Health and HIV*. London: Department of Health.

Department of Health (2002) *The National Strategy for Sexual Health and HIV Implementation Action Plan*. London: Department of Health.

Department of Health (2004) *Choosing Health: making healthy choices easier*. London: Department of Health.

fpa (2002) *Use of Family Planning Services: factsheet number 2*. London: Sexual Health Direct.

Government Statistical Service (2003) *Statistical Bulletin, Abortion Statistics, England and Wales: 2002, Bulletin 2003/23*. London: TSO.

Government Statistical Service (2004) *Statistical Bulletin, Summary Abortion Statistics, England and Wales: 2003, Bulletin 2004/14*. London: TSO.

Health Protection Agency (2004) *HIV and other Sexually Transmitted Infections in 2003, Annual Report 2004*. London: HPA.

House of Commons Health Committee (2003) *Sexual Health: third report of session 2002–03, volume I*. London: TSO.

LaMontagne DS, Fenton KA, Randall S *et al.* (2004) Establishing the National Chlamydia Screening Programme in England: results from the first full year of screening. *Sex Transm Infect.* **80**: 335–41.

Mawer C and McGovern M (2003) *Early Abortions: promoting real choice for women*. London: fpa.

National Assembly for Wales (2000) *A Strategic Framework for Promoting Sexual Health in Wales*. Cardiff.

Office for National Statistics (2001) *Health Services Quarterly 17 – report: conceptions in England and Wales, 2001*. London: ONS.

Office for National Statistics (2005) *Health Statistics Quarterly – conceptions: annual numbers and rates by area of usual residence for women aged under 18 at conception (England and Wales residents)*. London: ONS.

Scottish Executive (2005) *Respect and Responsibility: a strategy and action plan for improving sexual health*. Edinburgh: Scottish Executive.

Silver Ring Thing: www.silverringthing.com/index.html.

Social Exclusion Unit (SEU) (1999) *Report on Teenage Pregnancy*. London: SEU.

Teenage Pregnancy Unit (TPU) (2005) *Progress Report March 2005*. London: TPU.

True Love Waits: www.lifeway.com/tlw.

Chapter 18

Mental health

Lionel Joyce

The continuing shame

Millions of lives are destroyed by the stigma of mental illness (*Guardian* 2004) with discrimination occurring at every level of society and in all professions. It was directly instrumental in at least two high-profile deaths (North London Strategic Health Authority 2003) and probably many more. This stigma is further compounded by active racism (Norfolk, Suffolk and Cambridge Strategic Health Authority 2003) in the statutory services.

Stigma is only one complication of mental illnesses that affect one in four people in the course of their lives. Circa 4,500 people commit suicide each year (Samaritans 2004), with a high but reducing representation among young men (National Suicide Prevention Strategy for England 2005); people suffering from depression and schizophrenia account for 25% of this number. Some 45,000 people attempt suicide each year and 20% of these will go on to be successful (Mental Health Foundation 2005).

Adults with mental health problems are one of the most disadvantaged groups in society. Although many want to work, fewer than a quarter actually do – the lowest employment rate for any of the main groups of disabled people. Too often they do not have other activities to fill their days and spend their time alone (Social Exclusion Unit 2004).

All this in addition to the experience of debilitating illness, the loneliness, bewilderment and other discomforts of symptoms, the side effects of many treatments, all compounded by the fear of compulsory detention.

History

The BBC history series on Colney Hatch (BBC Website 2003) describes how the asylum movement developed and played out in relation to this hospital as follows:

> *The great asylum movement of the late nineteenth century followed appalling scandals involving embezzlement, rape and murder at the York Lunatic Asylum and at Bethlem in London. The reforming physician and later the medical superintendent at Colney Hatch, John Conolly (1794–1866), reported widespread use of all manner of restraints in his 1842 report. He had found straitjackets, hand and leg cuffs, and 'coarse devices of leather and iron' used in most asylums. Although care and cure were among the aims of the more enlightened the key requirement of asylums was safe custody. (Colney Hatch) was originally designed for less than 1,000 patients. Before long this increased to 2,000 and by the First World War to 3,500. The front of the building was nearly 2,000 feet in length, with towers at each side, and had the longest*

corridor in Britain. Occupying 20 acres of the site was a 600-seat chapel, farm buildings, a workshop, yards and lodges. There was also a kitchen garden, cemetery and other land including a 160-acre farm. By the 1870s the whole area was so dominated by the presence of the Colney Hatch Asylum, that the very name, Colney Hatch, would strike dread into people's hearts and even blighted development in the area.

Hospitals reproducing this model were built in every county and to serve every city. Their chapels and main buildings are still visible in most parts of the country.

The number of patients in mental hospitals reached its peak in 1955 (350 per 100,000 pop), despite some attempts to achieve care in more normal settings such as the Maudsley Hospital in the 1930s. Three landmark events were the 1959 Mental Health Act, the Hospital Plan (Ministry of Health 1962) and Community Care (Ministry of Health 1963) papers of 1962 and 1963. Jed Boardman in *Beyond the Water Towers* (Bell and Lindley 2005) makes clear that although three forces were at work – the open-door policy, new medication and the drive to put care back into the community – new drugs were less significant than is popularly believed. The dramatic decline in hospital population was to be achieved by a significant growth in community facilities, but this was more noticeable by its absence and the inability of the professions to develop new ways of working.

The development of services in the community followed a model of patch-based community mental health teams (CMHTs), comprising a consultant psychiatrist, 2–4 community psychiatric nurses (CPNs), 2–3 approved social workers (ASWs approved to make decisions in relation to the Mental Health Act over detention of patients), serving a population of between 25,000 and 50,000. Psychiatric units on district general hospital sites (DGH units), where the admission wards of the old psychiatric hospitals were more or less reproduced, supported these teams.

Genuine innovation was rare – the Long Benton Project in North Tyneside sited a combined inpatient, outpatient and day patient facility in a centre of population – managing on many less beds and being popular with patients: in Bradford a CMHT managed with no inpatient beds. But these were few and far between with huge variation in the quality of services.

Several factors then came into play – a new Labour government, a clear evidence base for different ways of working emerged from New Zealand and Australia and a new agency was created to bring systematic improvement across the services.

The National Institute for Mental Health, England (NIMHE)

The National Institute for Mental Health (in England) was established to support health and social care communities to develop their services, in line with the vision outlined in the *National Service Framework for Mental Health* (Department of Health 1999, 2004). Although a national organisation, NIMHE was particularly structured to help achieve national policy by focusing on local solutions, through its eight regionally based development centres.

In a significant attempt to achieve a more 'joined up' approach, on 1 April 2005, NIMHE formed – along with seven other initiatives that have had a role in supporting service improvement – the Care Services Improvement Partnership (CSIP) (www.sourceuk.net/indexf.html?06013). CSIP will build upon NIMHE's locally focused approach but will broaden the agenda to support also service improvement in relation to children, the elderly, people with a learning disability and health in the criminal justice system.

The user movement

The rise of the effective user movement can be traced to the MIND conference at Brighton in 1985. This introduced the Dutch model of advocacy to the UK that was quickly adopted by Nottingham – which became a leader in the user movement – and Newcastle. Both of these developed strong groups of users and experimented with different types of representation (patients' councils, advocacy), and user-run services. Lambeth introduced the Clubhouse model from the US as a way of delivering user-run services and South-West London became (and remains) the leader in the employment of service users. It became first fashionable and then essential to engage users in service design and in some aspects of management. This remains variable, with Merseycare having users on all staff appointments and a full-time user executive director, while Sheffield has a broad-based user council that determines much of the culture (e.g. the managers should not wear ties).

Formal recognition of the role of users was given by the creation of the 'expert by experience' (www.nimhe.org.uk/networks/experts.asp), a national programme with a constitution giving a structured role for users and carers in:

- developing mental health services for service users and carers
- promoting the delivery of effective mental health services
- monitoring the effectiveness of mental health services
- identifying and evaluating tools to measure outcomes, which assess quality of life
- research into the desired outcomes for service users and carers.

However, the number of user-run services has not grown beyond the few clubhouses, and the days of the user-run crisis service seem to be well in the past.

The Social Exclusion Unit (SEU)

The Prime Minister established the SEU in 1997 initially as part of the Cabinet Office, but the unit was moved to the office of the Deputy Prime Minister (ODPM). In 2003 the SEU was given the remit to consider what more could be done to reduce social exclusion among adults with mental health problems. Following extensive consultation in 2003, the report was published in 2004 (SEU 2004). This contained a number of shocking statistics, with a focus on unemployment and associated social isolation as a factor in suicide, the gross costs of £77 billion per annum to the economy and the specific costs of sickness and invalidity benefits. Over 900,000 adults in England claim sickness and disability benefits for mental health conditions, with particularly high claimant rates in the North. This group is now larger than the total number of unemployed people claiming Jobseekers' Allowance in England (Office for National Statistics 2004). The report was accompanied by a series of fact sheets suggesting courses of action and further information. It may prove a watershed in focusing attention on the real issues for people with mental illness of:

somewhere to live
someone to love
something to do

which would serve as a greater prophylactic than yet another drug development or service re-organisation. Users have expressed the view that the support they need is closer to a life coach than a CPN (What a consumer driven service would look like 2005).

Stigma

Learning from both feminism and race awareness issues does not seem to have transferred across to mental health. There is no equivalent to Gay Pride – Mad Pride (www.ctono.freeserve.co.uk) is not yet a movement – or to the race and sex awareness training that is mandatory in many large organisations.

The government, while fully aware of the damage of stigma and its prevalence (*see* SEU 2004), has allocated only the same funds that were available in 1998 – £1 million per annum.

An obvious leader in this area would be the NHS, with around 200,000 members of staff a year suffering mental illness, but it is regarded by many of its staff as worse than the private sector (personal communication, conversation with senior occupational health director) and only equalled by the medical profession (*see also* North London Strategic Health Authority 2003) in its disinterest and disdain. The economic case for effective positive discrimination to help people with severe mental illness can be illustrated by reference to bipolar disorder. It is reasonable to estimate around 1,000 doctors have bipolar disorder. The combined cost of training this workforce is £50 million; the replacement costs are £50 million with a 10-year time lag. It is reasonable to ask why there is an almost total absence of effective support and help on the one hand and a climate that tolerates stigma on the other.

The workforce

The key workers in mental health are psychiatrists, psychiatric nurses, social workers and psychologists. Throughout the 1990s staff shortages became a key issue, so that by 2000, the Sainsbury Centre for Mental Health stated that there were vacancy levels of 14% for consultant psychiatrists, with 85% of trusts reporting difficulties in filling nursing posts, shortfalls of clinical psychologists and 10% vacancy levels for occupational therapists across the NHS. There was no central planning or information on the mental health workforce nationally and the seriousness of the situation only became apparent through the House of Commons Select Committee and independent reports. In addition to existing problems, the expansion of services required as a result of the National Service Framework (Department of Health 1999) created a potential shortfall in excess of 10,000.

There were few experiments with different types of worker throughout this period and none particularly radical – the Workforce Action Team (Workforce Action Team 2001) was established to consider the issues and eventually recommended the creation of the new posts of support, time and recovery workers (who are often recovered or recovering users who provide support), gateway worker (to help GPs manage and treat common mental health problems) and community development worker (to work with people from black and minority ethnic communities). These do not challenge the existing professional hierarchy or roles but seek to patch up a system which cannot meet its staffing needs.

The voluntary sector

It was MIND (the National Campaign for Mental Health) that did much to drive the changes in mental health treatment in the 1960s. It effectively harnessed the outraged liberal conscience to the cause of large numbers of people in psychiatric hospitals and a sloppy and arrogant psychiatric profession, with poor or non-existent evidence base for decision making. This enthusiasm dissipated in the 1980s in the 'me' generation and has not been harnessed so effectively since. MIND has become the leading user organisation, while Rethink reflects the views of many carers as well as sufferers. Campaigning has become an insider activity, with bodies like the Sainsbury Centre for Mental Health and the Mental Health Foundation using evidence and research to win arguments, rather than passion and fury.

The Tory policy of introducing the market to health was picked up wholesale by the Labour government in 2000, and this has opened the door to the voluntary sector becoming a genuine alternative service provider. The sector has not yet matured to the point where it can rise above its petty jealousies and viciously competitive nature to offer genuinely a different type and style of provision. Unless there is an extraordinary growth in organisational development leading to organisation maturity, it is unlikely that the voluntary sector will be anything more than peripheral for the next 10 years.

The NHS lacks the courage to create a genuine mental health service: the NHS mental health trusts, therefore, sit and watch as their growth money goes to fund waiting list initiatives in surgery and trolley waits in accident and emergency. The NHS continues to be dominated by the medical model, while the voluntary sector, slowly overcoming its anti-psychiatry bias, has yet to pioneer effective alternatives.

Legislation

On 20 December 2000 the government published the white paper *Reforming the Mental Health Act* (Department of Health 2000). An alliance of some 50 service user, professional, service provider, trade union and voluntary organisations quickly came together to campaign to improve the proposed legislation. They sought improvement on eight main issues (Mental Health Alliance 2001).

1 To reduce compulsory admissions – the Act would increase them.
2 Right to a comprehensive assessment of needs without being eligible for compulsory detention.
3 Rights of access to advocacy.
4 Urgent safeguards for people with long-term incapacity who need care and treatment for their mental health problems.
5 Legally enforceable advance statements on their care and those they want involved.
6 A specific duty for full information to be given and for the individual's informed consent to be sought.

7 Relevant representation on the new mental health tribunal.
8 A reconsideration of the policy that non-offenders could be detained under the proposed system, regardless of whether or not they can be treated (*see* below).

Dangerous and severe personality disorder (DSPD)

The phrase DSPD only entered the public consciousness in the last 10 years, and came to particular prominence with the idea that people should be detained indefinitely because they might commit crimes in the future. In December 2004 the UK government published a white paper for a new mental health act (Department of Health 2000) (*see* above). This provoked a response from many sources, including civil liberties groups and psychiatrists (Farnham and James 2001). The heart of the issue relates to the overlap between risk and personality disorder (PD). The problem is that the risk and personality disorder literatures speak to different audiences and with different languages. Hence people in the criminogenic/offending world focus on stable/dynamic risk factors, which people in health would construe as personality characteristics, while in health settings the clinical targets that are focused often relate to the 'criminogenic needs' of the individual but with a different language set.

The common factor underpinning both risk and PD is the patient's inflexible, maladaptive, rigid interpersonal style. It is the impulsivity, poor problem solving, and rigid patterns of interpersonal functioning which lead to crime or, in clinical parlance, these stable, dysfunctional patterns of functioning are the defining characteristics of personality disorder.

The dichotomy can be explored through the two literatures. There is the 'what works' literature (McGuire 1995), *Guidelines from Research and Practice* (*see* Bonta, Law and Hanson 1998) outlines issues and practice in correctional settings, together with risk factors and risk literature that focus on changing risk, and the PD literature (*see* Livesley 2001, 2003; Sperry 2003) on changing interpersonal functioning. The clinical issue is to identify for each individual the aspects of their personality disorder (e.g. callousness, impulsivity, affective instability), which relate to the criminogenic risk factor (e.g. lack of empathy, poor problem solving, anger problems).

Drugs

Drug treatment is still the first choice in both specialist and primary services. The evidence base for talking therapies has been growing steadily since the mid-1980s and these – particularly cognitive behaviour therapy (CBT) and its derivatives – are now part of most treatment plans. Unfortunately, there remains a shortage of practitioners and delivery arrangements are haphazard. There is a strong new movement, lead by Christopher Dowrick of Liverpool University, to persuade GPs to re-assess their approach to depression and anxiety and to devote more time to patients (Dowrick 2004). In part, this is a reaction to the excessive prescribing of SSRIs (selective serotonin re-uptake inhibitors) and signals a return to a more holistic role for general practice. It also acknowledges the evidence of exercise, and other lifestyle choices, as both a response and a prophylactic. SSRIs became the new panaceas in the 1990s, spawning an enthusiastic literature (*Prozac Nation*, Wurtzel 1994) and massive fortunes for the pharmaceutical industry.

Doubts, both about the medicalisation of life problems and the harmful nature of these drugs, have been emerging for some time, with serious doubts about both starting and stopping Seroxat (Paroxetine or Paxil) – prompting a Panorama programme (http://news.bbc.co.uk/1/hi/programmes/panorama/2310197.stm).

The most promising development for the more severe illnesses has been the creation of the atypical antipsychotic medication Clozaril (clozapine), which can only be prescribed with weekly blood tests – making it expensive – and risperidone. In the small number of cases for which these drugs work they transform lives. The real challenge is to find equally effective drugs for the remainder of those who suffer schizophrenia and bipolar disorder (manic depression).

Dual diagnosis

Dual diagnosis is the term applied to people with mental illness who also use drugs and alcohol. Some illnesses, such as bipolar, are correlated with alcohol abuse. There is a debate, with strong racial overtones, about the role of cannabis in psychosis. The NHS has been confused in its response, with dual diagnosis exemplifying the problem of professional specialisation, (are you drugs and alcohol trained – if not can you really treat?), and silo thinking – there are two different lead bodies, NIMHE and the National Treatment Agency (NTA), with different funding streams, beliefs and cultures. There is still not a well-described service response to this long-standing phenomenon.

Conclusion

Mental health is the term used for mental illness, rather than any attempt to promote mental wellbeing (though the arrival of emotional intelligence and the idea of emotional literacy give this approach new potency). Like much to do with mental illness it is an unconvincing attempt to conceal the indifference which characterises statutory bodies – national and local, social care or the NHS – towards the plight of millions. The effort needed to confront the messy, complex business of mental illness treatment, protecting and caring for difficult individuals and stigma, exceeds the will available.

Successive governments have acknowledged the social consequences of mental illness. There is some reason to believe that each press outrage about an atrocity committed by a person with mental illness is used to strengthen the right-wing, anti-libertarian agenda, and gives the government another ally for detention without trial, identity cards and the like. Some attempt to fashion a more humane response to these tragedies, to address the causes rather then seeking to blame, would signal a new seriousness. More explanation is needed for the absence of any meaningful attempt to tackle stigma when it is costing the taxpayer huge sums of money.

References

BBC Website (2003) *Beyond the Broadcast – making history.* www.bbc.co.uk/education/beyond/factsheets/makhist/makhist7.

Bell A and Lindley P (eds) (2005) *Beyond the Water Towers.* London: The Sainsbury Centre for Mental Health.

Bonta J, Law M and Hanson K (1998) The prediction of criminal and violent recidivism among mentally disordered offenders: a meta-analysis. *Psychological Bulletin*. **123**: 123–42.

Department of Health (1999) *National Service Framework for Mental Health: modern standards and service models for mental health*. LAC (99) 34. London: DH.

Department of Health (2000) *Reforming the Mental Health Act*. London: Stationery Office.

Department of Health (2004) *Framework (and the NHS Plan) Underpinning Programme: workforce, education and training*. London: DH.

Dowrick C (2004) *Beyond Depression – a new approach to understanding and management*. Oxford: Oxford University Press.

Farnham FR and James DV (2001) Dangerousness and the law. *The Lancet*. 8 December. **358**.

Guardian (2004) Report on social exclusion. Action on Mental Health. 14 June.

Livesley WJ (2001) *Handbook of Personality Disorders: theory, research, and treatment*. New York: Guilford.

Livesley WJ (2003) *Practical Management of Personality Disorder*. New York: Guilford.

McGuire J (1995) *What Works: reducing reoffending*. New York: Wiley.

Mental Health Alliance (2001) *The White Paper – Reforming the Mental Health Act – a briefing from the Mental Health Alliance*. www.mentalhealthfoundation.org.uk.

Mental Health Foundation (2005) *People and Issues – Statistics*. www.mentalhealth.org.uk.

Miller Dr L (2004) Private discussion. Doctors' Support Network.

Ministry of Health (1962) *Hospital Plan for England and Wales*. London: Ministry of Health.

Ministry of Health (1963) *The Development of Community Care*. London: Ministry of Health.

National Suicide Prevention Strategy for England (2005) *Second Annual Report*. London: Department of Health and NIMHE.

Norfolk, Suffolk and Cambridge Strategic Health Authority (2003) *Independent Inquiry into the Death of David Bennett*. Norfolk, Suffolk and Cambridge Strategic Health Authority.

North London Strategic Health Authority (2003) *Independent Inquiry into the Deaths of Daksha Emson and her daughter Freya*. North London Strategic Health Authority.

Office for National Statistics (2004) *Labour Market Statistics*. May. London: Office for National Statistics.

Samaritans (2004) *Information Resource Pack*. www.samaritans.org.

Social Exclusion Unit (SEU) (2004) *Mental Health and Social Exclusion – Social Exclusion Unit Report*. June. London: SEU ODPM.

Sperry L (2003) *Handbook of Diagnosis and Treatment of DSM-IV-TR Personality Disorders*. New York: Brunner-Routledge.

What a consumer driven service would look like (2005) Blackwell Grange Hotel, Darlington, 15 April. Workshop sponsored by Durham and Darlington MH NHS Trust.

Workforce Action Team (2001) *Adult Mental Health: national service*. London: Department of Health.

Wurtzel E (1994) *Prozac Nation: young and depressed in America – a memoir*. London: Quartet Books Ltd.

Chapter 19

Alcohol

Geof Rayner

According to the Royal College of Psychiatrists (2005) alcohol is 'our favourite drug' (www.rcpsych.ac.uk/info/factsheets/pfacalc.asp). For centuries alcohol has delighted and perplexed society in equal measure. For many it is an innocent and enjoyable pleasure, but for others – medical bodies, the police, public health campaigners – the easily identified positive aspects of alcohol are set against its adverse medical, criminal justice, and broader health and social consequences. While evidence on the scale of alcohol-related harm remains powerful the ultimate policy-defining reality, and the source of industry power and influence, is that the production, retail, export of alcohol is of major industrial significance, with massive benefits for the Exchequer. Through adept lobbying the alcohol drinks industry has been successful in normalising perceptions of the drug and shifting policy makers' attention away from rising patterns of consumption, particularly among vulnerable groups. Despite rising media attention given to alcohol-linked anti-social behaviour the power of the industry and its sway of government helps explain why public health considerations have been marginalised and interventions to curtail patterns of harm limited in their impact. This chapter sets out the health and social impact of alcohol, examines the economic position of the alcoholic drinks industry, and examines the recent evolution of alcohol policy.

Health and social impact

According to the World Health Organization, alcohol-related death and disability accounts for 4.0% of the global burden of disease, ranking it fifth within 26 separate factors, and, perhaps surprising for many, at a similar level to tobacco. In developed economies like Britain – and as with most of the rest of Europe – alcohol is the third most detrimental health risk factor, accounting for 9.2% of the disease burden (Babor *et al.* 2003). Unlike tobacco its major negative consequences are experienced by a limited subset of its consumers, albeit with a broad spread of those indirectly affected. Unlike tobacco, alcohol – as with some illicit drugs – does appear to have some beneficial health properties – provided it is consumed in moderation. Research in France – a high consumption country suggests that 2–5 glasses per day of wine is associated with a 24–31% reduction in all-cause mortality, chiefly due to reductions in heart disease (Renaud *et al.* 1998). The assumption of some beneficial aspect to the moderate consumption of alcohol – whatever its factual basis – contextualises contemporary alcohol policies in the UK, despite the long history of policy making focusing on its deleterious social, health and industrial consequences. In terms of the benefits of alcohol, it has been pointed out that the impact for individuals may differ substantially from benefits identified at the aggregate level (Rehm *et al.* 2003). The promotion of 'sensible drinking' – the core message of current policy – may indeed apply to the majority but in practice a significant proportion of alcohol consumption occurs among heavy drinkers (defined in terms of men consuming eight or more units and women consuming six or more units on at least one day) – or young people in the process of developing alcohol dependency. Heavy drinking is associated with a wide syndrome of medical harm, including increased risk of death from causes such as breast cancer, damaged heart muscle (cardiomyopathy), inflammation of the liver (alcoholic hepatitis), scarring of the liver (cirrhosis) and cancers of the mouth, throat, oesophagus and colon (Fuchs *et al.* 1995). Alcohol can produce memory loss and depression (Uekermann *et al.* 2003). It can induce direct physical harm from ingestion (poisoning) and substantially increases injury risks (Watt K *et al.* 2004). People who both drink and smoke have a much higher risk of throat cancers than those using tobacco or alcohol alone, accounting for around three quarters of all oral and pharyngeal cancers (Blot *et al.* 1988).

If there is less dispute on the link between *individual* consumption and harm – universally disapproved of in government and by the alcoholic drinks industry itself – there is much less attention directed at the rising levels of alcohol consumption. The consequences are nevertheless clear. The rising trends of alcohol consumption have occurred parallel to a rising burden of alcohol-related disease. The number of deaths in England directly attributable to alcohol misuse, such as heart disease and liver cirrhosis, rose sharply in the second half of the 1990s, from 3,853 a year in 1994 to 5,508 in 1999 (Department of Health 2001) (*see* Figure 19.1).

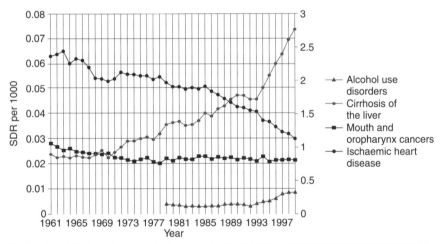

Note: Chronic mortality time-series measured on two axes. Ischaemic heart disease on right axis and the other causes on the left

Figure 19.1 Chronic mortality. *Source*: WHO Global Status Report on Alcohol (2004).

Industry arguments share the view that alcohol is an ordinary commodity which, like other ordinary commodities, can also be used inappropriately. An alternative public health perspective might be that, notwithstanding its common and everyday use, alcohol remains a drug with major health and social consequences and that this capacity for harm, and its minimisation, should assume the policy making centre ground (Babor *et al.* 2003). The resolution of this dispute largely in terms favourable to marketplace perceptions indicates both the economic power of the alcoholic beverage industry and conversely the relative political marginality of public health.

This does not result from a 'failure of evidence' but rather an expression of the fact that other practicalities determine the interpretation of evidence (Marmot 2004).

Evidence on the impact of alcohol is hardly in short supply; it has been documented, and for that matter legislated upon, for hundreds of years. Today we have a far more precise picture on the medical and social consequences of alcohol and of its field of effects. Older morality or disease-based models of understanding have largely been displaced by a more rounded view encompassing medical, mental health, sociological and physical risk dimensions. The public health perspective draws upon all of these.

Alcohol is implicated in sexual violence where both perpetrator and victim have been drinking (Finney 2004). It plays some part – often the major part – in road and industrial accidents, suicides, and other violent events. Alcohol is implicated in one in seven of road deaths and despite what has generally been observed as a sea change in public attitudes towards drink driving following on from successive social marketing campaigns, the number of drink-drive accidents rose from 10,100 in 1998 to 11,780 in 2000 (DETR 2000, 2001).

The consequences for families is also more nuanced than in the past. It has been suggested that the quality of parental interaction with children is more important than the frequency of parental drinking (Johnson 2002). Some researchers have suggested that mood and anxiety disorders among heavy drinking parents may have had a greater impact on the mental health of children than misuse of alcohol *per se* (Preuss *et al.* 2002). And while there appears to be a strong relationship between parental use of alcohol and family problems it is the latter that have greater impact in stimulating depression, anxiety, or loss of self-esteem in the later adult life of affected children than does alcoholism (Dooley 1997). This is not to minimise the corrosive impact of alcohol. A significant body of research shows that children in families with substance problems experience feelings of loneliness, social isolation, and chaos in the world around them (Watt 2002).

The government's alcohol strategy, *Drinking Responsibly*, confirms a picture of substantial alcohol related harm:

> In 2002/03, 1.2 million violent crimes were alcohol related and 44% of all violent crime was fuelled by alcohol. 35% of all attendances at hospital accident and emergency departments are related to alcohol as are 70% of those which occur between midnight and 5 a.m. One in five violent incidents take place around pubs or clubs. All this carries with it a high bill, with crime and disorder costs alone estimated to amount to £7.3 billion a year.

The total bill to society is estimated to be £20 billion (Department for Culture, Media and Sport *et al.* 2005). However, according to critics, the overall tenor of policy making, in which *Drinking Responsibly* is but one part, is considered to be highly accommodating to the industry, principally by understating the link between mounting harm and rising consumption levels – the latter being no more than a mark of the industry's success in marketing its products.

Alcohol use in the UK

Closer analysis suggests that the volume of alcohol consumed by a population only roughly approximates to the actual level of observed harm. Different groups consume alcohol in a variety of ways and drinking culture and mode of consumption have significant modifying effects. In the UK high consumption of alcohol over a short period (binge drinking), linked to antisocial behaviour, has largely displaced older images of alcohol misuse focused on street alcoholism. Binge drinking is not new and has been a feature of Britain and elsewhere in northern Europe for at least a millennia.

In recent decades the total volume of alcohol consumed in the UK has been moderate compared to some other European countries (Rayner 2003). This is changing. Whereas consumption has been falling steadily in France the UK saw the largest proportional increase in alcohol consumption in Europe between 1997 and 2004, moving up to ninth position (World Advertising Research Centre 2004). Increases in consumption has been paralleled by a shifting product mix; tradition-ally, the UK has been cast a 'beer-drinking' country. Figure 19.2 shows trends in household expenditure on different forms of drink. Recent industry data shows that by 2005 wine had overtaken beer in total sales (Modern Brewery Age 2005).

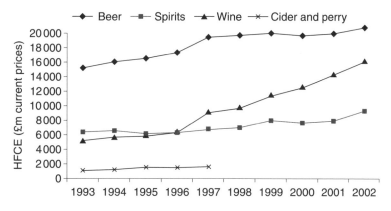

Figure 19.2   Household Final Consumption Expenditure (HFCE) at current prices on alcoholic drinks according to type (1992–2002). *Source*: *Consumer Trends*, ONS; *The Drink Pocket Book 2004*.

To these changing overall patterns of consumption can be added changing pat-terns of drinking varying by age, sex, or other demographic variables. In the UK abstinence is limited to around 11% for males and 14% for females (Hemström *et al.* 2002). According to the General Household Survey in 2002/03, around two thirds of adults aged 16 and over in Great Britain had consumed an alcoholic drink on at least one day during the previous week (74% of men and 59% of women). Of these nearly 30% exceeded the recommended daily benchmark (four units for men and three units for women) on at least one day during the previous week (General Household Survey 2004).

The issue which has most captured public attention has been the increase in teenage and youth drinking. A European-wide survey found that UK teenagers were near the top of the international league for binge drinking, drunkenness and experience of alcohol problems. Around half the boys and girls reported drinking five or more drinks in a row at least once in the previous month; 40% (42% boys, 38% girls) reported having been drunk at the age of 13 or younger; 48% of boys and girls reported having been drunk at least once in the last month. Young people under the age of 16 were drinking twice as much today as they did 10 years ago, and reported getting drunk earlier than their European peers. Not only was the purchase (although by law, not the consumption) of alcohol illegal, but the age of onset of drinking is occurring earlier (Grant *et al.* 2001). Early drinking tracked into young adulthood potentially leaves adolescents at increased risk of becoming long-term, heavy drinkers (Andersen *et al.* 2003; Bonomo *et al.* 2004).

The alcohol economy

A key element to the evolution of public policy on alcohol – and prominently featured in the opening pages of government reports – is the economic position of the alcoholic drinks industry. The alcoholic drinks market in the UK is worth around £27 billion, with the government netting £11.5 billion per annum in tax revenue. British registered Diageo, with more than 200 brands and presence in 180 countries, is the world's largest drinks company with a turnover of £10 billion a year. Scotch whisky is one of the United Kingdom's top five export earners with exports representing around 90% of sales and British distillers are among the largest in the sector. Over 70% of UK-produced gin and 30% of vodka is exported to over 200 countries (Gin and Vodka Association of Great Britain 2002). Alcoholic drinks production employs around 34,400 in direct manufacture and possibly half a million more in bars, pubs and other establishments. Such outlets have recently been identified as a force for regeneration in declining city centres. In London (while clearly not a declining urban centre) there was an estimated increase of 37% in London's bar jobs between 1995 and 2001, outstripping an overall growth of 16% in jobs in London over the same period (Roberts 2004).

The economic factors provide a powerful backdrop to drinks industry claims that alcohol is an ordinary commodity and that further restrictive 'moral' burdens from the past should be shed. These arguments have received a wide hearing. The government's Better Regulation Task Force (now Better Regulation Commission) argued that a more liberal licensing regime would have the effect of helping to take away *'some of the unnecessary burdens from this important industry and allow it to grow in the modern world'* (Cabinet Office 1998). Drinking was now to be viewed as purely a matter of consumer choice: *'Regulation should not be used – except through truly extreme constraints – to influence the volume and frequency with which the individual drinks'* (COI 1988). Underscoring the arguments for liberalisation has been the attractive view that easier access for consumers to alcohol in convivial settings would bring the UK closer to the ideal as found in the southern European countries, where binge drinking has been largely absent.

At least in part, the retail side of the drinks industry has moved in the opposite direction, away from the protectiveness of communal, intergenerational restraints and towards segmented markets. One factor explaining the rise in youth drinking has been the emergence of retail bar chains marketing nationally advertised youth brands, a trend which emerged as an industry response to the loss of market share to dance drugs and bottled water:

> *The marketing of alcohol products as recreational drugs, complete with the motifs of youth clubbing culture, became a staple of brewing industry advertising campaigns in the early to mid nineties and has continued as one of a range of market targeting strategies.* (Brain 2000)

This comes at the end of earlier trends first noted in the 1960s. National branding became an increasingly prominent factor in the decline of ale (a more localised product requiring time and skill) which, prior to 1960, commanded virtually all of the UK beer market. Accompanying the consolidation of ownership of production and brand management has been consolidation of ownership at point of sale. In 2002 it was estimated that in large provincial centres multiples controlled approximately two thirds of the pub market with corporate dominance a rising feature of the growing nightclub sector (Chatterton and Hollands 2003).

The Better Regulation Task Force is merely one conduit of industry influence. Another successful mode of engagement has been through the industry-funded Portman Group. This organisation was represented on the Advertising Standards Council (which adjudicates on alcohol advertising), the Better Regulation Task Force – now Better Regulation Commission – (which commended the Department of Health for 'downsizing' its functions and staffing in 2004), the Cabinet Office Strategy Unit's Alcohol Advisory Group (responsible for the national alcohol strategy) and the Scottish Advisory Committee on Alcohol Misuse. As a small organisation representing industry interest it was able to convert what might otherwise have been portrayed as self-interested industry arguments into palatable policy formulae and a lever for industry voluntary self control.

The new alcohol policies

Several competing policy drivers have been noted. These have included drinks industry pressure to deregulate and to 'normalise' alcoholic drinks consumption, exchequer income, the attractive prospect of inner-city regeneration, employment opportunities, rising concern over binge drinking and antisocial behaviour, and lastly evidence of harm. These drivers pull different ways, requiring the determinacy of some over others and the fragmenting of policy in pursuit of the different objectives. As noted, economic drivers carry more weight than public health concerns.

Certainly the first significant measure under the current government provided immediate evidence of the power of the drinks lobby. The licensing white paper *Time for Reform* (DCMS 2001) – subsequently delayed in implementation – promised the modernisation of alcohol licensing through abolition of the system of permitted hours alongside the claim – consonant with that of the Better Regulation Task Force – that this would bring about reductions in drink-related offences and in arrests for such offences and reductions in binge drinking and drunkenness on the streets. Limited evidence was presented to support this thesis. In essence the approach retained the characteristics of previous responses to alcohol problems (in classifying certain groups – binge drinkers – as 'the problem') but completely reversed the hitherto regulatory approach previously employed (in favour of the liberalisation of access). The Alcohol Harm Reduction Strategy for England appeared in early 2004, long after strategies for Wales, Northern Ireland and Scotland and 3 years after proposals to liberalise licensing. In his foreword the Prime Minister observed:

> alcohol misuse by a small minority is causing two major, and largely distinct, problems: on the one hand crime and anti-social behaviour in town and city centres, and on the other harm to health as a result of binge- and chronic drinking. (Cabinet Office 2004)

The impact of chronic drinking is acknowledged but it is said that such problems are limited to 'a small minority', a viewpoint which belies evidence found in the report of a broadening population profile of problematic drinking, only some of which could be categorised as binge drinking or which involved antisocial behaviour. The accompanying strategy was defined in four parts: better education and communication, improving health and treatment services, combating alcohol-related crime and disorder, and working with the alcohol industry. Critics of the policy noted that these four strategies were indeed required elements but that overall there was no concordance between the title of the report – *An Alcohol Reduction Strategy* – and strategies for the reduction in the consumption of alcohol overall. One critic drew attention to the statement in the report that there was no direct correlation *'between drinking behaviour and the harm experienced or caused by individuals'* (Plant 2004). (Plant omits the word 'behaviour' from this attribution.)

Alcohol harm prevention, primarily through reducing the exposure to alcoholic drinks among young people, can be an effective measure for reducing harm later in life. Public health measures, properly structured and integrated, have the potential to give high benefits for low returns. These range from drink-driving programmes, providing they are integrated with detection, the reduction of physical availability and taxation (Babor *et al.* 2003). On the other hand educational campaigns, the central element of the Alcohol Harm Reduction Strategy, have poor results, presumably because alcohol advertisers have a much stronger message, far greater resources, and an enticing product. And in the European context, some of the levers of prevention are now subject to agreement with other member states, particularly in the case of the harmonisation of excise duties and any potential measures around the restriction of advertising.

In the strategy reference is also made to *Choosing Health* (Secretary of State for Health 2004), the overall public health strategy for England, to follow, and complement, the alcohol strategy and in which it is stated that this will provide *'an excellent opportunity to learn more about how government can motivate individuals, and how individuals can motivate themselves to make responsible choices about drinking'*. When *Choosing Health* appeared one of the commitments made therein was to *'Work with the Portman Group to cut down binge drinking, including a new information campaign'* (Department of Health 2004).

Drinking Responsibly, a consultation on measures to restrain antisocial behaviour, followed on from these earlier reports and strategies and continued much of their individualistic emphasis, but it also returned to themes first aired in *Time for Reform*. The recommended actions focused on 'alcohol disorder zones', increased fines for licensed premises, and the French-style abolition of fixed closing times – this last measure on the grounds that fixed times encouraged binge drinking and resulted in *'large numbers of young people hitting the streets simultaneously causing the Police significant difficulties'*.

The emerging approach was fully in accordance with the views of the Portman Group, whose response to *Choosing Health* included the following: *'any prevention interventions in respect of health-specific issues should involve a strong emphasis on individuals taking personal responsibility for their drinking choices'* (Portman Group 2004). The Advertising Association (in its response to the Alcohol Harm Reduction Strategy) put it slightly differently: *'Responsibility for ending the binge drinking culture must also lie with the individual just as much, if not more, than it lies with the industry and licensed premises'* (Advertising Association 2003).

The implication which emerges from the recent evolution of alcohol policies for England, is consonant with, if not fully derived from, the views put forward by the alcoholic drinks industry and its marketing associates – this being that overconsumption of alcohol is an individually hedonistic trait; in effect a behaviour pathology within an otherwise blameless consumer trend of easier access to alcohol, albeit exacerbated by some rogue suppliers.

Conclusion

The social and health problems of alcohol are hardly limited to Britain but Britain has a profile of problems, influences and policies which are mostly unique. Though for much of the last century Britain has occupied the lower parts of the European range of consumption, problematic consumption has increased – while those of our nearest Continental neighbour have been in decline. Binge drinking is not a distinctively British 'vice', as noted this is shared with other northern European countries. The attempt to induce a cultural shift in the mode of consumption from the northern to the southern European type (implying drinking with meals, group and community pressure to restrict binging or antisocial behaviour) appears, for the present at least, to have been unsuccessful, as has the industry-modelled, social marketing-based, re-education programme to induce 'sensible drinking'. For critics, what emerges is less a public health strategy for reducing alcohol-related harm than an industry strategy to contain negative public perceptions of alcohol, to limit the purview of government regulation, and to refocus attention on the consumer rather than the provider of alcohol drink.

References

Advertising Association (2003) *Response to the Department of Health and Strategy Unit National Alcohol Harm Reduction Strategy Consultation Document.* 15 January. London: Advertising Association.

Andersen A, Due P, Holstein BE and Iversen L (2003) Tracking drinking behaviour from age 15–19 years. *Addiction.* **98**(11): 1483–4.

Babor TF, Caetano R, Casswell S *et al.* (2003) *Alcohol: no ordinary commodity – research and public policy.* Oxford and London: Oxford University Press.

Blot WJ, McLaughlin JK, Winn DM *et al.* (1988) Smoking and drinking in relation to oral and pharyngeal cancer. *Cancer Research.* **48**(11): 3282–7.

Bonomo YA, Bowes G, Coffey C *et al.* (2004) Teenage drinking and the onset of alcohol dependence: a cohort study over seven years. *Addiction.* **99**(12): 1520–8.

Brain KJ (2000) *Youth Alcohol and the Emergence of the Post Modern Alcohol Order.* Occasional Paper No. 1. London: Institute for Alcohol Studies.

Cabinet Office (1998) *Better Regulation Task Force Welcomes Liquor Licensing White Paper.* Press release. London: Cabinet Office.

Cabinet Office (2004) *Alcohol Reduction Strategy for England.* Prime Minister's Strategy Unit. March. London: Cabinet Office.

Central Office of Information (COI) (1988) *Better Regulation Task Force.* July. London: COI, p.7.

Chatterton P and Hollands R (2003) *Urban Nightscapes: youth cultures, pleasure spaces and corporate power.* London: Routledge.

Department for Culture, Media and Sport, Home Office, Office of the Deputy Prime Minister (2005) *Drinking Responsibly, the Government's Proposals.* London: DCMS.

Department for Culture, Media and Sport (2001) *Time for Reform.* London: DCMS.

Department of Health (2001) *Statistics on Alcohol: England 1978 onwards.* Statistical Bulletin 2001/3. London: Department of Health.

Department of Health (2004) *Summary of Intelligence on Alcohol.* London: Department of Health.

Department of the Environment, Transport and the Regions (DETR) (2000) *The Casualty Report.* London: The Stationery Office.

Department of the Environment, Transport and the Regions (DETR) (2001) *Road Accidents Great Britain*. London: The Stationery Office.

Dooley SY (1997) Comparison of adult children of alcoholic families with adult children from non-alcoholic families: a replication. *Dissertation Abstracts International*. **57**(7): 2875-A–2876-A.

Finney A (2004) Alcohol and sexual violence: key findings from the research. *Home Office Findings 215*. London: Home Office.

Fuchs CS, Stampfer MJ, Colditz GA *et al*. (1995) Alcohol consumption and mortality among women. *N Engl J Med*. **332**(19): 1245–50.

General Household Survey (2004) London: Office for National Statistics.

Gin and Vodka Association of Great Britain (2002) *2002 Budget Submission: the case for reducing excise*. London: Gin and Vodka Association of Great Britain.

Grant BF, Stinson FS and Harford TC (2001) Age at onset of alcohol use and DSM-IV alcohol abuse and dependence: a 12-year follow-up. *Journal of Substance Abuse*. **13**(4): 493–504.

Hemström Ö, Leifman H and Ramstedt M (2002) The ECAS survey on drinking patterns and alcohol-related problems. In: T Norström (ed.) *Alcohol in Postwar Europe: consumption, drinking patterns, consequences and policy responses in 15 European countries*. Stockholm: Almqvist and Wiksell International.

Johnson P (2002) Predictors of family functioning within alcoholic families. *Contemporary Family Therapy*. **24**(2): 371–84.

Marmot M (2004) Evidence based policy or policy based evidence? *BMJ*. **328**: 906–7.

Modern Brewery Age (2005) Wine sales overtake beer in Great Britain. *Modern Brewery Age*. **29 August**.

Plant M (2004) The alcohol harm reduction strategy for England. *BMJ*. **328**: 905–6.

Portman Group (2004) *Choosing Health, a Consultation to Improve People's Health: response of the Portman Group*. London: Portman Group.

Preuss UW, Schuckit MA, Smith TL *et al*. (2002) Mood and anxiety symptoms among 140 children from alcoholic and control families. *Drug and Alcohol Dependence*. **67**(3): 235-42.

Rayner G (2003) Global consumption of alcohol. In: E Millstone and T Lang (eds) *The Atlas of Food*. Brighton: Myriad Editions.

Rehm J, Room R, Graham K *et al*. (2003) The relationship of average volume of alcohol consumption and patterns of drinking to burden of disease: an overview. *Addiction*. **98**(9): 1209–28.

Renaud SC, Gueguen R, Schenker J and d'Houtaud A (1998) Alcohol and mortality in middle-aged men from eastern France. *Epidemiology*. **9**: 184–8.

Roberts M (2004) *Good Practice in Managing the Evening and Late Night Economy: A Literature Review from an Environmental Perspective*. London: University of Westminster/The Office of the Deputy Prime Minister. September.

Royal College of Psychiatrists (2005) *Alcohol: our favourite drug. Fact sheet*. www.rcpsych.ac.uk/info/factsheets/pfacalc.asp (accessed 9 September 2005).

Secretary of State for Health (2004) *Choosing Health: making healthy choices easier*. Cm 6374. London: The Stationery Office.

Uekermann J, Daum I, Schlebusch P *et al*. (2003) Depression and cognitive functioning in alcoholism. *Addiction*. **98**(11): 1521–9.

Watt K, Purdie DM, Roche AM and McClure RJ (2004) Risk of injury from acute alcohol consumption and the influence of confounders. *Addiction*. **99**(10): 1262–73.

Watt TT (2002) Marital and cohabiting relationships of adult children of alcoholics: evidence from the National Survey of Families and Households. *Journal of Family Issues*. **23**(2): 246–65.

World Advertising Research Centre (2004) *World Drink Trends 2004*. Henley on Thames: published in association with Commissie Gedistilleerd.

Chapter 20

Transport

Harry Rutter

Increasing recognition of the public health importance of transport in recent years has been accompanied by a shift in focus away from direct harms, such as those of injuries and air pollution, to a broader health-promotion perspective that considers issues such as physical activity, sustainability, and access to goods and services.

A modal shift away from cars to increased walking and cycling would improve health, reduce inequalities, and lessen the environmental impacts of transport. Many of the interventions required to achieve a modal shift of this sort, such as high-quality urban planning and design, lower speeds, and reallocation of road space, would be likely to improve health in other ways through reduced injuries, greater social cohesion, and better quality of life.

Transport patterns

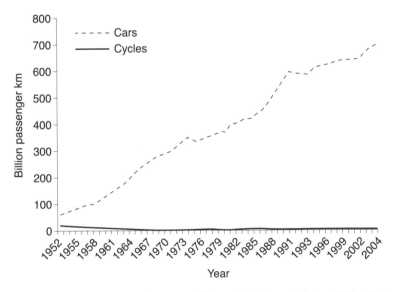

Figure 20.1 Passenger transport by car and bicycle in Great Britain 1952–2004. *Source*: DfT 2005a.

In the latter half of the 20th century car traffic increased over tenfold, while cycling fell by over 80% (*see* Figure 20.1) (DfT 2005a). Around 80% of journeys under one mile are made on foot, with an average walking journey distance of 0.6 miles (DfT 2003c). Cycling accounts for less than 1% of total distance travelled, an average of 39 miles per person per year (DfT 2003b). Almost two thirds of all trips are made by car, with an average trip length of just under nine miles (DfT 2003a). Adults living in households without a car both walk and cycle more than those in households with access to a car. Children in non-car-owning households walk over a third more than those in households with a car. In real terms, over the last 20 years the overall cost of motoring has remained roughly the same, while public transport fares have risen by over a third (DfT 2004a).

Air travel has grown enormously in recent years, from 46 million passenger movements in 1977, the year Sir Freddie Laker started the first low-cost airline, to 200 million in 2003. Department for Transport forecasts in 2000 predicted a rise in patronage to around 400 million passenger movements in 2020 (DfT 2005a).

Impacts of transport

Physical activity

Evidence for the health benefits of physical activity has been accumulating since Morris showed in 1953 that bus conductors had lower rates of heart attacks than bus drivers (Morris *et al.* 1953). There is now an extensive and reliable body of evidence on the health benefits of physical activity (Pate *et al.* 1995), ranging from reductions in heart disease (Berlin and Colditz 1990), high blood pressure (Paffenbarger *et al.* 1978), stroke (Hu *et al.* 2000), cancer (Thune and Lund 1996) and diabetes (Horton 1991), to improved mental health and wellbeing (Roth and Holmes 1987), and enhanced cognitive function (Kramer *et al.* 1999) and independence among older people (Province *et al.* 1995). These have been clearly outlined in a report from the Chief Medical Officer (Department of Health 2004a) and reinforced in the public health white paper, *Choosing Health.* (Department of Health 2004b). This has been followed up by an action plan (Department of Health 2005) which emphasises the importance of transport, especially active travel, in supporting physical activity.

Active travel, in the forms of walking and cycling, allows the integration of physical activity in the daily routine, but the cheapness and dominance of the car has encouraged living, working, education and commuting patterns that make it impossible for many people to use these modes to travel to work, go shopping, or drop their children at school. For those who can cycle to work the potential health benefits are appreciable: a study of around 30,000 people in Copenhagen followed up for almost 15 years, of whom around 7,000 were regular cycle commuters, found a relative risk of all-cause mortality among the cyclists that was over 25% lower than among the non-cyclists (Andersen *et al.* 2000).

Injuries

In 2004 there were 3,221 deaths, around 30,000 people killed or seriously injured, and over 200,000 injuries on UK roads. Cyclists made up around 4% of the total mortality, with 134 deaths, while pedestrians made up 20% with 671 deaths (DfT 2005b).

Hillman's work in the early 1990s showed that the number of life years gained as a result of the health benefits of regular cycling outweighed those lost through road deaths by at least 20:1 (Hillman 1993) yet the perception persists that cycling is a dangerous activity. This is not borne out by the facts: in 2004 in the UK there was one cyclist death per 37 million km cycled.

Deaths from traffic injury should be placed in the context of around a third of deaths from coronary heart disease being attributable to sedentary lifestyle (McPherson *et al.* 2002). With around 114,000 people dying each year of coronary heart disease this means that over ten times as many people die through lack of activity than on the roads. Improving safety, and making walking and cycling more appealing, could help to tackle both these problems at the same time.

There are many misapprehensions around injury data. Injury incidents are, fortunately, rare, and tend to be widely spatially distributed. Raw numbers of injuries do not reflect exposure to danger. Numbers may be low because pedestrian and cyclist traffic at a site is low, and their behaviour defensive, rather than because the true level of danger at a site is low. Appropriate denominators of exposure are rarely used in injury statistics.

Although deaths and serious injuries are well reported, minor injuries are not, and there is significant under-reporting of them. The official record may not accurately reflect what has happened at a particular location in terms of 'minor' injuries. 'Minor' injuries are, of course, unlikely to appear so to those who suffer them, even if they are not hospitalised.

When people make decisions on their travel behaviour it is almost invariably based on their perception of danger rather than the true level of risk. Thus it is the perception of danger that matters when trying to influence people's mode choices: if people believe walking and cycling to be dangerous, even if it is not, they are unlikely to use these modes. This sets up a vicious cycle when in fact what is needed is a virtuous cycle, as the more people who walk and cycle the safer it is for everyone. This has been shown in analyses of injury levels related to active travel levels in a range of different cities (Jacobsen 2003) (*see* Figure 20.2).

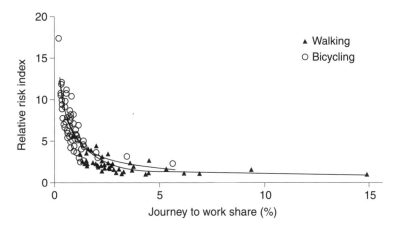

Figure 20.2   Walking and cycling in 68 Californian cities, 1998. *Source*: Jacobsen 2003.

The majority of drivers will exceed a 30 mph speed limit on a free-flowing road, and there is a close relationship between vehicle speed and likelihood of killing a pedestrian hit by a vehicle. If the distribution of speeds is plotted on the same graph as the speed–danger relationship it becomes apparent that at a population level the majority of the danger being imposed is by drivers travelling at or slightly above the 30 mph speed limit (*see* Figure 20.3).

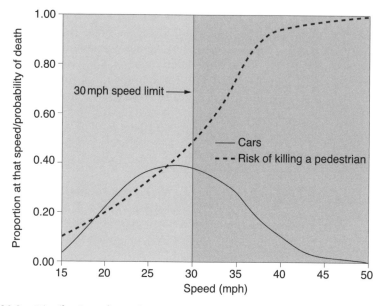

Figure 20.3 Distribution of speeds on 30 mph roads and risk of killing a pedestrian hit by a car. *Sources*: DfT 2002; Proctor 1991.

In 1997 Sweden adopted a road safety strategy known as Vision Zero. The Vision Zero approach treats traffic as a complex system which has to adapt to take better account of the needs, mistakes and vulnerabilities of road users: it places the onus on the system and its administrators to reduce injuries, rather than primarily on the individuals using the system. The four core principles of the strategy are (WHO 2004):

- **ethics**: human life and health are paramount and take priority over mobility and other objectives of the road traffic system
- **responsibility**: providers and regulators of the road traffic system share responsibility with users
- **safety**: road traffic systems should take account of human fallibility and minimise both the opportunities for errors and the harm done when they occur and
- **mechanisms for change**: providers and regulators must do their utmost to guarantee the safety of all citizens; they must cooperate with road users; and all three must be ready to change to achieve safety.

This approach, which places the vulnerability of the human body to injury at the heart of transport design and regulation, demonstrates a paradigm shift away from a transport system that is concerned with emphasising mobility to one that emphasises safety, and thus health.

Air pollution

Transport produces over 90% of carbon monoxide (CO) emissions, almost three quarters of nitrogen oxide emissions, and over half the PM_{10} particulates emissions[1] in Great Britain (DfT 2004a). Diesel vehicles are a major source of nitrogenous and particulate emissions, while petrol vehicles generate nitrogen oxides, CO, and volatile organic compounds. Catalytic converters can be quite effective at reducing these emissions once warmed up, but in urban areas, where there are many short journeys from cold starts, catalysts are much less effective. Both petrol and diesel engines produce carcinogenic emissions in varying proportions (COMEAP 1999a). Although modern emission tests are very stringent, questions have been raised about the degree to which they reflect real-world driving (Samuel *et al.* 2005a, 2005b) and engine management systems can be programmed to produce optimal emissions in the face of specific testing cycles.

Air pollution is associated with increased mortality and morbidity; there are over 8,000 premature deaths every year as a result of exposure to PM_{10}s, and around 3,500 due to sulphur dioxide (SO_2) (COMEAP 1998). It is not possible to quantify the effects of nitrogen dioxide and carbon monoxide but there is evidence to suggest that exposure to current levels of these pollutants affects health (COMEAP 1999b).

Social networks and community severance

Social networks tend to be good for health (Berkman and Syme 1979; House *et al.* 1988); busy roads may disrupt such networks, thus harming health. Widespread car use also results in fewer people interacting on the streets in the ways that pedestrians and cyclists are able to. Busy roads sever communities; a study of three streets in San Francisco in the 1970s elegantly demonstrated this by showing that the busier the traffic on a street the more fragmented the social networks, and the lower the satisfaction of residents (Appleyard and Lintell 1972). One aspect of this study, the number of neighbours known to residents in each street, is illustrated graphically in Figure 20.4 using lines to indicate social links between people in different properties.

This presents a challenge for planners, who are charged with reconciling the needs of residents, pedestrians and cyclists – local users – with those of people passing through an area. Research across Europe (ARTISTS 2005) has identified a range of ways in which these functions can be balanced, but shifting from a paradigm that sees streets as being primarily for cars to one that gives primacy to the needs of local users will take more than good practice guidance.

Inequalities and access

Some groups of people are disproportionately affected by the health impacts of traffic, especially children, the elderly, the poor and those who are otherwise marginalised (Bly *et al.* 1999). At the same time these groups are the least likely to have access to a car or bicycle. There are major socio-economic differences in car access and distance travelled: less than 40% of households in the lowest income quintile have a car compared to over 90% in the highest income quintile (DfT 2004a). In 2002/03 people in the highest household income quintile travelled, on average, nearly three times as far (11,000 miles) as those in the lowest income quintile (3,800 miles).

---

[1] PM_{10}: particulate matter generally less than 10 micrograms in diameter.

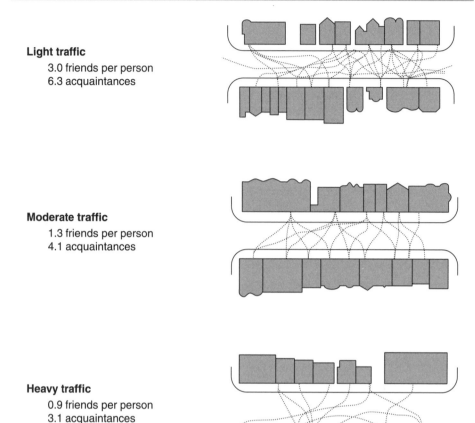

Light traffic
3.0 friends per person
6.3 acquaintances

Moderate traffic
1.3 friends per person
4.1 acquaintances

Heavy traffic
0.9 friends per person
3.1 acquaintances

Figure 20.4 Social networks in three San Francisco streets with differing traffic flows. Reproduced from Rogers (1997), and in turn based on Appleyard and Lintell (1972).

There are also socio-economic gradients for injuries, with children in social class V five times more likely to die as pedestrians than those in social class I (Abdalla *et al.* 1997). Children and young people suffer a disproportionate amount of deaths and injuries, peaking in the early teens (*see* Figure 20.5).

Transport does, of course, have a very positive side: people travel in order to gain access to goods, services, employment, friends and family, leisure pursuits, and healthcare. But the freedom cars bring has encouraged social developments that have resulted in increasing car dependence. Policy and planning trends over the last 40 years, since the publication of the Buchanan report (Buchanan 1963) in 1963, have favoured the private car over all other modes. Most motoring expenses (such as depreciation, tax and insurance) are paid up front, so the marginal costs of car use are low, and drivers don't pay for the externalities they impose (i.e. the health, environmental and social costs imposed by drivers on others). The increasing cheapness and accessibility of driving, in conjunction with planning decisions based around expectations of car use, have driven societal changes that have resulted in the need for many people to travel much greater distances than they previously would have done.

Many supermarkets, for example, are now situated outside or on the edge of towns, many rural areas have lost their shops, and it is normal even in cities for people to drive to work.

Access is a particular issue for health services, which are required most by the young and the old: groups that have limited use of cars. This is an issue for primary as well as secondary care facilities, and may be a particular problem in rural areas. Almost half of people without cars find it difficult to get to hospital (*see* www.dft.gov.uk/stellent/groups/dft_transstats/documents/page/dft_transstats_026297.hcsp). Accessibility planning is increasingly being used by local authorities, and to some extent healthcare organisations, to address these problems. It is a concept that arose from a Social Exclusion Unit report (www.social exclusionunit.gov.uk/publications.asp?did=229) in 2003 in an attempt to tackle the social exclusion associated with poor access to jobs, healthcare and other services. It has four stages: an accessibility audit; an audit of resources; an action plan; and monitoring (DfT 2003d). Accessibility planning is a requirement in the 2004 guidance on local transport plans.

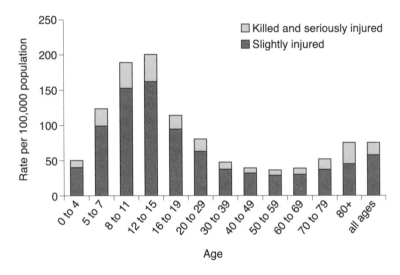

Figure 20.5   Pedestrian casualty rates by age. *Source*: DfT 2005b.

Environment

Emissions of CO_2 from transport in the UK increased from 26 to 35 million tonnes of carbon between 1980 and 2002. The share of CO_2 emissions attributable to transport increased from 16% in 1980 to 24% in 2002. The conclusions of the Expert Group on Climate Change and Health in the UK (Department of Health 2002) are that the likely effects of climate change on health in the UK include an increase in heat-related and a decrease in cold-related deaths, as well as a range of other effects due to more extreme weather, changes to patterns of disease-causing organisms and vectors, problems of access to services resulting from flooding, and global impacts resulting from population migration elsewhere in the world. Measures taken to reduce the rate of climate change by reducing greenhouse gas emissions could produce secondary beneficial effects on health, such as increases in zero-emission active travel.

The 2003 energy white paper set a target of a 60% reduction in CO_2 emissions by 2050. This stringent target is based on a target concentration of CO_2 of 550 parts per million (ppm), although it seems increasingly likely that lower limits around 400 ppm will be required (International Climate Change Taskforce 2005). This will mean that much greater cuts in CO_2 are needed. But even the 60% target poses a major challenge, and if it is to be achieved will almost certainly require huge reductions in motorised travel, especially aviation. Low or zero emission fuels, notably hydrogen, are only zero emission at the tailpipe; the energy that produces them has to come from somewhere. Although we may yet see the majority of our power being generated in nuclear power stations this, and renewables such as biofuels, replaces the environmental problem of climate change with a range of other environmental problems.

Cars produce road noise, engine noise, and other noise, such as slamming doors or loud car stereos at night. Around a third of people report that road traffic noise has worsened in the last 5 years, while only around 15% feel it has improved. There is a substantial loss of amenity from road building across attractive countryside, road signs in urban and rural areas, and the appearance of vehicles themselves. Over the period 1991–2000, a net total of about 10,600 hectares of land in England was changed to transport use; this is roughly equivalent in size to the urban area of the City of Leicester. In addition to the loss of land, and the danger and disruption caused by construction itself, road building also affects health through quarrying and other methods of extracting the raw materials (DfT 2004b).

Although motor manufacturers are often keen to promote the benefits of apparently 'clean' forms of transport, such as electric cars, these vehicles generally have little if any public health advantage over others apart from moving the production of polluting by-products away from the vehicle to the power station. While this is beneficial in highly polluted urban environments, it does not, of course, reduce any of the other impacts of cars on individuals, communities or the environment.

Challenges for the future

Reducing the amount of motorised travel that is undertaken would help reduce all the negative impacts of transport – congestion, pollution, injuries. Even accessibility problems could be lessened by this in the long term as reduced travel overall would act as a pressure on spatial planning to reduce the need to travel. But all the trends point in the opposite direction with people making more trips and travelling greater distances.

The challenges for the future lie in reconciling the enormous demand for travel that now exists, across all modes, with the need to support healthier lifestyles and ensure sustainable development. The growth in car usage cannot be justified in terms of its human or environmental impact. But many people are used to being able to travel how they like and when they like, and many of them live in places where maintaining their existing lifestyles would be difficult if not impossible without a car. In a culture that values the notion of 'choice', even if those choices are illusory, or narrowly framed, any perception that choice will be reduced or removed (such as through traffic restrictions, or road user charging) is likely to be fiercely resisted.

Rising to the challenge will require concerted action across a wide range of domains and disciplines. If public health professionals are successfully to improve health through transport we need to engage with a range of sectors that we may not be terribly familiar with: transport and spatial planners, architects, developers, employers. Learning to do this involves developing an understanding of different cultures, different approaches, and different sets of evidence. But if we do it well we have the potential to tackle a range of upstream measures with enormous potential to improve health and reduce inequalities.

References

Abdalla I, Barker D and Raeside R (1997) Road accident characteristics and socioeconomic deprivation. *Traff Engin Control.* **38**: 672–6.

Andersen LB, Schnohr P, Schroll M *et al.* (2000) All-cause mortality associated with physical activity during leisure time, work, sports, and cycling to work. *Archives of Internal Medicine.* **160**: 1621–8.

Appleyard D and Lintell M (1972) The environmental quality of city streets: the residents' viewpoint. *American Inst of Planners Journal.* **38**: 84–101.

ARTISTS (2005) *Arterial Streets Towards Sustainability.* Available from: www.tft.lth.se/artists/ (accessed 1 July 2005).

Berkman LF and Syme SL (1979) Social networks, host resistance, and mortality: a nine-year follow-up study of Alameda County residents. *American Journal of Epidemiology.* **109**: 186–204.

Berlin JA and Colditz GA (1990) A meta-analysis of physical activity in the prevention of coronary heart disease. *Am J Epidemiol.* **132**: 612–28.

Bly P, Dix M and Stephenson C (1999) *Comparative Study of European Child Pedestrian Exposure and Accidents.* London: DETR.

Buchanan CD (1963) *Traffic in Towns.* London: The Stationery Office.

Committee on the Medical Effects of Air Pollutants (COMEAP) (1998) *The Quantification of the Effects of Air Pollution on Health in the United Kingdom.* London: The Stationery Office. Available from: www.dh.gov.uk/PublicationsAndStatistics/Publications/Publications PolicyAndGuidance/PublicationsPolicyAndGuidanceArticle/fs/en?CONTENT_ID=400 6323&chk=s%2BUa%2Bx (accessed 1 July 2005).

Committee on the Medical Effects of Air Pollutants (COMEAP) (1999a) COMEAP statement on diesel v. petrol engined light vehicles. June. Available from: www.advisory-bodies.doh.gov.uk/comeap/statementsreports/diesel.htm (accessed 1 July 2005).

Committee on the Medical Effects of Air Pollutants (COMEAP) (1999b) COMEAP statement on *Transport and Health in London* by Stephen Glaister, Dan Graham and Ed Hoskins, October. Available from: www.advisorybodies.doh.gov.uk/comeap/statementsreports/ transport.htm (accessed 1 July 2005).

Department for Transport (DfT) (2002) *Vehicle Speeds in Great Britain 2002.* London: DfT. Available from: www.dft.gov.uk/stellent/groups/dft_transstats/documents/download-able/dft_transstats_508344.pdf (accessed 1 July 2005).

Department for Transport (DfT) (2003a) *Car Use in GB.* DfT personal travel factsheet. Available from: www.dft.gov.uk/stellent/groups/dft_transstats/documents/page/ dft_transstats_508295.pdf (accessed 1 July 2005).

Department for Transport (DfT) (2003b) *Cycling in GB.* DfT personal travel factsheet. Available from: www.dft.gov.uk/stellent/groups/dft_transstats/documents/page/ dft_transstats_508296.pdf (accessed 1 July 2005).

Department for Transport (DfT) (2003c) *Walking in GB*. DfT personal travel factsheet. Available from: www.dft.gov.uk/stellent/groups/dft_transstats/documents/page/dft_transstats_508289.pdf (accessed 1 July 2005).

Department for Transport (DfT) (2003d) *What is Accessibility Planning?* London: DFT. Available from: www.dft.gov.uk/stellent/groups/dft_localtrans/documents/divisionhomepage/032400.hcsp (accessed 1 July 2005).

Department for Transport (DfT) (2004a) *Transport Trends*. Available from: www.dft.gov.uk/stellent/groups/dft_control/documents/contentservertemplate/dft_index.hcst?n=9381&l=3 (accessed 1 July 2005).

Department for Transport (DfT) (2004b) *Transport Trends 2004: Section 8: Health and the environment*. London: DfT. Available from: www.dft.gov.uk/stellent/groups/dft_transstats/documents/page/dft_transstats_026311.hcsp (accessed 1 July 2005).

Department for Transport (DfT) (2005a) *Transport Statistics Great Britain*. London: Department for Transport. Available from: www.dft.gov.uk/stellent/groups/dft_transstats/documents/page/dft_transstats_041485.hcsp (accessed 8 June 2006).

Department for Transport (DfT) (2005b) *Road Casualties in Great Britain: main results: 2004 data*. London: DfT. Available from: www.dft.gov.uk/stellent/groups/dft_transstats/documents/page/dft_transstats_038553.hcsp (accessed 1 July 2005).

Department of Health (2002) *Health Effects of Climate Change in the UK*. London: Department of Health. Available from: www.dh.gov.uk/PublicationsAndStatistics/Publications/PublicationsPolicyAndGuidance/PublicationsPolicyAndGuidanceArticle/fs/en?CONTENT_ID=4007935&chk=aPZEuj (accessed 1 July 2005).

Department of Health (2004a) *At Least Five a Week: evidence on the impact of physical activity and its relationship to health*. London: Department of Health. Available from: www.dh.gov.uk/PublicationsAndStatistics/Publications/PublicationsPolicyAndGuidance/PublicationsPolicyAndGuidanceArticle/fs/en?CONTENT_ID=4080994&chk=1Ft1Of (accessed 1 July 2005).

Department of Health (2004b) *Choosing Health: making healthier choices easier*. London: Department of Health. Available from: www.dh.gov.uk/PublicationsAndStatistics/Publications/PublicationsPolicyAndGuidance/PublicationsPolicyAndGuidanceArticle/fs/en?CONTENT_ID=4094550&chk=aN5Cor (accessed 1 July 2005).

Department of Health (2005) *Choosing Activity: a physical activity action plan*. London: Department of Health. Available from: www.dh.gov.uk/PublicationsAndStatistics/Publications/PublicationsPolicyAndGuidance/PublicationsPolicyAndGuidanceArticle/fs/en?CONTENT_ID=4105354&chk=ixYz2B (accessed 1 July 2005).

Hillman M (1993) Cycling and the promotion of health. *Policy Studies*. **14**: 49–58.

Horton ES (1991) Exercise and decreased risk of NIDDM. *N Engl J Med*. **325**: 196–8.

House JS, Landis KR and Umberson D (1988) Social relationships and health. *Science*. **241**: 540–5.

Hu FB, Stampfer MJ, Colditz GA *et al.* (2000) Physical activity and risk of stroke in women. *JAMA*. **283**: 2961–7.

International Climate Change Taskforce (2005) *Meeting the Climate Challenge: recommendations of the International Climate Change Taskforce*. London: IPPR. Available from: www.americanprogress.org/atf/cf/{E9245FE4-9A2B-43C7-A521-5D6FF2E06E03}/CLIMATECHALLENGE.PDF (accessed 1 July 2005).

Jacobsen PL (2003) Safety in numbers: more walkers and bicyclists, safer walking and bicycling. *Injury Prevention*. **9**: 205–9.

Kramer AF, Hahn S, Cohen NJ *et al.* (1999) Ageing, fitness and neurocognitive function. *Nature*. **400**: 418–19.

McPherson K, Britton A and Causer L (2002) *Monitoring the Progress of the 2010 Target for Coronary Heart Disease Mortality: estimated consequences on CHD incidence and mortality from changing prevalence of risk factors*. London: National Heart Forum.

Morris JN, Heady JA, Raffle PAB *et al.* (1953) Coronary heart disease and physical activity of work. *Lancet.* **2**: 1053–7.

Paffenbarger R, Wing AL and Hyde RT (1978) Physical activity as an index of heart attack risk in college alumni. *Am J Epidemiol.* **142**: 889–903.

Pate RR, Pratt M, Blair SN *et al.* (1995) Physical activity and public health. A recommendation from the Centers for Disease Control and Prevention and the American College of Sports Medicine. *JAMA.* **273**: 402–7.

Proctor S (1991) Accident reduction through area-wide traffic schemes. *Traffic Engineering and Control.* **32**(12): 566–73.

Province MA, Hadley EC, Hornbrook MC *et al.* (1995) The effects of exercise on falls in elderly patients. A preplanned meta-analysis of the FICSIT Trials. Frailty and Injuries: Cooperative Studies of Intervention Techniques. *JAMA.* **273**: 1341–7.

Rogers R (1997) *Cities for a Small Planet.* London: Faber and Faber.

Roth DL and Holmes DS (1987) Influence of aerobic exercise training and relaxation training on physical and psychologic health following stressful life events. *Psychosom Med.* **49**: 355–65.

Samuel S, Morrey D, Fowkes M *et al.* (2005a) Real-world fuel economy and emissions of a typical EURO-IV passenger vehicle. Proceedings of the I MECH E Part D. *Journal of Automobile Engineering.* **219**(6): 833–42.

Samuel S, Morrey D, Fowkes M *et al.* (2005b) Real-world performance of catalytic converters. Proceedings of the Institution of Mechanical Engineers, Part D. *Journal of Automobile Engineering.* **219**(7): 881–8.

Social Exclusion Unit (2003) *Making the Connections.* London: Social Exclusion Unit. Available from: www.socialexclusionunit.gov.uk/publications.asp?did=229 (accessed 1 July 2005).

Thune I and Lund E (1996) Physical activity and risk of colorectal cancer in men and women. *Br J Cancer.* **73**: 1134–40.

World Health Organization (WHO) (2004) *Sweden's Vision Zero: no fatalities or serious injuries in road traffic.* WHO World Health Day 2004 website. Available from: www.euro.who.int/eprise/main/WHO/Progs/WHD4/20040212_2 (accessed 1 July 2005).

Chapter 21

Work and health: what direction for occupational health practice?

Kit Harling

The practice of occupational health has always been, and continues to be, concerned with the two way relationship between work and health (Faculty of Occupational Medicine 1998). It deals as much with the impact of work and working conditions on causes of ill health as it does with illness, injury or disability of the individual in determining a person's capacity for work activities.

The origins of the specialty of occupational health undoubtedly lie in the detection and prevention of the classical occupational illnesses. The lung diseases of coal miners (such as pneumoconiosis) and cotton workers (byssinosis) have largely disappeared: this is often through the disappearance of the industry as much as any improvements in hygiene at the workplace. However, diseases due to workplace exposures are still seen regularly and continue to exert their toll. Noise-induced hearing loss numbers millions among those afflicted and hand arm vibration syndrome, formerly known as 'vibration white finger', continues to affect hundreds of thousands of people in diverse industries. The prevention and identification of such diseases remains an important function of occupational health practice.

General improvements in safety at work have led to a reduction in accidents and death in the workplace with the current UK figure of around 220 deaths per annum (HSE) in a working population of approximately 30 million (HSE 2005). The industrial legacy of asbestos-related illness, although the material is rarely used at work now, kills nearly 3,000 people a year.

Despite undoubted improvements, a new generation of occupational diseases has emerged in the last two decades including work-related upper limb disorder and 'stress' characterised by less obvious or structural pathology.

In parallel with a concern for occupational diseases, occupational physicians have also been concerned with fitness for work – the impact of illness, injury or disability of whatever cause on employability and the ability to undertake work activities.

Historically, 'certifying doctors' were established nearly 200 years ago under the Factories Act 1833 and were initially employed to ensure that children applying for work had the 'ordinary strength and appearance of a child exceeding 9 years': in reality, the issue of a certificate by a certifying doctor absolved the employer of possible prosecution under the Act for employing underage children. It may be seen, however, as the start of one strand of 'Industrial Medicine' in Britain which came to play its part in the giant social reforms of the 19th century.

In the 20th century, the occupational health professional has always had the return of the ill or injured worker to their own job at the top of their list of functions. Indeed, Stewart in 1946, discussing the then new Disabled Persons

(Employment) Act 1944, said that rehabilitation and the supervision of the return of the sick or injured worker to work is one of the primary duties of an occupational physician.

The descriptions and terminology given to this strand of occupational health practice have often obscured this role from those not versed in the activity. Such clinical activity is often described (in the typical way of verbal shorthand) as 'company referrals' or 'managing sickness absence consultations'. These terms give no clue as to the underlying intent. However, it must be recognised that the terminology has seduced even some of the practitioners who may in reality focus on the short-term perceived needs of the employer rather than the broader advantages to all concerned of the successful rehabilitation of the worker.

By no means all, or even the majority, of those at work in the UK has access to an occupational health service. Research published in 2002 (Pilkington *et al.* 2002), on behalf of the Health and Safety Executive in Britain, showed that even on the broadest definition of occupational health (OH), only an estimated 40% of those in work could count on any OH support. The most prevalent provision was essentially a 'health and safety' service, focused on prevention of risks and compliance with the law. This reflects the balance between 'health' and 'safety' inherent in the application of the Health and Safety at Work Act 1974 over the last 30 years. It is of interest to note that the research was undertaken and reported in terms of the number of companies (of different type and size) that provide OH support, rather than the number of employees with access to services, again emphasising that OH was seen centrally as a matter exclusively for employers.

Separation of roles

Towards the end of the 19th century a small group of enlightened philanthropic employers provided healthcare for their employees, and sometimes their families, in the days before a national health service. So in the years running up to the Second World War there was, for a small number of employees at least, the provision of a comprehensive health service that dealt with the prevention of occupational disease, the treatment and management of both occupational and non-occupational disease and the rehabilitation of ill or injured workers back to employment. Thus, a model of integrated services existed, though it should be recognised that only a very small number of people had access to such services.

In the aftermath of the Second World War the NHS was created. This is not the place for a description of the creation of the NHS, which is in any event well known. Even then there were concerns about the costs of the service with Bevan apologising to Parliament when presenting the first annual budget for the NHS. He expressed the hope that the cost would reduce in future years as the health of the population improved with such a comprehensive healthcare provision.

At this point we see the separation of treatment services of all types from other healthcare provision. From the occupational health point of view, the NHS was not going to concern itself with the prevention of occupational disease, nor in large measure would it concern itself with returning ill or injured workers back to work – occupational rehabilitation. It would treat illness and injury such as lung disease, skin disease and back pain – whether caused occupationally or not – but the other matters such as prevention or occupational rehabilitation were rigorously excluded from its purview.

In my view this separation was the single most important factor shaping the development of occupational health services for the following 50 years. This separation of treatment from the other aspects of occupational health care led to an ever-widening divergence and lack of communication between those responsible for treatment services and those responsible for prevention and occupational rehabilitation. This gap stifled, with very few exceptions, the routine communications between those in the NHS treatment services and those outside.

This separation between those services provided by the state and those services funded by employers had an implicit assumption that matters pertaining to the relationship between work and health would be exclusively the concern of the employer. Who else would be interested in the prevention of occupational disease and its management in the workplace and what would the point of vocational rehabilitation be unless the employer, who controlled the workplace, willed it? It is only now with a recognition of the importance of social inclusion (SEU 2004) and legislative changes such as the Disability Discrimination Act that it is becoming acknowledged that those without current employment may have needs that fall within the field of occupational health.

The public health

What then of the relationship between health and work in the context of the public health? The latest UK review of public health was published as a white paper in November 2004. *Choosing Health: making healthy choices easier* (Department of Health 2004) marked the starting point for action to improve the health of the population. One chapter out of the six was devoted to work and health.

Workplaces have long been seen as an ideal setting for promoting health. For many years this has meant a focus on delivering 'standard' health-promoting messages – smoking cessation, improved diet, and more exercise – to the workforce. The target population was well defined and captive; cynics noted that employers were expected to pay for this service despite a lack of any specific benefit to the company. Nevertheless, the workplace remains a locus to get across health-promoting messages.

Choosing Health for the first time recognises that work and the workplace may play a very different role in promoting health. As I will discuss below, work itself has positive benefits on health and unemployment causes poor health. The workplace can be designed not only to prevent occupational illness or injury but can positively influence health in the broader sense. Much more work is needed in this area because as yet most of the evidence is of an association between workplace design and poor health: we need to prove that changing these features will improve health. The white paper commits the UK government to producing this evidence.

The evidence that lack of work results in poor health is also set out in the work and health chapter of *Choosing Health*. At the time of writing, only about 76% of the working-age population (WAP) is in work in the UK. Given a working-age population of about 38 million (ONS 2004) over nine million people could never have access to any occupational health support.

The figure of 76% of the WAP in work is derived from the whole population. For those individuals with disabilities, the figure is only about 50%: where the disability is of mental health, the percentage in work falls to about 20% (Labour Force Survey 2004).

About 2.7 million people in the UK are in receipt of incapacity benefit (long-term state benefit for those who are unable to work for health reasons): the figure has tripled in the last 25 years during which time the health of the UK population by most other measures has improved. Although there were structural reasons why the figure increased early in the quarter century when there was a rapid rise in unemployment, those features no longer operate. Looking at the declared causes of incapacity, around two thirds of the total is ostensibly caused by medical conditions like lower back pain, mild to moderate mental ill health and simple cardio-respiratory conditions such as hypertension and angina.

Careful consideration of the figures in the mental health category shows that the number of individuals with severe and enduring mental health problems has remained relatively static during this period. The growth has been entirely in what might be called mild to moderate mental ill health. There has been an enormous growth in the use of the term 'stress' to mean, among its other meanings, a long-term, work-preventing condition. These are conditions which should be relatively straightforward to manage from the medical point of view and as such should not, according to the medical model of work incapacity, prevent employment.

What then are the consequences of this lack of work? Those without employment have worse health, more illnesses, die younger and engage in riskier health behaviour; return to work is associated with improvements in health (quoted in *Choosing Health*, chapter 7).

Of course, not all work is good for health. The Whitehall II study for example has shown an association between certain features of work organisation and the risk of coronary disease. Occupationally caused diseases remain a threat with even traditional diseases such as noise-induced hearing loss still affecting millions of individuals.

Nevertheless, those in work enjoy a higher standard of health in general. However, the prevalent popular view, supported by lurid stories in the tabloid (and other) media, is that work is inevitably 'toxic', and thus to be avoided at all costs. This view combines in a risk-averse society with a concept that 'someone' must be to blame for any adverse event and avoidance of work is the only option.

Patients therefore come to primary care already conditioned by family and friends to the view that a return to work in the presence of any continuing symptom will inevitably result in rapid deterioration or relapse. It is little wonder then that general practitioners, in their role as patient advocate and to avoid any risk of making a condition worse, will readily comply with a request for a 'sick note'.

But it is clear that signing a patient off sick is not a health-neutral act. The longer an individual is off work, the less likely they are to return to employment. With lower back pain only 50% of those off work for 6 months are likely to resume work; by 12 months the proportion returning to work is 25%. The rest are condemned to a life of unemployment, poverty, poor health and social exclusion. Why then is the NHS not more focused on getting people back into work?

The UK government, and others, have recognised the dangers to society of having a large group of citizens excluded from the benefits of progress and forced into poverty, poor health and social exclusion. One way of alleviating such effects is through the provision of help to support those ill, injured or disabled back into employment. In a major shift in policy, the UK government launched *Pathways to Work* in 2003. This provided occupation-focused support to those claiming incapacity benefit; the process included health interventions directed at the psycho-social model of incapacity rather than duplicating treatment normally provided by the NHS.

Rehabilitation and occupational health

There has long been a recognition of the benefits of improving occupational health services (HSE 2000). Curiously, the approach to improving support to those who have work and are on long-term absence has been less focused. The *Framework for Vocational Rehabilitation* (DWP 2004) spent much time looking at terminology and titles without signalling a clear way forward or building on the approaches known to work: others, such as the British Society for Medical Rehabilitation in 2000, published a clear approach which commanded widespread support.

Traditionally the medical model of disability and incapacity for work has held sway. In this model the presence of disease pathology physically prevents an individual from undertaking work activities. That underlying condition is treated and the symptoms abolished. In this model the cure of illness and the resumption of 'health' will lead to the individual returning to work: all that is necessary is successful treatment and the abolition of symptoms. This model leads to the oft-repeated question of whether a particular absence is 'genuine' or if the individual is a 'malingerer'.

And yet this model is known to be incorrect. The changes associated with absence from work due to illness are complex. Simple matters such as loss of confidence and self-esteem are well known and are evident after only a few weeks. Many of those away from work through illness or injury develop depressive symptoms irrespective of the original cause of their absence. As described above, they may be receiving no doubt well-intentioned messages from family and friends who themselves believe that a return to work is positively dangerous and should be avoided.

A focus not only on the illness but on the psychological consequences and the social environment in which these changes take place is necessary for a rehabilitative approach to be effective. This so-called bio-psycho-social model is well described and the evidence is accumulating of its efficacy (Waddell and Burton 2004).

Even if this model was enthusiastically embraced by all those providing OH services, only a minority of WAP would get the support they need. Many workers will go on to long-term incapacity and even lose their jobs. To this group may be added the nine million people of working age who are not in employment.

It is unreasonable to believe that in the current (or indeed any reasonable future) climate the addition of occupational health services, free at the point of delivery, to the NHS would be politically acceptable. In the 'mixed economy' that is today's NHS, it is not necessary that occupational health – and the vocational rehabilitation that is an essential component – should be part of the NHS; there is no reason, however, why parts of the provision of occupational health services should not be within the NHS. What I believe is required is a new relationship between the NHS, employers and the providers, whether public or private, of occupational health type services. In addition, some way has to be found of providing services for those without a current employer.

Rather more importantly, the model used to underpin such rehabilitative services must change. The medical model implies a sequential approach. Treatment is undertaken until its completion at which point residual dysfunction is assessed. The remaining deficit is 'dealt with' by rehabilitation. The effectiveness of the bio-psycho-social model lies in its concurrent approach.

From the beginning of treatment, a message of likely return to work should be given. Features such as loss of training, loss of self-confidence and the emergence of depressive symptoms must be discussed and addressed. Even negative non-verbal communication will be seized on by patients and their families as confirmation of the dangers and improbability of a return to work. We do not administer medication with the message that it is unlikely to work and that the outcome is going to ruin future function. Why do we so often take this approach with return to work?

Treatment should be accompanied with a realistic view of what can be achieved. Recovery should be accompanied with measures to overcome barriers to returning to work. Employers can be involved from an early stage. Clinical confidentiality belongs to the patient, not the healthcare professional. With consent, and omitting unnecessary detail, the employer should be aware of progress and the changes that might be needed, if only on a temporary basis, to facilitate a return to work.

This may be seen by some as an increase in work for the healthcare professional. But if the result is an improved outcome for the patient, who would object?

At present there are no high-quality studies showing the positive cost benefit of such an approach: this reflects the difficulty of doing such studies as the *a priori* position is that there would be a large benefit over the myriad of costs associated with continuing ill health and unemployment.

The studies so far have been relatively short term and focused on direct costs rather than an integrated view of the total cost. The financial health of any country depends on tax from its population. Those on long-term incapacity pay less tax and receive benefit – that is to say they are a cost to society. The provision of appropriate help and support, returning such people to productive work, has the effect of reducing financial costs. Detailed work is already underway looking at the cost benefits of such approaches. This argument of course takes no account of the moral imperative or maximising an individual's inclusion within their society.

It is often argued that there would not be enough staff to develop a comprehensive occupational health and rehabilitation service for all those who are in employment, let alone those who currently have no work. If we were to use the traditional model of provision of services this may be true. There is no great reserve of either medical, nursing or other healthcare staff that can be suddenly deployed to make such an extension of service and the project figures for new healthcare workers over the next one or two decades does not give great optimism.

What is required is for those within the occupational health profession to look closely and critically at the work we do. We should ask whether or not all the tasks currently undertaken by a doctor, or a nurse, require the level of skill and expertise currently deployed. What are the possibilities of extending the roles of other healthcare professionals? What work indeed can be done by those without a healthcare background, but for whom we have identified the appropriate skills and competencies and delivered those by appropriate training? An unbiased look at the work of some in the voluntary sector would show examples of excellent practice.

The profession must show leadership. We must move away, as others have done, from doing everything oneself to recognising the importance of teaching, training, supporting and supervising the work of others. We must recognise the contribution that those with or without healthcare qualifications can play. We require a new approach to the delivery of services and a new emphasis. We must recognise that this will require new skills and competencies. Such change is essential if we are going to, as a prerequisite of improvement, change the attitude of the public and our colleagues in other healthcare work to the fundamentally beneficial relationship between work and health.

References

Department for Work and Pensions (DWP) (2004) *Building Capacity for Work: a framework for vocational rehabilitation*. London: DWP.

Department of Health (2004) *Choosing Health: making healthy choices easier*. Cm 6374. London: HMSO.

Faculty of Occupational Medicine (1998) *Core Curriculum for Occupational Medicine Training for Undergraduates* (2e). London: Faculty of Occupational Medicine.

HSE (2000) *Securing Health Together*. London: HSE Books.

HSE (2005) www.hse.gov.uk/statistics/index.htm.

Labour Force Survey (2004) www.statistics.gov.uk/CCI/nscl.asp?ID=6595.

ONS (2004) Website – population estimates 2004. www.statistics.gov.uk/CCI/nugget.asp?ID=6&Pos=1&ColRank=1&Rank=374.

Pilkington A, Graham MK, Cowie HA *et al.* (2002) *Survey of Use of Occupational Health Support*. Contract Research Report 445/2002. London: HSE.

Social Exclusion Unit (SEU) (2004) *Mental Health and Social Exclusion*. June. London: HMSO.

Stewart D (1946) Report of a discussion on the clinical consequences of the Disabled Persons (Employment) Act 1944. *Proc Roy Soc Med*. **39**: 158–62.

Waddell G and Burton K (2004) *Concepts of Rehabilitation for the Management of Common Health Problems*. London: The Stationery Office.

Chapter 22

Work and health: an overview of policy

Lord Hunt of King's Heath

As any health professional will tell you, people who work are more likely to be healthy and people who are healthy are more likely to work.

So getting people back into work and staying in work is vital if we are to reduce health inequalities and offer improved opportunities.

Both communities and the economy benefit from such an approach.

In the UK, we have one of the best health and safety records in the world and since 1997 have seen a 10% reduction in accidents at work.

Yet 35 million working days are lost every year to occupational ill health and injury. It is estimated that absence due to sickness costs around £12 billion a year – with costs to the public sector at around £4 billion.

As well as the impact on the health and wellbeing of employees and their families, unplanned absence puts additional pressure on those colleagues who pick up the extra work. It also has a significant impact on productivity.

While much good work, both inside and outside government, is already going on to improve the health and wellbeing of working-age people, a strategy was required to bring together all the elements.

So in October 2005 the Department for Work and Pensions launched a joint strategy with the Department of Health and the Health and Safety Commission/Executive to improve the health of working-age people.

The strategy has been structured around three key themes: engaging stakeholders, improving working lives and the healthcare of working-age people.

We want to implement the strategy, not by central government dictat, but through collective effort. So the success of our strategy depends on the support and participation of key people who have a role to play in improving and promoting the health and wellbeing of people of working age.

To generate awareness of our messages and to learn from the experts, we are creating national and local Stakeholder Councils. These bodies will involve a group of individuals, eminent in their field, whose experience and influence will help support the strategy.

We will be holding a Stakeholder Summit to determine the role of each stakeholder in helping achieve the vision.

Following the summit, we hope stakeholders will sign a charter setting out their role and the contribution they will make towards achieving our vision.

Of course, we need the views of everyone affected by the strategy – the entire working-age population. So we are planning to generate a national debate to help inform and change our thinking.

This will help to develop realistic and innovative proposals for the future direction of occupational health and wellbeing, and explore the funding issues that may arise from such proposals.

On the issue of improving working lives, we want to promote the benefits of a healthy and supportive working environment to all organisations and employees.

There are many organisations that already protect the health and wellbeing of employees. Yet we know that only 15% of all British firms provide basic occupational health support, and only 3% provide comprehensive support.

That is why we will launch Workplace Health Connect – a new service for small and medium-sized enterprises offering free and impartial advice on occupational health, safety and return to work issues.

The service will consist of an advice line covering England and Wales, and involve five regional pilots delivering free workplace visits to offer advice and support. This service will be delivered in partnership with the Health and Safety Executive (HSE) and in coordination with NHS Plus.

We recognise that the role of stakeholders, including health and safety representatives and GPs, is key if we are to achieve our goals.

We need to ensure effective links between GPs, occupational health professionals and employers are developed. We also need to improve the education of GPs in relation to health and work, and to assist them in providing better fitness-for-work advice to patients.

In order to ensure people take these issues seriously, the public sector needs to be seen as an exemplar in healthy workplaces and good occupational health practice. In other words, we need to practise what we preach.

The public sector employs approximately five million people, 1.3 million within the NHS alone. This equates to 20% of the workforce. Sickness absence rates in the public sector currently average 10 days per person per year, costing around £4 billion per year.

To address these issues, we have established a Ministerial Task Force for Health, Safety and Productivity, a cross-government Ministerial Forum tasked with driving improvements in sickness absence management in the public sector.

The HSE is also working with organisations across the public sector to deal with work-related stress through its management standards approach.

Our final theme is 'healthcare for working-age people'. We know that health problems can have a major impact on people's lives and their ability to work; even relatively common health problems such as musculoskeletal disorders can have a disproportionate effect if investigation and treatment are delayed or appropriate forms of rehabilitation are not available. This can lead to long-term absence, loss of self-confidence and even job loss.

We are now in a situation where once a person has been claiming incapacity benefit for a year, they are likely to continue claiming for a further 8 years – after 2 years they are more likely to die or retire than return to work.

So healthcare services need to be designed and delivered in a way that will help people to remain in work or support their return to work more quickly.

A key way of doing this is to support and engage healthcare professionals so they recognise the importance of work to their patients' wellbeing, and ensure they can fulfil their key role in making it easier for patients to remain in and return to work.

We also want to develop new ways of ensuring that employees can access investigation and treatment for health problems so they can stay in work and avoid unnecessary absences.

This could include the establishment of a clearer evidence base for decisions on assessment and prioritisation of clinical need – to build on recognition of the negative health impact of being away from work.

We will also look at ways of improving the management of common mental health problems as these can lead to long-term ill health.

On rehabilitation, we will build on the plans outlined in the *Framework for Vocational Rehabilitation*.

We know that rehabilitation brings benefits to individuals, employers and to society as a whole. The business argument for good health and safety management is crystal clear.

Businesses that develop programmes to promote good health and safety management have enjoyed benefits to the tune of £11 million of savings through reduced sickness absence and a reduction in health insurance spending of £200,000 a year.

But we recognise there are significant barriers to ensuring that rehabilitation is taken seriously.

A workshop organised by the Department for Work and Pensions (DWP) highlighted that creating the right environment where vocational rehabilitation can be offered goes wider than simply putting in place actual physical services.

This is a challenge almost unrivalled in terms of its complexity and sensitivity – for example, balancing the pressures of reforms in the NHS and any potential demand for health professionals to deliver vocational rehab.

We are beginning to address these issues by taking forward the *Better Routes to Redress* (2004) report and the DWP's *Framework for Vocational Rehabilitation* (2004).

Rehabilitation has taken on increasing importance in recent years. The Better Regulation Task Force report and recent review of Employers' Liability Compulsory Insurance highlighted the interest in rehabilitation as an alternative form of redress and the real appetite among insurers and legal professionals to explore how rehabilitation can become an accepted or preferred part of the litigation process.

Certainly, vocational rehabilitation has the potential to place the individual at the heart of the compensation process.

But regulation can only take you so far. What we need is a step change in attitudes both around returning to work, and approaches to compensation and risk in society.

The Compensation Bill will introduce legislation to enable claim-management companies to be effectively regulated. It will also clarify the existing common law on negligence to make clear that those who take reasonable care or exercise reasonable skill cannot be held liable for untoward incidents.

But it is important to put this into context. Between 2000 and 2005 the overall number of accident claims fell by 5.3%. Over the same period, accident claims against local authorities, schools, volunteering and other public sector bodies fell by 7.5%. In 2000, the cost of litigation in the UK as a percentage of GDP (gross domestic product) was less than a third of that in the United States.

Nonetheless, the 'compensation' issue is a major one that we need to address. It links to the nature of risk in society and people's approach to sensible risk management. We need a sensible debate to help inform the public of the truths behind some of the fiction.

So our agenda is an ambitious one – far more stretching than commitments of previous governments and more wide ranging.

To ensure the strategy progresses and actions make a real difference, we are placing responsibility with a Joint Ministerial Group involving ministers across government.

We also have, with the Department for Health, jointly appointed a National Director to focus on the health and wellbeing of working-age people.

The strategy will help us to break the link between ill health and inactivity. It will encourage good management of occupational health, and transform opportunities for people to recover from illness while at work, maintaining their independence and their sense of worth.

References

Better Regulation Task Force (2004) *Better Routes to Redress*. London: Better Regulation Task Force, www.brc.gov.uk/downloads/pdf/betterroutes.pdf.

Department for Work and Pensions (2004) *Building Capacity for Work: A UK Framework for Vocational Rehabilitation, ELCI 3*. London: Department for Work and Pensions, www.dwp.gov.uk/publications/vrframework/dwp_vocational_rehabilitation.pdf.

Chapter 23

Public health and genetics

Mark Kroese, Ron Zimmern and Simon Sanderson

Introduction

The Human Genome Project (HGP) was a 13-year-long project coordinated by the USA and involving groups from other nations. The project goals included identifying all the genes in the human DNA and determining the three billion base pairs that make up human DNA. While the project was completed in 2003, the analyses of the data obtained and the full results will take many more years (Collins *et al.* 2003). It has already been a catalyst for a dramatic advance in our knowledge of molecular science and the development of novel genomic technologies. As a result, new applications for healthcare have become available such as genetic testing and the ability to better define diseases. It has also led to improved management and care of patients with or at high risk of certain diseases, for example familial colorectal cancer (Burke 2004; Nabel 2004; Rappuoli 2004; Vogelstein and Kinzler 2004). In the UK, clinical genetic services are based in regional centres providing services for populations of between two to six million. These centres include molecular genetics, cytogenetic and biochemical genetic laboratories. All the departments in a centre work closely together providing clinical care (Donnai and Elles 2001). As knowledge and the number of clinical applications have increased, medical genetics has now extended beyond specialist clinical genetics services into other medical specialties and primary care. This will continue in the future as human genetics becomes an integral component of the practice of medicine. Genetics has its own terminology and some key terms are presented in Box 23.1.

> **Box 23.1 Genetic terms and definitions**
>
> **DNA** (deoxyribonucleic acid): the molecule that encodes the genes responsible for the structure and function of an organism and allows for transmission of genetic information from one generation to the next.
> **Gene**: the basic unit of heredity, consisting of a segment of DNA arranged in a linear manner along a chromosome. A gene codes for a specific protein or segment of protein leading to a particular characteristic or function.
> **Chromosome**: physical structure consisting of a large DNA molecule organised into genes and supported by proteins called chromatin.
> **Genome**: the complete DNA sequence, containing all genetic information and supporting proteins, in the chromosomes of an individual or species.

Public health genetics

The interaction between the development of new genome-based sciences and technologies and society is complex, with many important ethical, legal and social implications. The application of the methodologies and understanding of the population sciences, the humanities and social sciences will need to be considered in tandem with emerging biological knowledge. In parallel with the improved understanding of human molecular science, a new field of public health has been established to investigate and implement the fruits of this scientific endeavour in order to improve the health of the population. This field is called public health genetics or public health genomics.

Public health genetics has been defined as *the impact of genetics on the art and science of promoting health and preventing disease through the organised efforts of society.* It is a new field within public health that combines the insights of genetic and molecular science with epidemiology and the other population sciences as a means of preventing disease and of protecting and improving the health of the population. Its scope is wide, requiring an understanding of molecular genetics, the practice of clinical genetics, epidemiology, public health, the principles of ethics, law and the social sciences.

At its core is the notion that genetic factors, like the classic environmental exposures that have been shown over many decades to be causally implicated in disease, are themselves important determinants of health. Genetic factors play as important a role in influencing the risk of disease as do physical and biological agents, or social and structural factors such as poverty and unemployment. Genes do not act on their own; their expression and influence are the result of their interaction with a host of other factors, including other genes in the genome and the range of environmental exposures (Hunter 2005). The complexities of these relationships mean that, while genetic factors are at work in all diseases, they are rarely sufficient on their own to predict whether disease will develop.

Genetic epidemiology

Epidemiology is the core science of public health practice and is defined as the study of the distribution and determinants of disease frequency in human populations (Rothman 2002). Genetic epidemiology is a hybrid discipline that seeks to establish the role of genetic factors in disease occurrence in populations and families (Khoury *et al.* 1993). There are four key questions for the genetic epidemiologist.

Is genetic variation between individuals important in determining disease susceptibility?

There is a spectrum of causality from single-gene (or Mendelian) disorders, which are relatively rare, through to common complex diseases where genetic variation is only one of many risk factors (Beaty and Khoury 2000). Initial evidence for the impact of genetic factors is usually based on observing disease clustering in family, twin and adoption studies. Additional information can be sought on the relative contributions of genetic and environmental factors and by establishing a specific mode of inheritance (known as heritability and segregation analysis respectively).

Which genetic variants confer altered disease susceptibility?

Initial successes in gene discovery were in Mendelian diseases such as cystic fibrosis. In recent years, greater attention has been paid to unravelling the genetic basis of common complex diseases, which cannot be described by such simple genetic models. The two main tools for gene discovery are linkage analysis and association analysis. Linkage analysis looks for the co-*inheritance* of genetic variants with diseases in families. Association analysis looks for the non-random co-*existence* of genetic variants with diseases, usually in population-based case-control studies or in family-based studies.

What are the characteristics of these variants?

This question is about determining the prevalence of genetic variants in human populations and identifying interactions between genes, and between genes and environmental factors. These tasks will be greatly helped by large, population-based cohort studies, such as the UK Biobank project, where a large number of people will be followed for many years, contributing information about their genes, health and lifestyle.

How can the role of genetic information in health and disease be evaluated?

This is concerned with how genetic information can be used in practice and in particular two key tasks: integrating evidence from primary studies and evaluating the validity and utility of genetic tests in clinical diagnosis and risk prediction. International collaborations such as the Human Genome Epidemiology Network (HuGENet™) are key to integrating evidence from the many primary studies that have already been completed (Khoury 2004; Little *et al.* 2003).

Future challenges for genetic epidemiology

1 *Understanding common and complex diseases.* Single-gene disorders have been understood with comparative ease. However, diseases such as coronary heart disease and many cancers are far more difficult to understand. This is because the genetic variants discovered so far only confer a low risk of disease, the diseases themselves can be caused by multiple factors, and because these can vary both within and between different population groups. This means that epidemiological studies need to be very large and must be able to account for the impact of multiple risk factors if they are to be meaningful.

2 *Interactions between genes and between genes and the environment.* The methodology for the study of interactions is still at an early stage of development. We are only just beginning to understand how genetic variants in complex metabolic pathways interact with other genes and with environmental factors through advances in molecular science. New approaches, such as using the concept of Mendelian randomisation, may help achieve some of these objectives (Davey and Ebrahim 2005).

3 *Genetic association studies: separating the wheat from the chaff.* Genetic association studies are widely used for the study of complex diseases because they have

a number of advantages over other approaches. However, the literature is full of associations that have not been replicated or that do not have a sound biological foundation. The problem is deciding whether these conflicting results are due to real differences between populations or due to chance, bias or confounding. Improved design, reporting, analysis and integration of these studies are required if we are to move forward in our understanding of complex diseases.

4 *Knowledge integration.* Given the volume of primary studies, integration of current knowledge is key to the practice of public health genetics. The development of greater international collaboration will hopefully ensure that synthesis can keep pace with primary research.

Genetic tests

The development of new genetic tests has been an early application of the improved understanding of human genomics (Burke 2002). *GeneTests*, a US database, lists available genetic tests for over 1,000 diseases (www.geneclinics.org). Genetic tests should be evaluated like other medical interventions or technologies and not be treated differently. However, the methodology for genetic test evaluation is still under development. The ACCE framework for the evaluation of genetic tests was developed by the Office of Genomics and Disease Prevention, CDC, USA (www.cdc.gov/genomics/activities/fbr.htm). ACCE stands for analytical validity, clinical validity, clinical utility and the ethical, legal and social implications of genetic testing. The analytical validity of a genetic test defines its ability to measure accurately and reliably the genotype of interest. Clinical validity defines its ability to detect or predict the presence or absence of the phenotype or clinical disease. Clinical utility of a genetic test refers to the likelihood that the test will lead to an improved outcome and includes financial costs.

The exact definition of a genetic test is still debated but the term 'genetic test' should be regarded as a shorthand to describe a test to detect (a) a particular genetic variant (or set of variants), (b) for a particular disease, (c) in a particular population and (d) for a particular purpose (Kroese *et al.* 2004). The specification of all these factors is essential for test evaluation since validity will be to a large extent determined by them. The predictive value of tests will be dependent, for example, on the prevalence of the disease in the population; it is also well known that many individual variants on a gene (allelic heterogeneity) or that variants in more than one gene (locus heterogeneity) may give rise to the same disease. A genetic test should also be considered as part of an integrated package of care rather than as an isolated investigation.

The UK Genetic Testing Network (UK GTN), a national network of molecular genetic laboratories, has developed a tool to evaluate genetic tests based on the ACCE framework called the *Gene Dossier* (www.genetictestingnetwork.org.uk/). Experience so far has shown that the main difficulties in the area of genetic test evaluation include the lack of research data on how genetic tests perform especially in relation to clinical validity and the inability to evaluate predictive genetic tests. The focus of most genetic test evaluations so far has been on 'single gene' disorders where a genetic abnormality results in a high probability of developing disease rather than the common complex disorders such as coronary heart disease and diabetes.

The rapid expansion in the number of available genetic tests over recent years has exceeded the capacity to evaluate them. In order to use resources efficiently, healthcare systems will have to prioritise which tests to evaluate depending on the public health impact of the test. The internet allows access to genetic tests across national boundaries and depending on uptake may in the future have a significant impact on local health service delivery.

Policy implications of genetics

Genetics has provoked considerable public interest. This is reflected in the large number of newspaper and journal articles, media interviews and internet websites focusing on the various aspects of genetics. In some cases bold statements from research scientists making predictions based on their most recent research findings have provoked public concern. This situation illustrates the importance of the ethical, legal and social issues (ELSI) related to genetics. These issues are extensive in number and detail and will influence policy. Some of the broad areas are summarised in Box 23.2.

Box 23.2 Ethical, legal and social issues

- Privacy and confidentiality
- Informed consent and data protection
- Genetic testing
- Insurance
- Eugenics
- Discrimination
- Stem cell research
- Intellectual property rights
- Health inequalities
- Patenting of genetic information

Public concern about emerging technologies is not new. There have been similar responses in the past and it acts as a reminder that the public needs to be informed and engaged in the debate about research and its applications – more so when public funds are used to support such research. Experience so far has shown that to do this properly, communication between the science community and the public has to improve. Human genetics is not a new specialty and therefore the impact of what has occurred in the past cannot be underestimated, for example the eugenics movement and mandatory sickle-cell screening in the USA (Reilly 2000).

Concepts that contribute to public anxiety about genetics include *genetic determinism* and *genetic exceptionalism*. Genetic determinism describes the view that the genotype definitely predicts the phenotype irrespective of the impact of environmental factors. Apart from the rare 'single gene' disorders this is false. Genetic exceptionalism is the claim that genetic information is sufficiently different from other types of health information that it deserves special protection or other exceptional measures. This remains a controversial claim with diminishing evidence to support it. There has been extensive ELSI research and reports

(Burke *et al.* 2001; Cornish *et al.* 2003; European Commission Expert Group on the Ethical, Legal and Social Aspects of Genetic Testing 2004; European Society of Human Genetics 2003; Hodge 2004; Knoppers and Chadwick 2005; Tutton and Corrigan 2004). Despite this work there continues to be large gaps in our understanding and there is a need for further studies and discussion across all parts of society. It is only by addressing these areas that the maximum public health benefit can be achieved from the applications of human genetic research.

The policy issues that form much of the practice of public health genetics include:

- legal and regulatory frameworks in genetic testing
- the funding of science and the prioritisation of relevant research
- attitudes to the pharmaceutical and biotechnology industries
- education and training of health professionals and the public in the implications of genetic science
- development of the workforce capacity needed to carry out genomic research and translate the findings into healthcare applications and services.

In the UK, considerable progress has been made in these areas. One of the first surveys of policy issues was provided by the report from the Genetics Scenario Project *Genetics and Health* that was carried out by the Public Health Genetics Unit in Cambridge with support from the Nuffield Trust (Zimmern and Cook 2000). More recently, the government genetics white paper, *Our Inheritance, Our Future* in 2003 emphasised the importance of genetics within the health agenda and gave political support (Department of Health 2003). It provided an important stimulus for further research and service development. The white paper also provided a programme of investment in NHS clinical genetic services.

An infrastructure has been put in place to advise the UK government on genetic matters relating to health. The different committees, which provide specialist advice on human genetics and health issues, include the Human Genetics Commission (HGC), the Genetics and Insurance Committee (GAIC), Genetics Commissioning Advisory Group (GenCAG), Gene Therapy Advisory Committee (GTAC), Human Fertilisation and Embryology Authority (HFEA) and the UK Genetic Testing Network Steering Group (UK GTN). GenCAG and UK GTN are both Department of Health advisory committees, which are concerned with the development and quality of NHS clinical genetic services. The UK National Screening Committee has also informed decisions concerning screening programmes such as those planned for cystic fibrosis and haemoglobinopathies. The Genetic Interest Group (GIG), which is a national alliance of patient organisations for people and families affected by genetic disorders, is represented on many of these groups.

The Public Health Genetics Unit was established in 1997 in Cambridge to focus on many of these issues and to bring together the science with epidemiology and the ELSI implications of genetics. Six genetics knowledge parks (GKPs) were later created in England and Wales in 2002 with aims that include: improving public understanding of genetics, accelerating the transition of research findings into practice and developing economic, ethical, legal and social frameworks for human genetics. The GKPs also contribute to the training and education of health professionals. The NHS Education in Genetics Centre was formed in 2004 and has the lead role in the education and training of health professionals. Regulation in the field of genetics testing is not limited to statutory regulation but also includes the use of resource allocation mechanisms and clinical governance (Burke and Zimmern 2004). UK human genetic policy cannot be limited to the national only but also takes into consideration and requires collaboration with other countries and international organisations such as the European Union (EU), United Nations (UN), World Health Organization (WHO) and the Organisation for Economic Co-operation and Development (OECD).

In April 2005, an international expert meeting was held in Bellagio, Italy, which proposed that an international network be established in order to facilitate worldwide collaboration in the area of public health genetics. The network will be known as GRAPH *Int* (Genome-based Research and Population Health International Network). Its aim will be to *facilitate the responsible and evidence-based integration of genome-based knowledge and technologies into public policy and into services for improving the health of populations.* At its core will be the integration, both within and between disciplines, of genome-based knowledge with population science, the humanities and social science. This integrated and interdisciplinary knowledge will underpin four sets of activities in order to effect improvements in population health – namely (a) informing public policy, (b) developing and evaluating health services – both preventive and clinical, (c) communication and stakeholder engagement and (d) education and training. The proposed mechanism is illustrated in Figure 23.1.

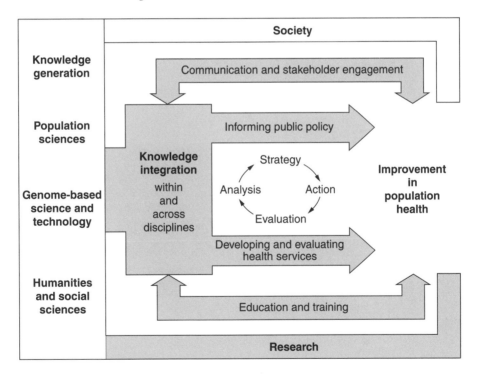

Figure 23.1 The enterprise of public health genetics.

There is now unanimous agreement among those who work in public health genetics or genomics that the enterprise in which they are engaged can be represented as the tinted components of the model set out in Figure 23.1.

Conclusion

Biomedical sciences have now the potential to really make differences to human health and it is inevitable that DNA-based tests and therapies will become part of routine medical practice and will have wider impacts on society as a whole. This will not happen suddenly but incrementally over time. While the advances in recent years have been extraordinary, major gaps still remain in our understanding of human genetics and obstacles persist to the translation of research findings into practice. The public health community has a critical role in building the evidence base for the use of valid genomic applications in population health, for evaluating these in practice and developing the workforce capacity to allow widespread implementation. In addition, it must inform and stimulate the development of the necessary infrastructure through education and the establishment of an appropriate policy and regulatory framework. Genetics will in time completely transform medical practice and could deliver major population health benefits if the infrastructure and frameworks are in place. The key to achieving this will be the support and engagement of the public.

References

Beaty TH and Khoury MJ (2000) Interface of genetics and epidemiology. *Epidemiol Rev.* **22**: 120–5.

Burke W (2002) Genetic testing. *N Engl J Med.* **347**: 1867–75.

Burke W (2004) Genetic testing in primary care. *Ann Rev Genomics Hum Genet.* **5**: 1–14.

Burke W, Pinsky LE and Press NA (2001) Categorizing genetic tests to identify their ethical, legal, and social implications. *Am J Med Genet.* **106**: 233–40.

Burke W and Zimmern RL (2004) Ensuring the appropriate use of genetic tests. *Nat Rev Genet.* **5**: 955–9.

Collins FS, Green ED, Guttmacher AE *et al.* (2003) A vision for the future of genomics research. *Nature.* **422**: 835–47.

Cornish WR, Llewelyn M and Adcock M (2003) *Intellectual Property Rights. A study into the impact and management of intellectual property rights within the healthcare sector.* Cambridge: Public Health Genetics Unit.

Davey SG and Ebrahim S (2005) What can Mendelian randomisation tell us about modifiable behavioural and environmental exposures? *BMJ.* **330**: 1076–9.

Department of Health (2003) *Our Inheritance, Our Future: realising the potential of genetics in the NHS.* London: HMSO.

Donnai D and Elles R (2001) Integrated regional genetic services: current and future provision. *BMJ.* **322**: 1048–52.

European Commission Expert Group on the Ethical, Legal and Social Aspects of Genetic Testing (2004) *25 Recommendations on the Ethical, Legal and Social Implications of Genetic Testing.* Brussels: European Commission.

European Society of Human Genetics (2003) Population genetic screening programmes: technical, social and ethical issues. *Eur J Hum Genet.* **11**(Suppl 2): S5–S7.

Hodge JG Jr (2004) Ethical issues concerning genetic testing and screening in public health. *Am J Med Genet C Semin Med Genet.* **125**: 66–70.

Hunter DJ (2005) Gene–environment interactions in human diseases. *Nat Rev Genet.* **6**: 287–98.

Khoury MJ (2004) The case for a global human genome epidemiology initiative. *Nat Genet.* **36**: 1027–8.

Khoury M, Beaty TH and Cohen BH (1993) *Fundamentals of Genetic Epidemiology.* Oxford: Oxford University Press.

Knoppers BM and Chadwick R (2005) Human genetic research: emerging trends in ethics. *Nat Rev Genet.* **6**: 75–9.

Kroese M, Zimmern RL and Sanderson S (2004) Genetic tests and their evaluation: can we answer the key questions? *Genet Med.* **6**: 475–80.

Little J, Khoury MJ, Bradley L *et al.* (2003) The human genome project is complete. How do we develop a handle for the pump? *Am J Epidemiol.* **157**: 667–73.

Nabel GJ (2004) Genetic, cellular and immune approaches to disease therapy: past and future. *Nat Med.* **10**: 135–41.

Rappuoli R (2004) From Pasteur to genomics: progress and challenges in infectious diseases. *Nat Med.* **10**: 1177–85.

Reilly PR (2000) Public concern about genetics. *Ann Rev Genomics Hum Genet.* **1**: 485–506.

Rothman KJ (2002) *Epidemiology: an introduction.* Oxford: Oxford University Press.

Tutton R and Corrigan OP (eds) (2004) *Genetic Databases: socio-ethical issues in the collection and use of DNA.* London: Routledge.

Vogelstein B and Kinzler KW (2004) Cancer genes and the pathways they control. *Nat Med.* **10**: 789–99.

Zimmern R and Cook C (2000) *The Nuffield Trust Genetics Scenario Project Genetics and Health.* London: The Stationery Office.

Public health in practice

Introduction

In this section of the book we look at public health in practice and focus on developments in the intervening years between editions. Obviously, these do not stand alone. The impact of white papers, the Wanless reports and successive Blair governments shape the way in which professional structures and healthcare systems participate in delivering better health. One of the key recommendations in the English white paper, *Saving Lives: our healthier nation*, was that the public health workforce should be strengthened and its multidisciplinary potential developed.

Jenny Wright charts the progress of specialist public health through its UK-wide progress to a competency-based approach and voluntary registration. Within England, the most recent policy statement, *Choosing Health*, formally recognised the need for an infrastructure to underpin the delivery of the public health programmes to reduce obesity and tobacco-related harm and improve sexual and mental health. Strengthening the workforce was one of three key underpinning strands which also included developing information and intelligence systems and ensuring an appropriate strategy for research and development. And the workforce referred to was not just public health doctors but people with the right skills at all levels across the wider workforce, including public health practitioners and specialists and those in leadership positions within organisations who contribute to health improvement.

Historically public health leadership has resided with those carrying the legacy of Medical Officers of Health, described in our first edition. The history of this legacy within the NHS has been chequered, and it is only now that the circle is being completed and Directors of Public Health (DsPH) are bridging health and local authority organisations in newly created joint posts. Such posts have been on the increase in England in recent years. Paul Redgrave describes recent experiences in England where DsPH are appointed to coterminous organisations – not only the positive but also the problematic aspects of such a role, also referred to in the Welsh case study (*see* Chapter 3).

Recent policy in England has brought public health and primary care closer together and the chapters by Ken Aswani and Yinglen Butt describe the potential roles of GPs, community nurses and primary care teams in the delivery of public health. The potential of new policies, contracts and extended roles of the wider team is drawn out – particularly that of pharmacists and also dentists as described by Rowena Pennycate and Sara Osborne. The English white paper on 'out of hospital' care, *Our Health, Our Care, Our Say,* as well as the development of practice-based commissioning offer further opportunities to bring a public health perspective to primary care.

But it is not only through primary care that the health service can contribute to improving health. Diane Gray and Nicholas Hicks review the historical tension between those academics such as McKeown and Ilich on the one hand who question the contribution of healthcare to better health, and Bunker on the other hand who points to the important contribution of health services to saving lives. At a time when the English NHS is moving towards a plurality of providers this reminder of the many ways in which acute hospital settings can contribute to the public's health is timely. This is not, as they remind us, only through the three domains of health improvement, health protection and health service quality but also through the strength of the image of the hospital as the front end of health and healthcare, hosting many of the elite of the medical world, providing them with power, capable of lobbying for change and influencing decisions. While this power is often coupled with an inpatient mentality and directed towards self-interest, it can be redirected and extended effectively beyond hospital walls.

Another aspect of public health practice which has both seen rapid change and extends way beyond hospital walls is health protection. Angus Nicoll picks up the story of the development not only of the Health Protection Agency but also of the growing awareness of the global nature of communicable disease and the need for effective systems to protect the public's health. The experience of SARS and the threat of avian flu coupled with the need to respond to both natural disasters such as the tsunami (December 2005) and Hurricane Katrina (October 2005), and to bioterrorism as demonstrated by the London bombs (July 2005), demonstrate the importance of surveillance and preparedness. But it is not only the acute issues which need to be addressed. The long-term impact of pollution on the environment, the need to achieve and maintain immunisation rates that protect the public and the problems of chronic infectious disease such as multiresistant TB and HIV/AIDS underline the need for public health systems which are strong, robust and supported.

Support for public health systems can be drawn from a variety of sources but both academic institutions and the process of performance management have a role to play. Selena Gray describes the progress made in developing academic public health so far but also highlights its fragility. Public health, by its inclusion within the medical framework of performance assessment, is disadvantaged by not fitting the medical paradigm and being concerned with a wider, less biomedical framework than mainstream medicine. Using the same criteria as those applied to biomedical or genomic research, areas of public health often lose out. While in the past this has had an impact on academic funding, recent policy moves to support academic public health, not least within *Choosing Health* in England, will hopefully move some way to redressing the problems both of academic capacity and career paths and of what is deemed worthy of research.

The potential shift within academic performance assessment has been mirrored by an actual shift in performance management of delivery of public health programmes within the NHS and local authority frameworks. Public health is now included in the need to meet performance management standards in both the NHS and local authorities. Tony Jewell describes the emergent frameworks for both systems and the role that public health directors can play across the interface.

Chapter 24

Developing the public health workforce

Jenny Wright

This chapter describes the development of the public health workforce, including the progress from a medically dominated to a multidisciplinary specialist profession. It describes the emergence of competency-based training and the creation of the voluntary register. A number of different initiatives and influences has converged to bring about fundamental changes to public health across the United Kingdom, leading to a broader-based professional and regulated workforce. The chapter will outline how and why this has happened and reflect on the implications of the unique opportunity to take an integrated strategic approach to development of the whole of the public health workforce and not just specific sectors within it. The challenge for future years is to make an integrated workforce a reality.

Until 10 years ago the public health workforce tended to be polarised between the 'haves' and the 'have nots'. The Chief Medical Officer of England, in his project to strengthen the public health function (Department of Health 1997) outlined for the first time in 1997 three levels within the public health workforce.

- *Specialists* – consultants working at strategic levels whose core function is public health and who have specialist knowledge and skills.
- *Practitioners* – those who spend some or a major part of their practice working with individuals and groups on public health. These groups included health visitors, environmental health officers, health promotion staff, information teams.
- *The wider workforce* – those who have a role in health improvement and reducing inequalities such as chief executives, voluntary sector staff, health service managers.

The increasing clamour during the 1990s for professional recognition and a career structure from others working in public health from backgrounds other than medicine was channelled through national groups such as the Multidisciplinary Public Health Forum. Groups such as epidemiologists, intelligence experts, health promotion specialists, and senior public health managers were without registration because doctors were the only professional group to have access to higher specialist training and thereby accreditation onto the General Medical Council (GMC) Specialist Register. The needs of practitioner groups such as health visitors and environmental health officers were also largely ignored.

Change did not take place until promoted as part of the Labour government's health strategy for England, *Saving Lives: our healthier nation* (Department of Health 1999). This introduced a number of key policy shifts without which development, and change within the workforce, would not have been possible. First, it openly recognised the existence of health inequalities in society and also that these inequalities were worsening over time as evidenced in differential life expectancy for different sectors of society depending upon a complex web including deprivation, social and educational attainment. Second, it called upon health and local government to work together to address the broader determinants of health and set in train policy initiatives to make this happen. Lastly, it announced the introduction of a new category of specialist in public health, with equivalence to consultant in public health (medicine), and open to those from backgrounds other than medicine.

This policy change promoted a more holistic view of the professional workforce which embraced those not working within the health service. The then Faculty of Public Health Medicine, the professional standard-setting body for public health, in response to the government's new strategy started to open up its higher specialist training schemes to those from backgrounds other than medicine. Consultant level appointments in England began to be advertised to suitably qualified and experienced public health professionals from either a medical or non-medical background. This was followed in 2002 with the setting up of over 300 primary care trusts in England by the opening up of Director of Public Health posts to doctors and non-clinicians (Department of Health 2001). A small but significant minority of these posts went to non-clinicians from a range of backgrounds including local government. In 2001, the membership of the Faculty of Public Health voted to drop 'medicine' from its title.

A mechanism had to be found nationally, and quickly, for quality assuring this new breed of specialists from backgrounds other than medicine now starting to appear in senior public health posts in England. One further initiative in the development of a multidisciplinary specialist workforce was needed, that of assessment and subsequent registration of accredited specialists to provide public protection in the same way that the GMC specialist register provides public protection for consultants in public health medicine. The four UK health departments provided pump-priming funding to set up the UK Voluntary Register for Specialists in Public Health. The register was opened in May 2003 to accept applications via two routes, those starting to come through the higher specialist training route and, separately, for an initial 3-year period, those already working at a senior level in public health via retrospective portfolio assessment. The first specialists started to come through both these routes from early 2005.

The Faculty of Public Health had, in 2001, started work, in consultation nationally, on the ten key areas of public health practice which were to form the basis for professional standards. They also were used, via the development of sub-competencies within each key area, as the basis for assessment via higher specialist training. The ten key areas were formerly agreed by the four Chief Medical Officers across the United Kingdom in 2002 and have provided a unifying focus for describing public health practice (*see* Box 24.1).

Box 24.1 Ten key areas of specialist practice

1 Surveillance and assessment of the population's health and wellbeing.
2 Promoting and protecting the population's health and wellbeing.
3 Developing quality and risk management within an evaluative culture.
4 Collaborative working for health.
5 Developing health programmes and services and reducing inequalities.

> 6 Policy and strategy development and implementation.
> 7 Working with and for communities.
> 8 Strategic leadership for health.
> 9 Research and development.
> 10 Ethically managing self, people and resources.

These key areas were also the focus of expanded work by Skills for Health (2004) with Department of Health funding into national public health practice standards.

The ten key areas also formed the basis for the framework for retrospective portfolio assessment of competence of aspiring specialists. The framework requires applicants to demonstrate acquisition of the public health knowledge base ('knows and knows how') and its practical application ('shows how'), i.e. demonstrate competence across all the ten key areas of public health as generalist/specialists (UK Voluntary Register). A fundamental principle of this means of assessment has been its generalisability and accessibility to senior public health professionals working in different organisations and different geographical settings. A number of professionals coming through this route have, for example, come from local government settings.

It was recognised early on that, because they had not been able to have the benefit of higher specialist training, those aspiring for accreditation on the register via retrospective portfolio development would be likely to have some, albeit minimal, development needs in order to meet all competencies. The English Department of Health, therefore, from 2002 provided short-term funding for regional specialist top-up schemes to cover gap filling of selected specialists but also support them in the technique of portfolio preparation. Similar top-up schemes have followed in Wales, Scotland and Northern Ireland. It is anticipated that there will have been some 200 specialists registered via this retrospective route by the end of the initial 3-year 'window' in May 2006.

A side effect of this initiative has been the rapid development of the senior professional public health workforce into positions of leadership where they could give the benefit of their breadth of experience at a time when available senior capacity was at an all-time low, particularly in England. This was valuable during the organisational changes in 2002 when many of the senior public health staff previously in operational health authority roles went into board-level strategic posts in PCTs or into the newly established Health Protection Agency.

This fundamental change for specialists has not been without issues and problems. Medical resistance was expressed largely in concerns about whether the portfolio approach constituted real equivalence with higher specialist training and whether accreditation was merely entry to specialist status via a backdoor route, i.e. an easy alternative to higher specialist training. There were equally concerns from non-medics, principally about the fact that this route, in the end, could only apply to relatively few senior professionals leaving a disaffected and unsupported majority of the workforce in need of further training to reach levels of competence required. Integrated training programmes are now in place in all deaneries in England and Wales but have yet fully to be put in place in Scotland and Northern Ireland. Issues over integration have largely centred on the lack in some areas of pay equivalence between specialist registrars (medical) and specialist trainees (non-medical) and also some resistance from doctors to allowing non-clinicians full access to health protection and on-call training.

The changes to date, therefore, had not tackled either the full range of specialist public health practice or, particularly importantly, the bulk of the workforce, the practitioners. These had to wait for the next policy shift and subsequent raft of initiatives which came at the start of this century.

Derek Wanless was asked to review health services spending in England by the Treasury in 2002. His first report (HM Treasury 2002) highlighted the need to invest in reducing demand by enhancing promotion of health and disease prevention. His second report (HM Treasury 2004) went further and called for a review of attitudes to health by the development of what he called the 'fully engaged scenario'. He warned that if people did not take more responsibility for their health then costs would spiral out of control over the coming years. The government responded at the end of 2004 with its public health white paper, *Choosing Health: making healthy choices easier* (Department of Health 2004b). This had six key health themes:

- sexual health
- mental health
- tackling obesity
- smoking reduction
- reduction in alcohol intake
- reduction generally in health inequalities.

Behind this new programme was a focus on skilling up the workforce at specialist level but also, and importantly, at practitioner level with a focus on equipping people to bring about behaviour change. A key ingredient was to be the leadership role of the public health workforce. A further driver for change has been the underpinning of the government's health policy by the introduction of public health targets into the service's performance management structure in England. The national standards from which targets are drawn has a specific section on public health (Department of Health 2004d) with public health targets relating to life expectancy, some cancers, smoking and teenage pregnancy feature as key elements of PCTs' formal assessment framework (Healthcare Commission 2004). Some public service agreement targets are also shared with local government and there is pressure on local authorities to work collaboratively with the health sector.

What has also emerged from all these changes has been a range of players in the public health field. Nurses can now register as community public health specialists with the NMC (Nursing and Midwifery Council). Pharmacists have been encouraged to develop their roles through the public health strategy. The Chartered Institute of Environmental Health is refocusing its training to reflect better public health issues.

The final pieces in the jigsaw have come from two separate initiatives, one focusing on doctors' education, the other on the back of shifting the whole of the English NHS workforce, apart from doctors and dentists, onto a single pay framework.

Modernising Medical Careers (Department of Health 2004c) and the new PMETB (Professional Medical Education and Training Board) which replaces the Specialist Training Authority are driving changes to higher specialist training for doctors. This promotes competence-based assessment. It will also lead to more flexibility over training as GPs and other specialists are encouraged to formally develop public health competencies while remaining in their base specialties.

The Faculty of Public Health in response to these changes is proposing radical changes to its methods of assessment which will, following a revised membership examination, be via competencies measured by prospective portfolios. In this they will be learning from the non-medical Register retrospective portfolio approach. Indeed, it is proposed to use the Voluntary Register portfolio assessment framework for retrospective assessment of overseas doctors applying to work in public health in the UK. The Faculty's membership examinations have been changed to reflect the needs of a much broader public health workforce and will examine in all the ten key areas of public health.

Agenda for Change (Department for Health 2004a), although set up to bring the whole of the NHS workforce (apart from doctors and dentists) under a single system of pay bandings, is also serving to unify the approach to the public health workforce. Through the development of national public health profiles and pay bands at different levels of the workforce, rising from those entering the profession to the most senior levels, there will be a coherent approach to job definitions and pay scales for the first time. This will provide a framework for career progression and a structure which, it is hoped, will embrace 90% of the NHS public health workforce. This is the first time that the needs of practitioners as a whole have been addressed. It is anticipated that there will be approximate pay equivalence also between specialists and medical consultants in public health. It is anticipated that an NHS Public Health Career Framework, indicating competencies and training needs, linked to the Knowledge and Skills Framework (Department of Health 2004e), will be developed to permit horizontal and vertical progression in public health. This work is yet to be completed but the Skills for Health work on public health practice provide the National Occupational Standards on which competencies can be based (Skills for Health 2004).

In public health, therefore, for the first time one will be able to see, alongside the suite of job profiles' entry requirements, where Master's in Public Health will fit and where membership and higher specialist training and assessment will be required. The Faculty of Public Health is considering offering its membership examination in a series of papers at diplomate level (together they will comprise membership) which will help give a benchmark for practitioners at key job levels.

Both the new medical and *Agenda for Change* approaches lead to a more flexible approach to training, competency-based approach and work-based assessment.

In line with these changes, and also to meet continuing pressure from the workforce, the UK Voluntary Register's proposed next stage is to accredit and register senior professionals with expertise in specific areas of public health at consultant-equivalent level via retrospective portfolio assessment. Groups that have expressed an interest in such registration include health promotion, public health intelligence, health economists, public health pharmacy, public health nutrition, public health academics, health psychologists, environmental health and health protection staff. The Faculty of Public Health is already considering setting up a prospective training route for defined specialists in its domains of public health practice – service improvement, health improvement, health protection with the underpinning domains of health intelligence and academic public health. There may also be other players in developing higher-level training programmes for defined groups.

Both the Register and Faculty approaches to defined specialists are likely to centre round the concept of core and non-core competencies. All aspiring specialists, whether from medical or non-medical backgrounds, will be required to meet, in addition to the knowledge base in the ten key areas of public health, an agreed core set of competencies at generalist/specialist level then additional competencies at higher level in their chosen field. These competencies will continue to be derived from the ten key areas of public health practice which have shown remarkable robustness in continuing to define the overall approach but also flexibility in their capability of being adapted to suit changing circumstances. Having common core competencies will also support the *Agenda for Change* approach to development through its various levels.

These approaches will help several key groups in the public health workforce achieve formal recognition and regulation. It will, for the first time, for example, bring in non-clinicians working in academic public health and match the medical direct entry route for academics onto the specialist register. This approach will also support registration of specialists from non-medical backgrounds within the new Health Protection Agency which brings together all staff from a range of agencies dealing with health protection issues – field services, surveillance, chemicals and poisons, emergency response, etc. It will also support development and recognition of the health-promotion workforce, recent estimates of which number some 2,000 across England and Wales (Department of Health 2005).

There are still issues for further consideration, work and resolution. When will the UK Voluntary Register cease to become voluntary and registration become a statutory requirement for specialists from non-medical backgrounds? Should practitioners also be registered? How will the Register handle a potential range of organisations accrediting higher specialist training? What is the relationship with other councils and registering bodies, e.g. for nurses? Local government funding for training of its staff in public health and in providing equivalence are still issues to be tackled. Competencies at the different levels for practitioners, curricula and work-based assessments based on these have still to be developed.

The framework for development is there, however, and the policy and workforce drivers in place to make it happen. Development of the public health workforce has come a very long way in a very short space of time. Much of this has been driven by organisational change in England and Wales with less discernible change in Scotland and Northern Ireland.

Different parts of the system have shown that they are able to learn from each other and use the best of each other's material to move forward. There appears to be a will to make it work. There may be a way to go but building blocks are in place for developing a truly integrated public health workforce for the first time.

References

Department of Health (1997) *The CMO's Project to Strengthen the Public Health Function in England*. London: Department of Health.

Department of Health (1999) *Saving Lives: our healthier nation*. London: Department of Health.

Department of Health (2001) *Shifting the Balance of Power in England*. London: Department of Health.

Department of Health (2004a) *Agenda for Change: Final Agreement*. London: Department of Health.

Department of Health (2004b) *Choosing Health: making healthy choices easier*. London: Department of Health.

Department of Health (2004c) *Modernising Medical Careers: the next steps. The future shape of foundation, specialist and general practice training programmes*. London: Department of Health.

Department of Health (2004d) *National Standards, Local Action: Health and Social Care Standards and Planning Framework (2005/06–2007/08)*. London: Department of Health.

Department of Health (2004e) *NHS Knowledge and Skills Framework and Development Review Guidance*. London: Department of Health.

Department of Health (2005) *Shaping the Future of Public Health: promoting health in the NHS, project report*. July. London: Department of Health.

Healthcare Commission (2004) *Assessment for Improvement: our approach*. London: Healthcare Commission.

HM Treasury (2002) *Securing Our Future, Taking a Long Term View*. London: HM Treasury.

HM Treasury (2004) *Securing Good Health for the Whole Population*. London: HM Treasury.

Skills for Health (2004) *National Occupation Standards for Public Health Practice*. London: UKPHA.

UK Voluntary Register: www.publichealthregister.org.uk.

Chapter 25

Making joint Director of Public Health posts work

Paul Redgrave

This chapter describes the experiences of the newly created role of jointly appointed Directors of Public Health. It gives pointers from experience of what will make the posts work better and describes some of the challenges faced.

Introduction

Several local authorities (LAs) and primary care trusts (PCTs) across the country have appointed a joint Director of Public Health (DPH). In their most developed form these posts are jointly funded; the DPH is an executive director of the LA and a board member of the PCT. The public health function is accountable to both organisations and there are office accommodation and support staff in both organisations. In other parts of the country, there is strong commitment to joint policy making and co-operation but there are lesser degrees of integration. With the current structural changes many areas are reviewing their arrangements for the public health programmes for issues such as smoking, diet and exercise which have risen up the public and political agenda. LAs are coming under pressure to meet health-related public service agreement floor targets and PCTs are under more pressure to achieve targets to improve health and reduce health inequalities, which they cannot do by themselves.

This chapter briefly considers the historical context of the relationship between local government and health services before posing the question: what is the added value of going for a joint DPH post? The national and local drivers for change will be reviewed and the structures and processes needed to set up a joint post outlined. The potential problems associated with joint posts are described along with suggested solutions. The focus of this chapter will be the practicalities of establishing joint posts, but it should be read in conjunction with Tony Elson's chapter (*see* Chapter 11).

In writing this chapter, the experience gained from negotiating the establishment of a joint post and shared public health directorate in Barnsley has been drawn upon, as has the experience from working in the post. Other information has been obtained from a more systematic review of joint posts and from informal communications with colleagues around the country who are grappling with this exciting but complex and, on occasions, daunting work environment. The overall conclusion is that these posts provide a great opportunity to practise public health in a more effective way. The critical factors for making such posts work successfully and challenges for the future are discussed.

Local government and health services – a relationship with a history

Early public health pioneer and general practitioner, Dr William Duncan, was employed by Liverpool City Council as its Medical Officer of Health (MOH) in the 1830s. The population was faced with serious health problems which medical practice could not prevent and had little to offer in the way of treatment. By working within the local government of the time Dr Duncan was better placed to influence policies, such as the introduction of clean water and better housing that dramatically improved health. The work of Duncan and other early MOHs led to the National Public Health Act of 1845. Ashton describes the development of the public health movement in the mid-19th century and charts its high and low points through to the end of the 20th century (Ashton 1999; Ashton and Seymour 1988). For more than a century until their abolition in 1974, LAs employed MOHs who were responsible for providing a range of community-based health and social services.

For the past two decades successive governments have stated their commitment to improving health and reducing health inequalities. Despite many positive policies, too little has been done to stem the increase in inequalities in health and life expectancy, which are strongly correlated to widening inequalities in income (Hunter 2003; Shaw, Davey Smith and Dorling 2005). Nonetheless the recent and somewhat unexpected surge of interest in public health suggests a tipping point has been reached. Concerns over the effects of second-hand smoke, childhood obesity, junk food and school meals are constantly receiving media attention. The second Wanless report, addressed to the government, makes a strong economic case for increased investment in the public health agenda (Wanless 2004). The report has been influential in creating a more positive environment in which public health can operate. However, like Dr Duncan and the early MOHs, we will have to continue to argue for legislation to ban smoking in all workplaces, for curbing junk-food advertisements for children and for more progressive, redistributive taxation policies.

Why go for a joint DPH? National and local drivers for change

What is the added value of having a joint DPH post over maintaining a PCT-based DPH and with strong partnership working? The most powerful and basic argument for joint posts is that LAs have more influence over the key determinants of health. If public health is part of the LA as well as the PCT it has many more opportunities to influence decisions that improve health.

The English public health white paper *Choosing Health* (Secretary of State for Health 2004) and associated Delivery Plan (Department of Health 2005) attempt to address the central issues of how to support people to smoke as little as the Californians, eat like people in Mediterranean countries and exercise as much as the Finns. Other important issues centre around keeping children and young people safe, healthy and engaged in the education system and how to support people to practise safe sex and reduce unwanted pregnancies. The role alcohol and drugs play in mental and physical health and crime and antisocial behaviour is also undergoing increasing scrutiny. The health service clearly does have a role to play in addressing these issues but the stronger levers lie with local authorities (LAs), the voluntary and community sector and communities themselves. *Choosing Health* specifically mentions the appointment of joint DsPH as an opportunity to support the health improvement agenda.

The government has raised the stakes by setting LAs and PCTs targets to improve health and reduce health inequalities. This growing pressure on LAs is manifested through the Comprehensive Performance Assessment processes, public service agreement floor targets and local public service agreement (LPSA) targets. Valuable star ratings will be affected and reward money for LPSAs lost if health targets are not achieved. There are opportunities, but also added pressure, for around 70 of the more disadvantaged LAs who have been awarded 'Spearhead' status to be early implementers of the *Choosing Health* white paper and for around 20 LAs who also are Communities for Health pilots. It is planned that local area agreements (LAAs) will fundamentally alter the relationship between central and local government. The 21st wave and 42nd wave pilots are negotiating local targets and also freedoms to pool budgets and reduce bureaucratic duplication of reporting. A jointly appointed DPH and a jointly accountable public health directorate have the opportunity to be at the heart of these leading edge new arrangements.

In a similar way, PCTs are under increasing pressure to deliver on health inequalities targets through local delivery plans. Currently, these public health-related targets are not of the same status as those relating to waiting lists and waiting times but, nevertheless, for some of them star ratings are at stake. PCTs are aware that inequalities targets can only be met by collaborative work with local partners and that a strong, shared public health function will be beneficial. Joint work across PCTs and LAs is essential to reach the most marginalised groups suffering the greatest health inequalities, e.g. travellers.

In many of the more disadvantaged areas of the country addressing health is an important component of social and economic regeneration. A joint DPH is able to develop sophisticated information on health needs at LA, ward, neighbourhood and general practice level. In these areas, health equity audits are tools to redress the inverse care law and strengthen health services (Tudor Hart 1971). Public health is well placed to establish links with the Department of Work and Pensions' Job Centre Plus and Pathways to Work programmes. Community development programmes, community health educators and efforts to maximise the effect of the NHS's economic footprint locally are all important ways of helping people obtain employment and move out of poverty.

Influence can be brought to bear on resource allocation within both the LA and PCT to reduce health inequalities locally. In autumn 2004 several DsPH undertook an important, and at least partially successful, piece of work with the Special Interest Group of Metropolitan Authorities (SIGOMA). This group represents 46 of the most disadvantaged LAs outside London. Arguments were developed to lobby for an increase in the 'pace of change' for the resource allocation formula to enable poor PCTs to reach their fair share target sooner (Barnsley MBC and Barnsley PCT 2004). By being part of LAs, DsPH have better access to a range of government departments and to lobby groups such as SIGOMA.

Structures and processes needed to set up a joint DPH post

In order successfully to establish a joint DPH post there needs to be a level of enthusiasm within the LA to tackle health issues in a more overt way. All LA directorates need to be prepared to consider their strategies and policies and assess the impact they have on the health of the population. PCTs need to be prepared to shift the paradigm in which they operate to focus more upstream on health, as well as downstream on healthcare.

Developing a shared set of values which LA officers and members and the PCT board sign up to is an important step. In Barnsley the Fit for the Future Strategy has been agreed and is '*a bold long term strategy to improve health and reduce health inequalities in the Borough*'. Fit for the Future has become the strap line for preventive health work in Barnsley with a high recognition rating among the local population.

Negotiations must take place to agree a DPH job description, person specification and how the post will be funded and supported. Agreement must be reached on the degree of collaboration between the organisations. In some areas PCTs and LAs have drawn up specifications for the provision of a common service for public health (Barnsley MBC and Barnsley PCT 2003).

Agreement must be reached regarding at what level the DsPH and other members of the public health team operate. There are examples where the DPH is an executive director of the LA and is seen as an equal member of the senior management team as well as being a board member of the PCT. Deputy DPH and public health consultant posts tend to operate at assistant director level in the LA. Practicalities such as office accommodation, support staff and good IT support in both organisations need to be addressed.

Information from around the country indicates considerable variety in arrangements and degrees of 'jointness'. In some areas there is joint funding of the DPH post, a strong commitment to joint policy making and co-operation but there are lesser degrees of integration of the public health function. Some areas have joint posts but the funding is not shared.

Potential problems with joint DPH posts – and suggested solutions

Information in this section is based on personal experience of almost a year of working as a joint DPH, from a systematic review of joint posts (Roberts 2005) and from personal communication with other jointly appointed DsPH.

Joint DPH posts are necessarily big jobs with many different relationships that must be established and maintained. There are significant practical issues related to attending all the important meetings – the PCT board, full council, the LA cabinet, two senior management teams and away days of the different groups. There are inevitable clashes. This problem will be made worse if there is more than one PCT relating to an LA, if there is lack of coterminosity or if there is a non-unitary LA – for example, the county and district model of local government characteristic of the shires. The solutions must be to have authorised deputies, ensure colleagues in all organisations have a clear understanding of the arrangements and encourage the sympathetic timetabling of meetings.

If public health is to exert influence in LAs as well as PCTs then it has to be fully involved in strategy development and financial planning in both organisations. It must also be prepared to take its share of responsibility in performance management arrangements. Inevitably there has to be a degree of duplication of the bureaucracies in the LA and PCT. By having a shared and agreed public health programme this can be minimised but still can seem a heavy burden. Rationalising risk management procedures, HR functions, and other functions to one organisation can help diminish the burden of bureaucracy.

Among jointly appointed DsPH there is concern over managing the balance between strategic and operational work. The consensus is that with such a broad scope to these joint posts, they just cannot work if you get drawn into managing operational issues. The public health directorate will still have some operational responsibilities, for example, information provision and analysis, emergency planning, advice to commissioners and other such activities. An infrastructure of competent public health staff will be needed to carry out these functions. Inevitably joint DsPH will take a share of the responsibility for managing multi-agency functions, for example, older people's boards, children's trust boards, or the Drug Action Teams, but they should keep their involvement at as strategic level as possible. Several joint DsPH have expressed concerns that they have difficulties maintaining the role of public health in their PCT and health services generally. The solution will again be found in building public health capacity and the use of competent deputies, including the strengthening of public health networks.

The cultural differences between LA and PCT are marked, and need to be addressed. The 'democratic deficit' in the NHS is a constant issue for many LA members and some officers. Opening up the NHS to oversight and scrutiny committees is a significant step in addressing these concerns, as is ensuring LA representation on NHS trust boards. There is much to learn about the different cultures especially around managing financial issues and deficits.

Critical factors in enabling joint DPH posts to work

Probably the most important factor in making these posts work is the level of understanding in both organisations about the role and function of public health. Support from chief executives and the leader of the LA is crucial and support from director colleagues important. Agreement across both organisations as to what are the priority issues and an agreed joint programme for public health is vital. Coterminosity between the LA and PCT boundaries is very helpful indeed.

Many jointly appointed DsPH, who will have gained most of their experience in health authorities and PCTs, will initially be on a steep learning curve. It is important that they have the political awareness and ability to operate outside their 'comfort zone'. They must be prepared to lead, challenge, persuade, cajole and influence and recognise that they will be influencing mainstream budgets rather than managing them.

Future challenges for joint DPH posts

Probably the biggest challenge is achieving the targets for which public health is increasingly taking responsibility. For example, in many disadvantaged areas reducing teenage pregnancy is proving difficult. Reducing the health inequalities gap is also going to be very tough unless inequalities in income distribution are reduced. Opportunities to become part of an effective lobby arguing for this are more possible within the more political environment of LAs. Making LAAs work is also going to be challenging, but is an opportunity for public health to have greater impact. While developing work within LAs and local strategic partnerships, joint DsPH have to keep their eye on the ball for their health service responsibilities. Primary care services and the public health role of many health service staff do need developing, particularly in some of the most disadvantaged areas, and the potential of health-promoting hospitals needs to be realised. The training needs of joint DsPH, their staff and public health trainees must be addressed to ensure a competent workforce is available for this new and challenging environment.

Joint DsPH can already point to a range of examples of where their position has helped forward sound, preventive public health work. These include steering a paper though full council on tobacco control measures, building on the Healthy Schools programme to improve food for school children and working on the health aspects of local transport plans. They may also have worked with environmental services on pollution issues leading to local cancer scares, or influenced a local alcohol strategy better. The early MOHs 150 years ago faced seemingly intractable public health problems. The modern threats to health may carry different challenges, but the need to address the key determinants of health remains as powerful today. Joint post working offers the greatest opportunity to date in addressing this challenging public health agenda.

References

Ashton J (1999) Past and present public health in Liverpool. In: S Griffiths and DJ Hunter (eds) *Perspectives in Public Health*. Oxford: Radcliffe Medical Press.

Ashton J and Seymour H (1988) *The New Public Health*. Milton Keynes: Open University Press.

Barnsley MBC and Barnsley PCT (2003) *Service Specification for the Provision of a Common Service for Public Health* (unpublished).

Barnsley MBC and Barnsley PCT (2004) *Fit for the Future – the strategy*. Barnsley: Barnsley PCT.

Department of Health (2005) *Delivering Choosing Health: making healthy choices easier*. London: Department of Health.

Hunter DJ (2003) *Public Health Policy*. Cambridge: Polity Press.

Roberts M (2005) *Joint Director of Public Health Posts – an overview of current experience and opinion* (unpublished).

Secretary of State for Health (2004) *Choosing Health: making healthy choices easier*. London: The Stationery Office.

Shaw M, Davey Smith G and Dorling D (2005) Health inequalities and New Labour: how the promises compare with real progress. *British Medical Journal*. **330**: 1016–22.

SIGOMA (2004) *Healthy Places, Healthy People: the case for fairer funding to tackle health inequalities*. Barnsley: SIGOMA, Barnsley MBC.

Tudor Hart J (1971) The inverse care law. *Lancet*. **I**: 405–12.

Wanless D (2004) *Securing Good Health for the Whole Population*. London: HM Treasury.

Chapter 26

Primary care as a gateway to public health

Ken Aswani

Introduction

There are various ways of defining primary care. Traditionally primary care was synonymous with the general practitioner (GP). Over the last 30 years, in addition to the GP, the core primary care team has included practice nurses, district nurse, midwives, professions allied to medicine, and receptionists. Over the last 5 to 10 years a wider definition of primary care has been used. At one level this can include health services provided outside the healthcare setting including social care. At the minimum it includes specialist nurses, allied health professionals, pharmacists, dentists and optometrists. Social workers may also be included. However, primary care is not only the gateway to health services but to health as well.

What can primary care provide?

One of the key benefits of primary care is that it is accessible and used by the majority of the population. Over a million patients visit their GP surgeries on each working day in the United Kingdom. Four million people visit a pharmacist each day. Accessibility to the population is important. GP surgeries and pharmacists are often no further than the local shop's premises and the people that work in them are very much part of the local community.

One of the key components of any public health message is that it has to be credible. Opinion polls still regard staff in primary care, in particular the GP, as somebody they would trust the most. Primary care can, therefore, have a powerful impact in improving public health.

Perhaps the most potent vehicle for public health is via the GP consultation. Patients consult their GP for a range of problems. GPs deal with the presenting problem but they also deal with ongoing problems, in addition to providing advice on prevention. A range of public health issues, including lifestyle issues such as smoking, are particularly suitable for GP advice. The main advantage is the one-to-one consultation with the patient, who is often receptive to advice. Quite clearly if patients are in a GP surgery, their concerns about their health have already been activated. If the GP and patient can reach an understanding and agree a course of action, the outcome is much more likely to be successful, e.g. smoking advice to a patient presenting with bronchitis. The GP is able to explore the patient's fears and concerns about giving up smoking and to address these. The GP can be very specific about the diseases the patient may be vulnerable to in the future, including cancer, heart disease and strokes.

Some patients may still not be ready to give up smoking but many will take positive action in the future and make a serious attempt to give up. If the consultation had not occurred then the patient may not have taken any further action regarding their smoking. Bearing in mind the huge number of GP consultations that occur daily, there are many opportunities a day to address the range of issues which can range from smoking, lifestyle measures, sexual health, falls prevention and so on.

Raising issues opportunistically is not the only advantage. Each consultation is carried out in the context of the patient's social, psychological and family circumstances. In ideal circumstances the GP/practice has an ongoing relationship with the patient and their family and accumulated knowledge about them over many years. The GP is, therefore, able to deliver relevant messages in the most appropriate way to the patient. This is key to the patient changing their behaviour. Generic health-promotion messages, such as take more exercise, will be given in different ways, depending on whether the patient is a librarian or a builder. Second, it may not be appropriate to ask the patient to lose weight, take more exercise, stop smoking and change their diet if they have many other problems. However, a follow-up consultation would enable these issues to be tackled. Approaching patients holistically is a key component of primary care. Although many of the first consultations in primary care are still with the GP, members of the primary care team play a key role in combining the health-service role with giving key health-promotion messages. For example, practice nurses – who undertake a range of activities in primary care including the management of long-term conditions, family planning, cervical cytology and a range of other interventions – play a crucial role in promoting the health of the population. Practice nurses have a range of advantages including more time in the consultation. In addition, from the patient's perspective, the practice nurse may potentially be more approachable, particularly for certain groups, such as teenagers. They often run specific clinics, e.g. men's health, teenage health, older people. Targeted interventions by the multiprofessional staff in primary care are one of the most underused interventions to improve health. At one of our local surgeries the practice nurse organises Tai Chi classes for their older people to help them keep mobile and improve their balance. Health visitors and midwives have also key roles linking with essential groups in the community, especially women and children. Educating mothers allows not only them to benefit but also their children and family. Messages given at a time when mothers are most receptive can have impact. A mother may not have wanted to give up smoking before being pregnant but if her newborn baby is going to be more susceptible to asthma and bronchitis and the effects of passive smoking, she may be persuaded to change her mind. Such messages need to be integrated as part of a holistic care package.

Health visitors are often described as public health professionals. Crucially the health visitor visits the family at home and becomes aware of the social, psychological and family setting. She can not only link with the rest of the primary care team and attend primary healthcare team meetings but also link to social services and all the range of community services that is available, in particular Sure Start. For example, in many areas, particularly inner-city areas, there is a high turnover of patients and local services are simply not visible to many patients. Health visitors play a crucial link between linking the patient's needs to the services that are available. With the advantage of the whole of the primary care team working together, any of the practitioners can link and use the other as a resource, either directly, or as a resource to signpost patients to the most appropriate setting. In doing this the distinction between health service and promoting health becomes blurred.

The wider primary health team

Given the significant advantages of the core primary health team the benefits of the wider primary healthcare team have only more recently been realised. The team includes school nurses, specialist nurses, and allied health professionals, pharmacists, dentists and optometrists. Patients may well be in regular contact with many of these professionals. Pharmacists are likely to have contact with patients on at least four million occasions daily. This is a massive opportunity for promoting public health and is very much underused. With the advent of the new pharmacy contract there is a golden opportunity to make an impact on the public health of the United Kingdom. The evidence on smoking cessation has demonstrated that the crucial role played by pharmacists is supporting a significant number of smokers to quit. Pharmacists can also target public health messages to their population and intervene where appropriate, e.g. if they are dispensing a prescription for somebody with obvious heart disease and notice that they are not taking aspirin, they could take this further and, if there is no contraindication, they can offer advice that this essential preventive measure is undertaken. Emergency hormonal contraception availability via a pharmacist is a mechanism by which unplanned teenage pregnancy can be reduced. Signposting to local services, whether this be to local leisure facilities or a range of self-help groups, voluntary organisations both for older people or other local community groups, is a key role that can also be played by pharmacists.

Challenges

The challenges for public health have been well described in the government document *Choosing Health* (Secretary of State for Health 2004). Life expectancy is falling for example in the London Borough of Waltham Forest for women and is well below the national average for men (*see* Figure 26.1).

This is an outer borough in North-East London with a significant number of inner-city challenges. The 2005 public health report (Li 2004, 2005) shows poor health outcomes in terms of circulatory disorders, cancer, neonatal and perinatal mortality and HIV. Severe mental illness rates are above the national averages. Life expectancy for women is falling now at the level of 1991. Traditional inequalities such as deprivation and social class are factors; however, the main challenge is associated with ethnicity and associated health issues. Unfortunately if we do not understand the links between ethnicity and health we shall fail to make the impact we need. The specific health needs of the ethnic minorities are many and varied. Some examples of these are as follows:

- cardiovascular disease – particularly in the black and South Asian population
- sickle cell – in the Afro/Caribbean population
- diabetes – particularly in the South Asian population

- women and child health – poorer health in the black and ethnic minorities group.

Primary care and public health need to work together to target these areas.

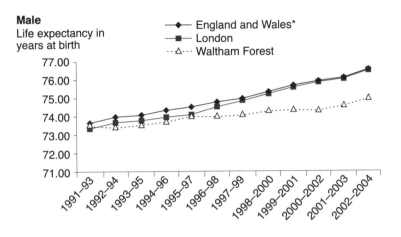

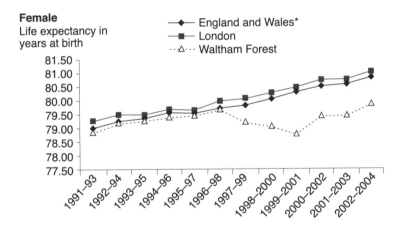

Figure 26.1 Life expectancy at birth. *Source: Compendium of Health and Clinical Indicators 2004.* *Non-resident deaths excluded.

Partnership working

It is clear that public health is not improved by one agency alone but is most effective when working through partnerships. Primary care professionals can be very effective in working with the local community in terms of getting key messages across. Being part of the community for a number of years also gives primary care professionals the knowledge and credibility to take on this role.

National priorities and the roles of primary care

Table 26.1 highlights the expected roles of primary care, primary care organisations and partnership working in delivering the health improvement agenda as laid out in *Choosing Health*.

Table 26.1 National priorities – primary care roles

Area	Primary care	Primary care organisation	Working with partners
Coronary heart disease (Read and Ramwell 2004)	Prevention in terms of health and lifestyle advice, particularly diet and exercise. Patients who have established heart disease given specific and effective modification receptors including blood pressure and cholesterol control. Management of long-term conditions.	Supports primary care. Establishes strategic links between all partner agencies. Supports and provides locality and borough wide information to allow targeted intervention.	Local authority, local strategic partnership, schools and businesses work together to enable coronary heart disease and diabetes prevention to be given priority.
Sexual Health (Burack 2000; Mawer 1999; Seamark and Lings 2004)	Opportunistic advice, screening, family planning. Specific targeted clinics, e.g. teenagers. Provision of more specialised sexual health services.	Identifying local needs. Wider health promotion. Engagement and targeting of the population.	Schools, colleges, youth groups, other groups, e.g. local football organisations.
Smoking (Butler *et al.* 1999; Coleman 2004; Haslam 2000; Lennox *et al.* 2001)	Recording smoking status, offering smoking cessation advice. Undertaking smoking cessation programmes (in particular pharmacists).	Publicity and support for primary care training of professional groups, wider health promotional activities.	Working with all at-risk groups. Non-smoking policy. Working with businesses.
Obesity	Lifestyle advice, particularly diet and exercise. Targeting of high-risk groups, e.g. those with coronary heart disease and diabetes. Providing more specialised intervention for those at particular risk.	Taking a strategic approach and linking with all key agencies to adopt a more proactive approach to tackling obesity.	Particularly schools and local authority.
Drugs	Prevention and health advice. Running young people's clinics or specialised drug addiction services.	A more strategic approach in prevention and provision of drug services.	Local authority, police and key organisations.
Alcohol	Recording alcohol consumption and advising safe drinking. Specialist support and signposting for those requiring a high level of service. Employment – working with those on incapacity benefit and linking them with drug centre agencies to identify training opportunities.	Building partnerships between primary care and outside bodies.	

The GP contract

On 1 April 2004 a new GP contract was implemented in the United Kingdom. This is now followed by the pharmacists' and dental contracts. As well as the overarching national public health agenda in which GPs and primary care teams play a key role, the GP contract provides opportunity to integrate prevention into the payment system. The contract is divided into three areas.

1 Essential and additional services – this includes patients requiring a consultation.
2 Additional services – this includes immunisation and cervical cytology services.
3 Enhanced services – this includes a range of specialised services the practice may wish to provide including drug addiction services, mental health services and coil fitting. It can include a vast range of services determined by local need.

Quality and Outcome Framework (new GP contract – nGMS)

This part of the contract links to specific quality indicators and practice funding and is linked to the achievement of these. The quality indicators are broken down into points. A maximum of 1,050 can be achieved.

The ten clinical areas are:

- coronary heart disease
- asthma
- chronic obstructive pulmonary disease (COPD)
- hypertension
- stroke/transient ischaemic attacks
- mental health
- hypothyroidism
- epilepsy
- diabetes
- cancer (Austoker 1994).

The indicators are broken down on the basis of structure, process and outcome. Many of the areas require a smoking history to be recorded and, if the patient is a smoker, smoking cessation advice to be given. Already we are seeing significant improvements and indicators relating to secondary prevention and better outcomes for these patients. There is much discussion about how the Quality and Outcomes Framework can be modified to take on board key national priorities. Key areas for consideration in the future include obesity and sexual health.

Practice-based commissioning

From 1 April 2005 GP practices have a right to an indicative budget for services that need to be locally commissioned, e.g. hospital outpatients, day cases, inpatients. The scope of this can extend into mental health and emergencies and the budget may include prescribing. This represents huge opportunities and at the same time can present some threats. The opportunities exist for practices to be effective in managing demand by commissioning appropriate integrated, cost-effective services for their patients. This is particularly relevant for the significant percentage of our population who have long-term conditions. Commissioning can be applied widely and used in a very innovative way. There is nothing preventing practices commissioning preventive services such as smoking cessation support, exercise programmes, initiatives to reduce the incidence of sexual transmitted diseases, healthy schools programmes, tackling obesity and so on. However, certain aspects need to be addressed. One is the mindset of commissioners to think as widely as possible, to focus on health as well as health services, and take a longer-term view. Second, practice-based commissioning has to be efficient in order to release resources to invest in health prevention. Too often the will to address public health is there but funding is used to treat acute problems. This cycle can be broken by taking a more proactive approach to local health needs. Cost-effective analyses on effective interventions will confirm the areas to focus on. One of the most powerful mechanisms is to ensure that health professionals are strong advocates for promoting health and utilise all their opportunities they have in ensuring their patients stay healthy. There is some evidence that, in the area of case management (carefully coordinating the care of high-risk patients), taking a strategic approach for the longer-term conditions, redesigning services in the community in particular with greater skill mix, can release resources to invest in preventive health.

A joint approach with local authorities, voluntary organisations, acute trusts and private organisations is likely to prove to be more effective than working in isolation. Linking with the community is key and can be achieved through a range of groups including faith communities. Ethnic minorities are one of many groups that can be harder to access but one can nevertheless succeed through specific means.

The reality in practice is the Quality and Outcomes Framework of the new GP contract (nGMS) will incorporate a range of indicators, which will be targeted to tackle the major public health issues, e.g. obesity.

Long-term conditions

Another challenge to public health and general practice is how to ensure quality of life through effective secondary and tertiary prevention. Put another way – how do we make sure our patients who have chronic diseases are able to live healthy longer lives despite their conditions and disabilities? Up to 15 million people in the UK have a long-term condition. General practice has always managed up to 90% of care in many of the long-term conditions. The approach to long-term conditions has changed, particularly thinking of the chronic disease care model (Wagner). Organisations in the USA work on the three-tier pyramid model. The pyramid provides a very easy to understand way of intervening in the management of long-term conditions. The three levels are:

- Tier 1 – disease management
- Tier 2 – care management
- Tier 3 – case management.

An example of Tier 1 would be somebody with high blood pressure who was stable on medication. In respect of Tier 2, care management would be somebody with asthma who has had episodes of poor control. These can be managed in primary care or by a specialist nurse. In Tier 3, case management tends to be reserved for people at high risk of hospital admission, typically two or more admissions in the last 6 months and a number of co-morbidities.

The key focus in the management of long-term conditions is patient empowerment. There is a significant amount of evidence to show that if patients take control of their illness the health outcomes improve.

The impact of technology allows home monitoring to be undertaken and the data to be transmitted to professionals who can advise accordingly. Public health can support primary care by providing knowledge about effective interventions and strategic advice based on the health needs of the population. This will support both primary care teams in their treatment plans and also primary care organisations in their commissioning roles.

Having a vision for public health and primary care

Historically there have been clear links between public health and primary care, with primary care cast in the role of social entrepreneur in developing links across communities. Three examples of primary care taking the leader in improving the health of their local population are as follows.

The Bromley-by-Bow Centre (*NHS Magazine* 2002a) is a healthy living centre which has been in existence for many years and is a good example of the provision of primary care in a setting with a number of other activities, including training, employment and daily activities. Their approach demonstrates integration of health and health services into a broader approach, experimenting with new approaches – for example, the use of art to communicate more effectively in a diverse population than the traditional health-promotion leaflets. The centre is the focal point of the community and a good example of a public health approach to primary care.

The second example is in Leicestershire and provided by Dr Angela Lennox (*NHS Magazine* 2002b). Once again primary care is taking the lead in tackling some of the issues of our most deprived population.

Professor Chris Drinkwater's model of a Healthy Living Centre approaches health through involvement of the local population in a wide range of activities (West End Health Resource Centre).

The changing role of primary care organisations

Primary care organisations in England and Wales were set up with three main responsibilities (Dobson 2001):

* to improve the health of the population and reduce inequalities
* to improve and develop primary care
* to secure health services for the population.

A typical primary care organisation has a population base of between 200,000 and 250,000 allowing an overview of commissioning and provision at a local level with health needs identified on a local basis and action to address these needs coordinated across a range of agencies including primary care. Waltham Forest PCT in North-East London has made specific efforts to link the public health needs of the local population with primary care. The borough is divided into six community council areas. These are coterminous with the clusters of GP practices. A local team consisting of GPs, management staff and non-executives link with partners to provide leadership across these six areas of about 40,000 population to address local health needs.

Public health is everyone's business. Embedding this in primary care is one way of mainstreaming the public health agenda. However, we face a time of change with the introduction of new initiatives such as practice-based commissioning and payment by results as well as an impending white paper, *Care Outside Hospital*.

Primary care – care outside the hospital

Most of the initiatives in the 2000 NHS Plan and indeed the resources have been focused around hospitals particularly in relation to reducing waiting lists and accident and emergency waiting times.

The current major policies affecting hospital care are choose and book (a part of patient choice), allowing patients to choose four or five providers, and payment by results which means hospitals are paid a fixed national tariff price for each activity undertaken. One potential disadvantage of this method is that if a hospital suddenly increases its activity levels all the local resources would dry up resulting in limited ability to invest in primary care or public health.

The next phase of the reform is to provide choice for patients in primary care, to improve quality in primary care, and redesign traditional hospital services, e.g. minor surgery, outpatients, which can often be carried out in the community, in many cases using advanced skills of GPs, pharmacists, nurses and allied health professionals. The opportunity to use innovation in the care of patients and preventive health approaches is very significant. Patient choice and being much more patient-centred than ever before are key policy drivers. Increasing choice and contestability of providers does mean a range of providers will emerge including the private sector. Although this is partly a 'market', taking a positive approach to commissioning from different providers can allow quality and health improvement to defined.

There needs to be a balanced approach in terms of taking a longer-term view and the health service should not be defined as numbers treated. Communities, local authorities, voluntary organisations, patient groups, primary care, and specialist services could very effectively work together to improve the health of the population.

Waltham Forest in North-East London is an example of this with all local stakeholders working together to improve health. The National Service Frameworks in diabetes and coronary heart disease are a mechanism of the areas that can be tackled. The emphasis is on linking with a local population of 40,000, which allows closer dialogue between the implementation and the local community.

Acknowledgement

I would like to acknowledge thanks to Dr Pui Ling Li, Director of Public Health, Waltham Forest PCT, for her helpful comments.

References

Austoker J (1994) Cancer prevention in primary care: setting the scene. *British Medical Journal*. **308**: 1415–20.

Burack R (2000) Young teenagers' attitudes towards general practitioners and their provision of sexual health care. *British Journal of General Practice*. **50**(456): 550–4.

Butler C, Rollnick S, Cohen D *et al.* (1999) Motivational consulting versus brief advice for smokers in general practice: a randomized trial. *British Journal of General Practice.* **49**(445): 611–16.

Coleman T (2004) Cessation interventions in routine health care. *British Medical Journal.* **328**: 631–3.

Dobson R (2001) Primary care trusts to take lead on public health. *British Medical Journal.* **323**: 249.

Haslam C (2000) A targeted approach to reducing maternal smoking. *British Journal of General Practice.* **50**(457): 661–3.

Lennox AS, Osman LM, Reiter E *et al.* (2001) Cost effectiveness of computer tailored and non-tailored smoking cessation letters in general practice: randomised controlled trial. *British Medical Journal.* **322**: 1396.

Li PL (2004, 2005) *Public Health Report 2004 and 2005.* London: Waltham Forest NHS Primary Care Trust.

Mawer C (1999) Preventing teenage pregnancies, supporting teenage mothers. *British Medical Journal.* **318**: 1713–14.

NHS Magazine (2002a) All inclusive primary care. 1 May. Cover feature. www.nhs.uk/nhsmagazine.

NHS Magazine (2002b) Social works primary care. September. Feature article. www.nhs.uk/nhsmagazine.

Read A and Ramwell H (2004) A primary care intervention programme for obesity and coronary heart disease risk factor reduction. *British Journal of General Practice.* **54**(501): 272–8.

Seamark C and Lings P (2004) Positive experiences of teenage motherhood: a qualitative study. *British Journal of General Practice.* **54**(508): 813–18.

Secretary of State for Health (2004) *Choosing Health: making healthy choices easier.* Cm 6374. London: The Stationery Office.

Smeeth L and Heath I (1999) Tackling health inequalities in primary care. *British Medical Journal.* **318**: 1020–1.

Wagner E. *Improving Chronic Care Model.* www.improvingchroniccare.org/change/model/components.html.

West End Health Resource Centre. www.westend-health.co.uk.

Chapter 27

The role of public health nursing

Yinglen Butt

Background

There is renewed interest in the contribution that public health nursing can make in improving the future health of our nation. Nurses are innovators and public health nursing offers considerable scope for the budding innovator to explore new ways of enhancing practice, engage in research that evidences/redefines work and collaborate across professional boundaries to improve the health and wellbeing of the population. Nurses have responded and delivered on key policy initiatives. Therefore the re-emergence of interest in public health nursing has legitimised their ongoing inclusion in key policy development.

Recent government policies have specifically identified public health nurses as key contributors in addressing the public health agenda. The policy drivers have come at a time when the public's interest in improved health requires the professions to adopt innovative approaches to service delivery. The current political agenda therefore offers challenges as well as opportunities for nurses, midwives and health visitors as they position themselves alongside their other partners to create systems that will support improved health outcomes through the reduction of inequalities.

In the past public health was associated with public health medicine; however, nurses have their own unique contribution to make. An inclusive approach is now required that acknowledges the contribution that can be made by a wide number of professions including the nursing specialties in improving health. The wider family of nurses, regardless of the setting in which they work, have a key contribution to make. All nurses can contribute to health improvement; however, some will have this as a considerable part of their role.

This chapter explores what public health nursing means, identifies some recent government policies that have influenced practice, and highlights some of the current and future challenges/opportunities for nurses in public health practice.

Defining public health

Acheson (1988) defined public health as *'the science and art of preventing disease, prolonging life and promoting health through the organised efforts of society'*. While this definition has been in use for some time, and encompasses one of the broader definitions of public health, Sir Derek Wanless (2004), in a speech at the UKPHA Congress in Brighton, suggested that this definition could be further expanded, the new definition being: *'the science and art of preventing disease, prolonging life and promoting health through the informed choices and organised efforts of society'*. It acknowledges that society needs to have the appropriate knowledge to make choices in an informed way. It also marks a step towards a more person-centred approach, as individuals become more involved in decisions about their own health and that of their communities.

Defining public health nursing

The resurgence of interest in public health nursing has also created a need to debate the definition of public health nursing. Public health in nursing has been cited as a 'way of seeing' the needs of individuals and local populations in order to bring about health gain (Billingham and Perkins 1997). It has also been noted, *'in general, public health is a collective, or population view of the health needs and health care rather than one which focuses on individuals'* (Plews *et al*. 2000). Essentially, public health nursing is about choosing to improve health and wellbeing and using the creative energies that exist between and across individuals, organisations and communities to positive effect.

Policy agenda

Liberating the Talents (Department of Health 2002) sets out how the 2000 *NHS Plan* (Department of Health 2000) could be delivered within primary care and trust settings. It identified that the three core functions underpinning the work are:

- first contact – assessment, diagnosis, care, treatment and referral
- continuing care – rehabilitation, chronic disease management
- public health – health protection and promotion programmes that improve health and reduce inequalities.

The core functions epitomise public health practice through identifying the need for assessment, management of identified need and ongoing prevention and health promotion to ensure good health outcomes.

The consultative document, *Every Child Matters* (Department for Education and Skills 2003), highlighted that nurses, midwives and health visitors would need to deliver services that would enable them to make effective contributions to the five outcomes (be healthy; stay safe; enjoy and achieve; make a positive contribution; and enjoy economic wellbeing) expected for children and young people to make a positive transition into adulthood. It identified nurses, midwives and health visitors as essential collaborators in effecting positive outcomes for the most vulnerable. In addition, one of the document's recommendations was for the Chief Nursing Officer (CNO) to review the nursing and midwifery contribution to the health and wellbeing of vulnerable children and young people. The CNO's review (Department of Health 2004c) acknowledged the changes required in practice in order 'to take forward *Every Child Matters*'. One recommendation made was:

> *PCTs, children's trusts and local authorities are encouraged to work towards having a minimum of one full-time, whole year, qualified school nurse for each cluster or group of primary schools and its secondary school taking account of health needs and school populations* (Department of Health 2004c – *see* Chapter 16).

Similarly, the *National Service Framework (NSF) for Children, Young People and Maternity Services* (Department for Education and Skills, Department of Health 2004) acknowledged that a core set of skills was required for all practitioners working with children and young people. The standards identified in the NSF set out the vehicles that can be used by practitioners in their health improvement roles when working with children, young people and families. Evidence exists of such practice: Beverley Clarke (private fostering coordinator), has made significant progress in ensuring that the needs of privately fostered children and young people are incorporated into national and local policy. A population approach was taken, having initially identified clients on her caseload. Her work involves ensuring that a child-centred approach remains central to decision making. Collaborative practices have strengthened the basis of this work, enabling the needs of this vulnerable group to be embedded in legislation, professional practice and local planning.

The English public health white paper, *Choosing Health* (Department of Health 2004b), identified that, while the population's health had improved significantly, there remained huge inequalities and *'new challenges to ensure that as a society we continue to benefit from longer and healthier lives'*. It acknowledged that individuals were interested in improving their own health and that could be the impetus that advanced the development of the health-improvement work. When the population was consulted, key areas were identified that would enable sustainable changes in health improvement and these became the underpinning principles of the document which are: *'informed choice for all, personalisation of support to make healthy choices, and working in partnership to make health everyone's business'* (Department of Health 2004b). It identified the need for nurses to use every contact as a health-promoting opportunity, and the major contribution that nurses, midwives and health visitors can make in their health-improvement role to reduce smoking, obesity, alcohol intake and improve sexual and mental health.

These developments are built on in the 2006 white paper, *Our Health, Our Care, Our Say* (Department of Health 2006) which proposes a major shift in emphasis from downstream hospital-based healthcare to upstream health improvement and prevention. The proposals are not especially novel but, if successful, they will lead to new ways of working and providing services with a much greater emphasis throughout primary care on public health and prevention. The aim is to make primary care and community services much more accessible to users in terms of opening times and the range of services available.

Challenges and opportunities

Although earlier attempts to separate commissioning from provision were modified in order to allow integrated PCTs to continue if they so wished and if agreed to by the new strategic health authorities, the government remains keen to promote greater diversity in service provision in the belief that this can only improve quality and benefit users. It is claimed that increased capacity and contestability will allow people greater choice and convenience. In particular, the government is keen to encourage new social enterprises with a commitment to innovation. It is especially anxious to ensure that poor areas where there have been problems in attracting primary care practitioners will be opened up to new market entrants who can demonstrate real service improvements. In the new mixed economy of care, NHS providers will compete for business and work alongside new providers from the voluntary and independent sectors. All of these developments will have major implications for public health nurses both in terms of the skills they will need, and where (and for whom) they will be working. In many ways it will be a more complex and fragmented world which carries its own risks at a time when the government also wants to see closer joint working across primary care and local government.

References

Acheson D (1988) *Public Health in England*. London: Her Majesty's Stationery Office.

Billingham K and Perkins E (1997) A public health approach to nursing in the community. *Nursing Standard*. **11**(35): 43–6.

Department for Education and Skills (2003) *Every Child Matters*. London: Department for Education and Skills.

Department for Education and Skills, Department of Health (2004) *Change for Children – Every Child Matters. National service framework for children, young people and maternity services: core standards*. London: The Stationery Office.

Department of Health (2000) *The NHS Plan*. London: The Stationery Office.

Department of Health (2002) *Liberating the Talents: helping primary care trusts and nurses to deliver the NHS Plan*. London: The Stationery Office.

Department of Health (2004a) *A Career Framework for the NHS Discussion Document*. London: The Stationery Office.

Department of Health (2004b) *Choosing Health: making healthy choices easier*. London: The Stationery Office.

Department of Health (2004c) *The Chief Nursing Officer's Review of the Nursing, Midwifery and Health Visiting Contribution to Vulnerable Children and Young People*. London: The Stationery Office.

Department of Health (2006) *Our Health, Our Care, Our Say: a new direction for community services*. London: The Stationery Office.

Plews C, Billingham K and Rowe A (2000) Public health nursing: barriers and opportunities. *Health and Social Care in the Community*. **8**(2): 138–46.

Wanless D (2004) *UKPHA World Congress. Proceedings of Sustaining Public Health in a Changing World: Vision to Action*. 19–22 April. Brighton.

Chapter 28

Dental public health

Rowena Pennycate and Sara Osborne

Introduction

This chapter aims to give the reader a broad understanding of the key aspects of dental public health. It covers the diseases, the epidemiology, oral health inequalities, older people, fluoridation, and current challenges and opportunities in dentistry.

Many people take their oral health for granted yet good oral health is essential to everyday life. As described in the *Oral Health Strategy for England* (Department of Health 1994) oral health is a standard of health of the oral and related tissues which enables an individual to eat, speak and socialise without active disease, discomfort or embarrassment and which contributes to general wellbeing.

Not only is oral health important for day-to-day life, it is an indicator of other health and social issues. When you look at the rates of decay compared with other measures of deprivation, it is the same people suffering from both poor oral health and poor general health.

The diseases

There are two main dental diseases – tooth decay and gum disease. These diseases cause pain and discomfort in most of the population at some time during their lives but interestingly they are both preventable. Despite this, the majority of the population suffers decay and/or gum disease to some degree at some stage in their life. Tooth decay is the most common reason for general anaesthetics in children as the diseased teeth are often extracted.

Epidemiology

Over the last 30–40 years, dental health in the UK has improved dramatically. The Adult Dental Health (ADH) Surveys (Office for National Statistics 2000), carried out every 10 years, enable us to monitor the changes and identify patterns of disease. In 1968 the first ADH survey revealed that 37% of adults in England and Wales had no teeth. By 1998, this figure had dropped dramatically to 13%. The main reason for this is believed to be the introduction and use of fluoride mainly in the form of toothpaste.

The number of teeth an adult needs for functional dentition is 21 (the usual number of adult teeth is 32). Having 21 teeth is an indication of a good state of health generally. The ADH surveys have shown that the percentage of the population considered to have functional dentition has also increased from 73% in 1978 to 83% in 1998 although there is a general deterioration in the older age groups (over 55 years old).

Table 28.1 shows the general condition of teeth in the population according to the 1998 Adult Dental Health Survey. The table clearly indicates that there is a deterioration in oral health with age. Up to the age of 44, people are much more likely to have all their own teeth, fewer restorations and less wear generally.

Table 28.1   Adult oral health

Age (years)	% of all adults		% of dentate adults				
	Edentate	Dentate	Natural teeth and dentures	21 or more natural teeth	At least one artificial crown	At least moderate tooth wear	Exposed, worn, filled or decayed roots
16–24	0	100	1	100	7	2	20
25–34	0	100	3	98	24	5	50
35–44	1	99	10	94	41	8	71
45–54	6	94	20	82	49	12	86
55–64	20	80	43	57	48	18	90
65–74	36	64	54	46	39	}34	}97
75 and over	58	42	63	23	36		
All	13	87	18	83	34	11	66

Source: Adult Dental Health Survey, 1998 (ONS 2000).

The Child Dental Health Survey (Office for National Statistics 2004) is also carried out every 10 years. Like adults, there have been vast improvements in the dental health of children. According to the latest Child Dental Health Survey, in 2003, 43% of 5 year olds had obvious decay in the primary teeth. Forty per cent of 5 year olds had at least one primary tooth with decay into dentine and 12% had at least one filled primary tooth. Among 8 year olds, 57% had obvious decay in the primary teeth. Fifty per cent of 8 year olds had a least one primary tooth with decay into dentine and 26% had at least one filled primary tooth.

Decay in adult teeth in children has also decreased. The proportion of 8-, 12- and 15-year-old children with decay has gone down. The percentage of 15 year olds with decay in 1983 was 42%, in 1993 it was down to 30% and in 2003 it was only 13%.

Despite these dramatic changes, children still suffer unnecessary levels of tooth decay that can lead to pain and suffering and in some cases to children having teeth extracted under general anaesthetic.

Health inequalities

Dental health inequalities match other health inequalities. It has become widely accepted that dental decay is associated with social deprivation. Despite the improvements in dental health, there has been a polarisation of disease. The 1998 Adult Dental Health Survey clearly showed the dental health inequalities between socio-economic classes. Social classes I and II are more likely to have their natural teeth and have fewer restorations compared with social classes IV and V (*see* Table 28.2).

Table 28.2 Socio-economic class and adult dental health, 1998 (percentage with each condition)

Social class of head of household	% of all adults		% of dentate adults				
	Edentate	*Dentate*	*Natural teeth and dentures*	*21 or more natural teeth*	*At least one artificial crown*	*At least moderate tooth wear*	*Exposed, worn, filled or decayed roots*
I, II, IIINM	8	92	16	86	38	10	67
IIIM	15	85	20	79	30	14	68
IV, V	22	78	23	76	28	12	66

Source: Adult Dental Health Survey 1998 (ONS 2000).

The inequalities are the same for children. When you consider that the average number of decayed, missing or filled teeth (DMFT) for 5-year-old children in the UK is 1.6 but more than half of the child population have no decay, this means that the remaining 43% have the decay and the average number of teeth with decay is 3.7. This is unacceptable, especially when you consider that tooth decay is a preventable disease.

The interesting aspect of health inequalities is that they can appear in 5 years but also disappear in 5 years. Targeted water fluoridation has been shown to have dramatic effects on inequalities. Comparisons between Manchester (where the water is not fluoridated) and Birmingham (where the water is fluoridated) show marked differences in the average statistics for decayed, missing or filled teeth. Children in Manchester have three times the amount of decay than their peers in Birmingham. The populations are the same in all factors except for fluoride in the water. Programmes such as promoting tooth-brushing with fluoride toothpaste, and reducing the frequency of consumption of sugary foods and drinks, may well improve the dental health of a generation.

Older people

It is well documented that we have an ageing population. People are living longer coupled with a falling birth rate meaning that there is a growing older population. This population is more ethnically diverse and has more women in it; it has a broad spectrum of dependence ranging from those with a high level of disposable income who are able to fund their own healthcare to those who cannot. This population is living longer than previous generations but also they are living with serious health problems for longer.

There are three distinct cohorts of older people; those who are very old and likely to be edentulous; those entering old age who have maintained most of their teeth although they need a lot of work; and those in middle age now who have good oral health and are unlikely to need much complex treatment although they may choose to have cosmetic work carried out. The middle group is likely to present a challenge in respect of their future oral health needs. As the statistics above suggest, more people are keeping their own teeth but these teeth need a lot more care and attention. They are often heavily restored and require much maintenance (British Dental Association 2003).

Maintaining oral hygiene is the key to good oral health and the link between oral health and general health in older people is more significant than people might think. As people get older, they are more prone to diseases and may have impaired dexterity which can have a marked effect on oral health. The same factors can lead to changes in diet. For example, older people often eat little and often which may cause an increase in sugar intake frequency. The downward spiral that can occur when a person's diet changes can have catastrophic effects on quality of life. A decrease in nutrient intake can lead to a decline in general health. This can have a knock-on effect on independence. A change in diet can affect oral health which, if left untreated, can lead to problems eating, drinking, socialising and ultimately a much poorer quality of life.

Fluoride

Fluoride has been proven to be an effective and safe way to prevent dental decay. The improvement of dental health over the last 30–40 years has been attributed to the introduction of fluoride toothpaste. In the UK, only 10% of the population receives fluoridated water yet it is an effective and cost-effective way of tackling tooth decay (British Fluoridation Society *et al.* 2004). The World Health Organization has recognised that fluoridation is one of the top 30 public health initiatives yet, despite this, it still remains a controversial topic with numerous debates on the safety, efficacy and legality of fluoridating the water supply.

The history, issues and legislation around water fluoridation

The arguments on the safety of fluoridation are around the possible links to cancers, birth defects, fluorosis and issues around personal choice and mass medication.

There had been no new water fluoridation initiatives since the 1985 Water (Fluoridation) Act subsequently subsumed by the 1991 Water Industry Act. This Act gave power to the water companies to fluoridate the water supplies at the request of the local authority. Unfortunately the water companies refused to fluoridate on the grounds that they had no indemnity.

Since this ruling, there have been several research projects looking at the safety and efficacy of fluoridation. The York report (2000) concluded that the best available research evidence suggests that fluoridation of drinking water reduces tooth decay but it also found a link between the concentration of fluoride and levels of fluorosis. The lack of good quality evidence was also highlighted and York called for further research to improve the evidence base (NHS Centre for Reviews and Dissemination 2000).

The Department of Health commissioned the Medical Research Council (MRC) in 2002 to look at the risks and benefits of water fluoridation. The MRC ruled out many of the supposed health negative effects of fluoride but called for further research into the way natural and artificial fluoride is absorbed (Medical

Research Council 2002). The Chief Medical Officer and the Chief Dental Officer commissioned Newcastle University to undertake this research and the results show that there is no difference (University of Newcastle 2004).

In March 2003 work started on amending the Water Bill 2003 (formerly known as the 1991 Water Industry Act). The Water Bill 2003 progressed through both the House of Lords and the House of Commons. In March 2005, the draft regulations were passed by both houses and enacted. The new Act will enable local communities to decide whether they want their water supply fluoridated or not. Strategic health authorities will have to follow guidelines on how to consult with the population that will receive the water.

If strategic health authorities manage to successfully implement water fluoridation then we should see changes in the number of decayed teeth and a reduction in the number of children undergoing tooth extractions under general anaesthetic within as little as 5 years.

An example of an innovative campaign on water fluoridation was a postcard initiative. The postcard, supported by the British Dental Association, UK Public Health Association, Faculty of Public Health and the Royal College of Nursing, was designed so that dentists, members of the public and people interested in public health could send it to their MP encouraging them to support the amendment.

Health promotion campaigns

There are a number of oral health promotion campaigns including Mouth Cancer Awareness Week, Smile Week and Oral Health Month. Oral Health Month is a joint venture between the British Dental Association and Colgate. The 2004 campaign, 'Fighting together for better oral health', was quite a unique initiative. The campaign engaged dentists, Colgate, the British Dental Association and the public all working together for a month to promote better oral health. In addition to the usual instore promotions and media coverage, ten areas of the UK with the worst oral health were identified and targeted to receive health-promotion materials including oral hygiene literature, toothbrushes and toothpaste.

Looking ahead, challenges and opportunities

New contractual arrangements for dentists

Dentistry faces a challenging time. Legislation has been passed through the Westminster Parliament which will move the focus for dental provision to local level. Care is now commissioned by PCTs from independent contractor dentists, corporate bodies or provided by dentists employed directly by the trusts and allows PCTs to seek to meet the oral health needs of their population. Remuneration for general dental practitioners has moved away from payment for individual items of service to payments based on provision of care for a cohort of patients. Together with the proposed introduction of an oral health assessment, this is intended to change the emphasis of dental care to that of preventing disease. The oral health assessment focuses on lifestyle, diet and general health as well as on oral health and self-care. Guidance from the

National Institute for Clinical Excellence has called for changes to the 6-month recall. Historically patients have been called back to the dentist for 6-month check-ups as a standard procedure but now patients will be called back according to clinical need. This means that a patient could be seen every 3 months for an examination if they were considered to have poor oral health or up to 2 years if they had good oral health. The length between each visit would be dependent on a number of factors including risk of dental decay and/or gum disease (NICE 2004).

This change of legislation was enacted in April 2006 in England, with the Welsh Assembly Government also covered by the same powers to allow this move to take place in Wales. In Scotland proposals for a 3-year investment plan have been announced which will include support and enhancement to existing NHS dental services and dental public health programmes including tooth-brushing programmes and support for nursery- and schools-based oral health improvement initiatives. The changes are accompanied by additional funding but the extent to which the dental profession will be engaged with the changes is as yet unknown. Access to NHS dentistry is difficult in many parts of the country as a result of workforce shortages. Some dentists in England moved in advance of April 2006 to the new local contracts but others are changing the emphasis of the funding of their practice to private rather than NHS contracts. Patient charges have also been reviewed and a new system of payments was also introduced in April 2006. It remains to be seen whether the challenge to simplify the charges for dental care and retain the level of funding from these direct patient contributions, while ensuring that those in greatest need of care are not deterred from seeking it, has been met.

Skill mix

The regulations governing other dental professionals have also changed, allowing the registration of dental nurses and technicians and the regulation of all dental professionals, including hygienists and therapists, through ethical guidance and curricula rather than prescriptive lists of duties. The implementation of the PCD (professionals complementary to dentistry) regulatory reforms will mean that it is much easier for the General Dental Council to change the roles and duties of groups of PCDs (or indeed to create more new classes of PCDs). There is now far more emphasis on team-working, and skills and responsibilities are being delegated more and more within clinical teams. Dentistry cannot be immune to these trends and there are good reasons for welcoming this. Not least of these reasons are the continued workforce shortages facing the profession and the changing epidemiological and demographic context in which dentistry is being practised.

References

British Dental Association (2003) *Oral Health for Older People; 2020 vision*. London: British Dental Association.

British Fluoridation Society *et al.* (2004) *One in a Million – the facts about water fluoridation*. London: British Fluoridation Society, UK Public Health Association, British Dental Association and Faculty of Public Health.

Department of Health (1994) *Oral Health Strategy for England*. London: Department of Health.

Medical Research Council (2002) *Water Fluoridation and Health. Working Group Report*. London: Medical Research Council.

NHS Centre for Reviews and Dissemination (2000) *A Systematic Review of Public Water Fluoridation* (CRD Report No. 18). York: NHS Centre for Reviews and Dissemination, University of York.

NICE (2004) *NICE Guidelines on Frequency of Dental Check-ups 2004/044*. London: NICE.

Office for National Statistics (2000) *Adult Dental Health Survey: oral health in the UK 1998*. Edited by A Walker and I Cooper. London: The Stationery Office.

Office for National Statistics (2004) *Child Dental Health Survey 2003: preliminary findings*. www.statistics.gov.uk/downloads/theme_health/cdh_preliminary_findings.pdf.

University of Newcastle (2004) *Bioavailability of Fluoride in Drinking-water – a human experimental study commissioned by the Department of Health*. Newcastle: University of Newcastle.

Chapter 29

The contribution of the acute sector to promoting public health

Diane Gray and Nicholas R Hicks

In the minds of the public, hospitals tend to represent healthcare and health, a fact exploited by politicians and frustrating to many others, including public health practitioners. As reactive organisations, dealing with the effects of disease and unhealthy lifestyles on individual patients, hospitals' role in promoting population health may seem obscure. However, the acute sector absorbs over half developed countries' total spend on healthcare and therefore consumes significant proportions of their annual gross national product (GNP) (OECD 2005). Its contributions to the health of populations in these countries are therefore pertinent.

Health is (in the majority of cases) improved in hospitals by the very nature of the services and care provided there, although this is tempered by the negative contribution of iatrogenic and nosocomial illnesses. Healthy lifestyles can be promoted in, and by, hospitals both systematically and opportunistically to patients, staff and visitors who collectively comprise a significant proportion of the population. Furthermore, people in the surrounding community can derive benefit from hospitals without even stepping foot inside. Indeed, as this chapter will explore, hospitals hold a unique and key position in providing, promoting and protecting good health.

The past contribution of the acute sector

The debate on whether healthcare has had a positive, negative or neutral impact on population health has raged for many decades. On the one hand, in the 1960s, commentators such as McKeown and Illich asserted that iatrogenic disease, medical and surgical errors, and the 'medicalisation' of common conditions have worsened population health (Illich 1976; McKeown 1979). More recently, opponents of these views, such as Mackenbach and Bunker, have argued that advances in medical care, such as thrombolysis and the introduction of coronary care units in the treatment of heart attacks, have been responsible for a significant proportion of the increase in life expectancy since 1950 and for significant decreases in patient morbidity (Bunker 2001; Mackenbach 1996). The latest reviews have concluded that there is truth in both viewpoints – that while healthcare up to the mid-20th century may have had little overall impact on population mortality, advances in medical science coupled with the relatively recent advent of evidence-based medicine in the latter decades of the last century have dramatically improved outcomes for patients and therefore for populations. Indeed, Nolte and McKee have illustrated that, at the end of the 20th century, it has been improvements in *access* to effective healthcare (as well as healthcare *per se*) that has reduced mortality in infants in countries such as Greece and in middle-aged and elderly people in countries like the United Kingdom (Nolte and

McKee 2004). As the largest component of healthcare in terms of staff numbers and share of total annual budget, and as the sites for much of the research evidence produced, the acute sector must be credited with significant contributions to these improvements in the public's health over recent decades.

At the start of the 21st century, however, parts of the acute sector in the United States and United Kingdom are starting to move away from purely managing individuals (with impacts on population health a secondary benefit) towards a more holistic approach and including public health sentiments. For example, Kaiser Permanente, a large health maintenance organisation in the United States, is proud of the dual mindset it encourages and nurtures in its doctors, to improve both the health of the individual and that of the population (Ham *et al.* 2003).

Ensuring high-quality healthcare

As organisations delivering acute healthcare, perhaps the most natural public health role for hospitals is to ensure this care is of the highest quality. The emergence of clinical governance (with increased emphasis for risk management and patient safety) in England in the late 1990s has been a key example of developing this function, working in conjunction with guidance from the National Institute for Clinical Excellence and the national regulatory body (currently the Healthcare Commission) (Department of Health 1999). However, so far, clinical governance has not gained the same prominence as financial or corporate governance. In the future, acute hospitals' ratings in England will include performance against public health standards, although the level of detail required – and therefore, one might cynically comment, the degree of hospital participation in public health – is (at least to begin with) somewhat superficial (Healthcare Commission 2005).

The spread of foundation trust status among English hospitals, which further separates hospitals from commissioning and public health bodies, raises concerns that involvement in the public health agenda may slide back down the list of priorities for hospital management as they strive to gain the competitive advantage in the new NHS marketplace of 'payment by results' (Department of Health 2003a, 2003b). Similar market tools in the United States resulted in gaming and diagnosis-related group (DRG) creep – for example, classifying patients with more severe forms of illness or keeping them admitted just long enough to slip into a higher tariff band (Hsia *et al.* 1988). On the other hand, the drive to improve quality and cost-effectiveness of hospital care (and the break-up of public health teams during the move from health authorities to primary care trusts) has led to some hospitals (for example, Leeds Teaching Hospitals, Great Ormond Street Hospital for Sick Children and Oxford Radcliffe Hospitals) directly employing public health practitioners in senior positions. There is no single model of acute care public health, but successful post holders have had to be credible to both clinicians and managers, functioning as the 'honest broker' to ensure that local clinical policy is evidence based. They balance increasing clinical sub-specialisation with a population approach, and challenge the assumptions of management and clinicians on current organisation and practice (Proceedings of 'Public Health in Hospitals' conference 2003). From within hospitals, public health practitioners are well placed to disseminate public health skills to a wider body of healthcare professionals, many of whom would not view their jobs as including any public health but need to do so in order to push clinical governance and health improvement forward. The roles of in-house public health experts have also incorporated responsibility for establishing and maintaining clinical governance systems, implementation of National Service Frameworks, facilitating and conducting health service research, and using clinical epidemiology skills in analysing and interpreting the mass of available data collected by hospital information departments. They may be well placed to spot NHS 'DRG creep' and should be in a senior enough position to prevent its spread. On a more positive note, information such as hospital episode statistics, bed numbers, outpatient referral numbers, attendances at emergency departments, drug usage, staffing levels, and so on, especially when linked with primary care information, can inform the development of wider programmes of health promotion and creation of innovative services spanning primary and secondary care.

Protecting health

The acute sector's part in health protection has developed over recent years for several reasons. The increasing threat from covert chemical and biological terrorism means that the earliest indication of an incident could be the changing epidemiology of cases attending emergency departments (Heffernan *et al.* 2004). Second, reorganisation of Britain's public health structures has resulted in hospital laboratories taking over some of the responsibilities from the public health laboratory service in the screening and surveillance of infectious diseases, and hospital clinicians becoming more involved in contact tracing and treating as on-call public health becomes more centralised and remote (Department of Health 2002).

Hospitals also face specific health-protection problems. Methicillin-resistant *Staphylococcus aureus* (MRSA) and other nosocomial infections remain prevalent among inpatients, with around 0.15 cases of MRSA bacteraemia per 1,000 bed days in general acute trusts in England (Health Protection Agency 2005). Although the persistence of nosocomial infections is largely due to increasing patient turnover and complexity of cases (www.hpa.org.uk 2005), the solution to preventing its spread is probably the most simple public health intervention of all: hand washing. Yet, despite developing specialist infection control teams, the rise in nosocomial infection numbers and reinforcement of the 'clean hands' message still remain challenges for hospital public health.

Promoting good health

In 2003–04, there were 11.6 million admissions to NHS hospitals in England, 15 million attendances at emergency departments, and over 44 million outpatient appointments (Department of Health 2004b; Hospital Activity Statistics 2005). These patients were cared for by 81,000 doctors and a million non-medical staff (including nurses, allied health professionals, scientific and technical staff, and porters) (Department of Health 2005a, 2005b). A further unknown number of people came into contact as visitors, when delivering goods, and by using the NHS as a training site. Many of those passing through hospital doors each year are targets for health-promotion campaigns in the community and arrive at hospital at points in their lives when they are more receptive to advice on healthier lifestyle choices (Florin and Basham 2000).

Acute hospitals therefore provide a captive, receptive and appropriate audience for health promotion, which can be delivered both opportunistically and systematically. Evidence has shown that opportunistic advice to patients from healthcare professionals on smoking cessation, decreasing alcohol consumption and increasing physical activity is effective (Mulvihill and Quigley 2003; Mulvihill *et al.* 2004; Naidoo *et al.* 2004). Hospital policy can also act as a form of preventive risk management, whereby hospital food can set the example for patients, visitors and staff on producing healthy meals, and smoke-free hospital sites provide an impetus to staff and patients to quit (Health Development Agency 2004). Apparently competing priorities can also be creatively converged: smoking cessation and alcohol abstinence advice offered to patients on surgery waiting lists potentially advantage both patients and hospitals with speedier postoperative recovery and decreased risk of complications (Møller *et al.* 2002; Tønnesen *et al.* 1999).

In 1988, the World Health Organization launched the Health Promoting Hospitals project, in which hospitals are supported to provide health promotion, disease prevention and rehabilitation services. It now covers 25 countries and over 700 hospitals in Europe, including 83 in the United Kingdom (Health Promoting Hospitals 2005). Initially, its member hospitals undertook isolated projects to improve the health of a group of patients. More recent challenges have been to create a sea-change in the culture of hospital organisation to take greater responsibility for community health (Gröne 2004).

Pursuing health promotion in acute hospitals has had low priority compared with the pressure to meet clinical need or to meet other targets such as waiting times and financial balance. However, several recent events have started to encourage a role for the acute sector in improving population health. First, a clear manifesto pledge by the British Labour government to reduce inequalities in life expectancy across the country by 2010 has resulted in a focus on healthcare interventions, such as thrombolysis and inpatient care of patients with respiratory disease, which can delay the premature deaths of those already with disease (Labour Party Manifesto 2005). Second, the Wanless reports in England demonstrated that future costs of the NHS could drain the public purse unless the general public could be encouraged to take up primary prevention messages and lead healthier lifestyles, and the NHS move from a 'sickness service' to a 'health service'. By moving from 'slow uptake' to 'fully engaged', a healthier public (and a more responsive NHS) would save the NHS up to £30 billion by 2023 (Wanless 2002, 2004). The subsequent government response in England, *Choosing Health*, controversially placed the NHS – and therefore hospitals – at the centre of the drive to improve the population's health (Department of Health 2004a). As part of this move towards a 'health' service, hospital staff are now increasingly being seen as role models for the general public, with concomitant increases in health-promotion advice and support specifically for hospital staff through the *Improving Working Lives* initiative (Department of Health 2000). Some hospitals are also resurrecting strict disciplinary measures against staff seen smoking or drinking alcohol while in hospital uniform (North Somerset PCT 2003; Royal Surrey County Hospital NHS Trust 2003).

In addition, policy makers have recognised that large proportions of populations in developed countries – over one third in England – have at least one long-term condition such as asthma, diabetes or heart disease, and make up a significant proportion of the emergency inpatients in hospitals. For example,

Damiani and Dixon found that patients with chronic obstructive airways disease were almost solely responsible for the winter pressure on hospital beds in London (Damiani and Dixon 2002). Attempts are now being made to encourage people with long-term conditions to better manage their own health and prevent complications – traditional secondary prevention – as exemplified in England by the publication of a national model for the health and social care for people with long-term conditions (Department of Health 2005c).

Promoting healthier lifestyle choices is only one method the acute sector can use to improve the health of the people within them. The work of Ulrich and others has highlighted the relevance of creating health-promoting physical environments for patients and morale-boosting surroundings for staff and patients within hospitals (Waller and Finn 2004), now being encouraged through new architectural design as promoted by the CABE (Commission for Architecture and the Built Environment) 'Healthy Hospitals' campaign (www.healthyhospitals.org.uk 2005). Crowley and Hunter have argued that public health is too concerned with improving healthcare, to the detriment of tackling broader determinants of health, such as housing and employment, and developing communities, which could produce greater impacts in health improvement (Crowley and Hunter 2005). Yet hospitals also have the potential to impact on underlying determinants of health, acting as 'corporate citizens', in their day-to-day running. Routes of influences are as: a local employer; a bulk purchaser of foods (minimising the impact of 'food miles') and other goods (choosing sustainable producers); an energy consumer (promoting energy efficiency in new buildings and staff practices); a source of waste (using environmentally sound methods of disposal); and a popular local destination (developing green travel plans and alternatives to car transport) (Coote 2002). Through their immense commissioning and spending power, hospitals have the ability to demand changes towards more environmentally friendly and healthy modes of production, delivery and disposal of the goods they purchase. Furthermore, hospitals can be agents of social inclusion by having human resources and recruitment policies that make the most of and develop the skills of the local population.

The acute sector is therefore an opportune, and underutilised, site for health promotion. Its onward development depends, however, on greater acknowledgement of these opportunities and an expressed will from senior management and clinicians to work with other health and non-healthcare colleagues to incorporate health promotion into hospitals' everyday activities.

Future contributions

At present, the acute sector in England is being driven in two directions: first, the purchaser/provider split and introduction of patient choice mean developing higher quality and more cost-effective elective care in order to market services to and win contracts from commissioners (both in PCTs and general practices). Second, care for people with long-term conditions encourages closer links with primary and social care, to ensure that patients' emergency attendances at and admissions to hospital are as infrequent and short as possible. While there are some tensions between the two policy directions, both reinforce the need for good public health intervention in and by the acute sector: to prevent complications in elective care (primary prevention and robust clinical governance procedures) and to prevent emergency admissions (secondary prevention of relapses or acute deterioration). The refreshed emphasis on promoting healthier lifestyles creates a third tension for acute hospitals: as the population's concept of health moves away from simply the absence of disease and towards improving quality of life, the acute sector must accelerate the move to work with its community (including local authority and voluntary groups) to provide both a therapeutic and a more holistic service for its patients and the community from which they come.

Beyond the public health triad

Yet there is more to hospitals' role in promoting public health than contributions to the triad of public health components (health promotion, health protection, healthcare quality) (www.fph.org.uk 2005). The strength of the image of hospitals as the front end of health and healthcare, hosting many of the elite of the medical world, provides them with power as a local politician, capable of lobbying for change and influencing decisions. While this power is often coupled to an inpatient mentality and directed towards self-interest, it can extend effectively beyond hospital walls. For example, the Royal College of Physicians (as befits the parent organisation of the Faculty of Public Health) is actively working to reduce the harm caused by alcohol abuse, obesity and smoking through education of its members, the general public and policy makers (Working Party of the Royal College of Physicians *et al.* 2004; www.rcplondon.ac.uk 2005). If this degree of involvement in the 'health agenda' were replicated by district hospitals, then significant effects could be seen in local communities.

To the public, hospitals are a visible safety net. This is typified by the 'Kidderminster effect' of the 2001 British general election, when a Labour seat was lost to a local doctor standing as an independent candidate on a 'Save Our Hospital' ticket (Morgan 2001). The general public relish the knowledge that, should they ever need the services of a hospital, one is nearby. Hospitals create a sense of security and wellbeing, and as such have become part of the fabric of the community. This in itself promotes good public psychological health, and suggests that hospitals will remain, for the foreseeable future, symbols to the public of health and healthcare. The extent to which hospitals choose to exploit this status for the benefit of their local population depends on the relative merits of programmes such as Health Promoting Hospitals balanced against financial incentives and political targets. Until the latter reflect the aims of the former, local populations will not be best served by their hospitals, despite any perceptions otherwise.

In summary, hospitals can have a profound impact on the health of their surrounding population, through:

- the clinical care provided and the use of evidence to support this provision
- minimising the dangers of hospital-acquired infections and communicable disease
- using patient and public 'footfall' and individual contacts as an opportunity to promote 'healthy' messages
- using both staff and hospital as exemplars of 'health' (through the public behaviour of staff members and the policies of the institution)
- being a 'corporate citizen', through considerate use of economic power and sensitivity to the local community.

However, the distractions for hospital management and clinicians of the requirements to deliver healthcare in an increasingly competitive arena mean these opportunities to protect and promote public health are too frequently missed.

References

Bunker JP (2001) The role of medical care in contributing to health improvements within societies. *Int J Epidemiol.* **30**: 1260–3.

Commission for Architecture and the Built Environment (CABE) (2005) *Healthy Hospitals.* www.healthyhospitals.org.uk (accessed April 25 2005).

Coote A (2002) *Claiming the Health Dividend: unlocking the benefits of NHS spending.* London: King's Fund.

Crowley P and Hunter DJ (2005) Putting the public back into public health. *J Epidemiol Community Health.* **59**: 265–7.

Damiani M and Dixon J (2002) *Managing the Pressure: emergency hospital admissions in London 1997–2001.* London: King's Fund.

Department of Health (1999) *Clinical Governance in the New NHS.* Health Service Circular 1999/065. London: Department of Health.

Department of Health (2000) *Improving Working Lives Standard.* London: Department of Health.

Department of Health (2002) *Getting Ahead of the Curve: action to strengthen the microbiology function in the prevention and control of infectious diseases.* London: Department of Health.

Department of Health (2003a) *Payment by Results: preparing for 2005.* London: Department of Health.

Department of Health (2003b) *Short Guide to NHS Foundation Trusts.* London: Department of Health.

Department of Health (2004a) *Choosing Health: making healthier choices easier.* London: Stationery Office.

Department of Health (2004b) *HES Headline Data.* London: Department of Health. Available at: www.hesonline.nhs.uk.

Department of Health (2005a) *Hospital, Public Health Medicine and Community Health Services Medical and Dental Staff in England: 1994–2004.* Bulletin 2005/03. London: Department of Health.

Department of Health (2005b) *NHS Hospital and Community Health Services Non-medical Staff in England: 1994–2004.* Bulletin 2005/04. London: Department of Health.

Department of Health (2005c) *Supporting People with Long Term Conditions: an NHS and social care model to support local innovation and integration.* London: Stationery Office.

Faculty of Public Health: www.fph.org.uk/about_faculty/what_public_health/default.asp (accessed 29 June 2005).

Florin D and Basham S (2000) Evaluation of health promotion in clinical settings. In: M Thorogood and Y Coombes (eds) *Evaluating Health Promotion. Practice and methods.* Oxford: Oxford University Press.

Gröne O (2004) Beyond Health Promoting Hospitals: developing patient-centred networks of health and social care services. *HPH Newsletter.* December.

Ham C, York N, Sutch S *et al.* (2003) Hospital bed utilisation in the NHS, Kaiser Permanente, and the US Medicare programme: analysis of routine data. *BMJ.* **327** (7426): 1257.

Healthcare Commission (2005) *Criteria for Assessing Core Standards.* London: Healthcare Commission.

Health Development Agency, Pharmacy Health Link (2004) *The Case for a Completely Smokefree NHS in England.* London: Health Development Agency.

Health Promoting Hospitals (2005): www.euro.who.int/healthpromohosp (accessed 29 June 2005).

Health Protection Agency (2005) *Action to Strengthen the Microbiology Function in the Prevention and Control of Infectious Diseases*. Available at: www.hpa.org.uk/infections/topics_az/staphylo/MRSA_four_year.pdf (accessed 29 June 2005).

Heffernan R, Mostashari F, Das D *et al.* (2004) System descriptions: New York City syndromic surveillance systems. *MMWR.* **53**(Suppl): 23–7.

Hospital Activity Statistics: www.performance.doh.gov.uk/hospitalactivity/data_requests/ (accessed 20 April 2005).

Hsia DC, Krushat WM, Fagan AB *et al.* (1988) Accuracy of diagnostic coding for Medicare patients under the prospective-payment system. *N Engl J Med.* **318**(6): 352–5.

Illich I (1976) *Limits to Medicine*. London: Marion Boyars.

Labour Party Manifesto (2005). Available at: www.labour.org.uk/manifesto (accessed 29 June 2005).

Mackenbach JP (1996) The contribution of medical care to mortality decline: McKeown revisited. *J Clin Epidemiol.* **49**: 1207–13.

McKeown T (1979) *The Role of Medicine: dream, mirage or nemesis?* Oxford: Blackwell.

Møller AM, Villebro N, Pedersen T and Tonnesen H (2002) Effect of preoperative smoking intervention on postoperative complications: a randomised clinical trial. *Lancet.* **359**(9301): 114–17.

Morgan B (2001) *General Election Results, 7 June 2001*. London: House of Commons Library Research paper 01/54.

Mulvihill C and Quigley R (2003) *The Management of Obesity and Overweight. An analysis of reviews of diet, physical activity and behavioural approaches. Evidence briefing* (1e). London: Health Development Agency.

Mulvihill C, Taylor L and Waller S (2004) *Evidence Briefing: prevention and reduction of alcohol misuse: a review of reviews* (2e). London: Health Development Agency.

Naidoo B, Warm D, Quigley R *et al.* (2004) *Evidence Briefing: smoking and public health: a review of reviews of interventions to increase smoking cessation, reduce smoking initiation and prevent further uptake of smoking* (1e). London: Health Development Agency.

Nolte E and McKee M (2004) *Does Healthcare Save Lives? Avoidable mortality revisited*. London: Nuffield Trust.

North Somerset Primary Care Trust (2003) *Tackling Smoking: policy on smoking in the workplace*. www.northsomerset.nhs.uk/hr/policy/NSPCT%20Policy%20on%20Smoking.doc (accessed 18 May 2006).

Organisation for Economic Co-operation and Development (2005) *OECD Health Data*. Available from: www.oecd.org/document/30/0,2340,en_2649_34631_12968734_1_1_1_1,00.html.

Proceedings of 'Public Health in Hospitals' conference (2003) 30 October. Sponsored by the Faculty of Public Health, the British Association of Medical Managers and the Department of Health.

The Royal Surrey County Hospital NHS Trust (2003) *Substance, Alcohol and Drug Misuse Policy*. www.royalsurrey.nhs.uk/intranet/Royal-Surr/Freedom-of/The-Public/SAD-Policy.pdf (accessed 18 May 2006).

Tønnesen H, Rosenberg J, Nielsen HJ *et al.* (1999) Effect of preoperative abstinence on poor postoperative outcome in alcohol misusers. *BMJ.* **318**: 1311–16.

Waller S and Finn H (2004) *Enhancing the Healing Environment: a guide for NHS trusts*. London: King's Fund.

Wanless D (2002) *Securing Our Future Health – taking a long term view*. London: HM Treasury.

Wanless D (2004) *Securing Good Health for the Whole Population: final report*. London: HMSO.

Working Party of the Royal College of Physicians, Royal College of Paediatrics and Child Health, Faculty of Public Health Medicine (2004) *Storing Up Problems: the medical case for a slimmer nation*. London: RCP.

Chapter 30

Health protection and environmental public health in the UK and the rest of Europe

Angus Nicoll

Summary

Health protection is a new concept that has gained popularity as an area of public health activity in the last decade. Its core functions include the prevention and control of infections (the communicable disease function), protection against non-communicable environmental hazards (chemicals, poisons and radiological hazards) and emergency planning and the healthcare response to emergencies. The limits of health protection are less well defined. As a group of activities it has considerable overlap with the term *environmental public health*. Like other parts of public health, health protection is exercised by many people who would not view themselves as public health specialists though most if not all of these people are exercising public health skills. Health protection is concerned with both acute events and also long-term issues. The UK has the most explicit national approach to this area with the adoption of a health protection strategy (2002), the creation of the Health Protection Agency (2003) and the Health Protection Agency Act (2005). These developments are expected to deliver a series of improvements including strengthening surveillance, delivering surge capacity, and modernising public health pathology. Outside the health services sector there are important developments under the Cabinet Office system with the formation of national and regional resilience teams operating across sectors to ensure that services are sustained in emergencies and sectors are well coordinated. In response to a number of national and international events other countries in Europe and beyond are adopting variations on the UK model. At the European level there have been organisational arrangements for health protection for some years under the European Commission. However, these are limited by European Union law which has little to say on public health and mostly leaves this to member states. Because this is demonstrably an inadequate response to infectious disease threats which require coordinated response a European Centre for Disease Prevention and Control (ECDC) has been established in 2005, initially only dealing with infectious diseases and the emergency health response. Other important developments are the modernisation of the International Health Regulations which were adopted by the World Health Assembly in 2005, the creation a decade ago of a single UN body for dealing with HIV and AIDS and the creation of a UN coordinator for pandemic influenza.

Introduction

Delivering *health protection* is one of the core functions of public health (*see* Box 30.1).

Box 30.1 Definition and scope of health protection

Definition: the components of health protection

- The communicable disease function.
- Protection against non-communicable environmental hazards.
- Emergency planning and response (Regan 1999).

Scope

- Preventing and dealing with the threats to health from infectious diseases.
- Protecting against threats from chemicals and radiological hazards.
- The healthcare response to emergencies.
- Environmental public health.

However, those that deliver or contribute to health protection come from many specialties and disciplines both within and beyond the strict limits of the public health profession (Nicoll and Murray 2002; Regan 1999) (*see* Box 30.2).

Box 30.2 UK groups delivering the public health response

1 An influenza pandemic

- Public health – consultants in communicable disease control,* regional HPA teams and *Regional Directors of Public Health.*
- Specialist virology.
- General microbiology – public health *and clinical microbiologists.*
- *National Health Service – primary and secondary (hospital) care teams.*
- *Local, Regional and National Resilience Teams.*
- *National government and the Cabinet Office.*
- *Local government – Environmental Health Officers.*
- *Professional staff in training.*

Support services for the above (public health scientists, communication specialists, information technologists, administrative staff, etc.).

- *Other government sectors – education, transport, etc.*

Those in italics are usually or often outside the Health Protection Agency in England.

2 Controlling tuberculosis

- Public health – consultants in communicable disease control.
- Regional HPA teams and *Regional Directors of Public Health.*
- Specialist bacteriology.
- Microbiology – public health *and clinical microbiologists.*
- *Outreach and advocacy services for ethnic minority groups.*

- *Non-governmental organisations.*
- *National Health Service – primary and secondary (hospital) care teams.*

Those in italics are outside the Health Protection Agency in England and Wales.

3 Preparing for deliberate release of chemical and biological agents

- Health emergency planning advisers.
- Public health – consultants in communicable disease control, and regional epidemiologists and *Regional Directors of Public Health.*
- Microbiologists.
- Toxicologists.
- *Clinicians.*
- *The security services (army, police, intelligence).*
- *The emergency services (fire, ambulance).*
- *National government and the Cabinet Office.*
- *Local government.*
- *International agencies.*
- Professional staff in training.

Support services for the above (public health scientists, communication specialists, information technologists, administrative staff, etc.).
Those in italics are usually or often outside the Health Protection Agency in England

* These titles apply in England – the titles of this and some other posts will differ in other parts of the UK.

The United Kingdom (currently 2005) has the most explicit health-protection function in Europe. In 2002, England's Chief Medical Officer, Professor Sir Liam Donaldson published a health-protection strategy for controlling infections, and other environmental threats, as well as delivering the health services' response to emergencies (*see* Boxes 30.1 and 30.3). This confirmed infectious disease control and health protection as health priorities. As a central part of the strategy in April 2003 a Health Protection Agency was created for England and Wales with a broad remit. It combined four non-departmental public bodies with those professionals currently delivering health protection locally in Wales (*see* Boxes 30.4 and 30.5). In 2005 the strategy was given a statutory basis and the Agency extended to the whole of the UK with its Parliament passing the Health Protection Agency Act though there are important organisational differences between the four countries (*see* Table 30.1) (Department of Health 2002; HPA Act 2004; www.hpa.org.uk). There are many more similarities than differences; however, there are some important variations in the delivery of health-protection services, especially at the local level. With hindsight the production of the strategy and Agency can be viewed as extraordinarily timely, both nationally and internationally. A series of events has taken place that raised the profile of health protection in Europe and beyond (*see* Box 30.6) (Donnelly *et al.* 2004; Fleming 2005; Harling *et al.* 2001; Lightfoot *et al.* 2001; Morita *et al.* 1995; Mort *et al.* 2005; Nicoll *et al.* 2001; Okumura *et al.* 1998; Simms *et al.* 2004; Trotter and Edmunds 2002).

Box 30.3 Key elements of the UK Health Protection Strategy

- Creation of a Health Protection Agency.
- A local health-protection service.
- A national expert panel to advise on infectious disease strategy.*
- A strengthened and expanded system of infectious disease surveillance.
- New action plans to address infectious disease priorities.
- Rationalisation of microbiology laboratories and introduction of standards.
- An inspector of microbiology.
- A programme of new vaccine development and deployment.
- Strengthened clinical and preventive services for dealing with infection in childhood.
- Further development of plans to combat the threat to public health of deliberate release of biological, chemical or radiological agents.
- Better public information.
- Stronger professional education and training programmes.
- A research and innovation programme.
- A review of public health law.

* NEPNEI – Chief Medical Officer's National Expert Panel on Infectious Disease (First Chairman Professor Chris Bartlett).

Box 30.4 Functions of the Health Protection Agency

- To provide information, expertise and advice on infectious diseases, chemical and radiation hazards.
- To coordinate all systems of surveillance relevant to the prevention and control of infectious diseases in England.
- To develop and maintain a system of surveillance to protect the public health against the risks from chemical and radiation hazards.
- To identify gaps in surveillance and develop information systems to close them.
- To set standards and guidelines for the notification and reporting of infection by health professionals and by laboratories.
- To recommend changes to the statutory list of notifiable diseases and institute modern criteria for case definitions.
- To work with the Commission for Health Improvement where there are serious deficiencies in standards of infection control in hospitals, primary care or other health service premises.
- To work with the NHS and local authorities to provide a health protection and infectious disease control service.
- With the NHS and local authorities to investigate and manage outbreaks of infectious diseases, and chemical and radiation incidents in liaison with the appropriate authorities.
- To respond to new or emerging threats, including terrorism.

- To advise on national and local policy in relation to the prevention and control of infectious diseases and the protection of the public health from chemical and radiation hazards.
- To commission microbiology laboratories to provide specialist public health or reference functions.
- To review the current arrangements for provision of advice on chemical toxicology issues relating to clinical poisoning and chemical incidents to provide a robust, efficient system which meets the needs of both central government and the NHS.
- To provide agreed technical services.
- To advise the NHS Director of Research and Development on the use of a new research and innovation fund.

Box 30.5 Organisations and professional groups in the UK Health Protection Agency

National organisations:
Centre for Applied Microbiology and Research
The National Focus (Chemical Incidents)
The National Radiological Protection Board
The Public Health Laboratory Service
Communicable Disease Surveillance Centre
Central Public Health Laboratory (specialist and reference microbiology) and other reference laboratories
General public health microbiology

Professional groups:
Consultants for Communicable Disease Control
Health emergency planning advisers
Medical toxicologists and environmental epidemiologists and scientists
Public health microbiologists
Radiation scientists
Regional epidemiologists
Specialist microbiologists (reference laboratories)
plus support teams for all the above, public health scientists and nurses, environmental health officers, data managers, statisticians, IT specialists and administrative staff

Organisations encompassed by UK Health Protection Act 2005:
Communicable Disease Surveillance Centre – Northern Ireland
Health Protection Scotland
National Public Health Service Wales

Table 30.1 Organisational differences between the UK countries' health protection

	Central body's name	Have managed local staff	Includes general public health
England	Health Protection Agency	Yes	No
Northern Ireland*	Communicable Disease Surveillance Centre (NI)	No	No
Scotland	Health Protection Scotland	No	No
Wales	National Public Health Service Wales	Yes	Yes

*The arrangements in Northern Ireland are currently under review (November 2005) and are therefore subject to change.

Box 30.6 Recent 'acute' health-protection events of international importance

- Employment of biological and chemical agents by terrorists (1990s onwards).
- The foot and mouth epidemic in the UK (2000).
- Terrorist attacks in the USA (2001).
- Deliberate releases of anthrax in the USA and 'copycat' releases internationally (2001).
- SARS outbreaks in multiple countries (2003).
- Avian influenza (H5N7) in The Netherlands (2003).
- Avian influenza (H5N1) in the Far East and South East Asia and rising threat of a human pandemic (1997 onwards).
- Terrorist attack in Madrid (2004).
- Tsunamis in the Indian Ocean (2004).
- Terrorist attacks in London (2005).
- Flood rendering a whole city in an industrialised country unliveable – New Orleans (2005).

However, health protection addresses important strategic issues as well as immediate events (infection outbreaks, natural disasters and other emergencies). Given its scope a number of ongoing priorities also fall under the ambit of health protection (see Box 30.7). The list is long and includes the resurgence of previous threats to health: tuberculosis, gonorrhea and syphilis, rising levels of HIV (Nicoll and Hamers 2002) as well as heightened public expectations over safety of medical products (Baxter 1990; Brown 2000), concern over the health risks from chemicals and radiation in the environment (Health Protection Agency www.hpa.org.uk; National Radiation Protection Board 2004), emerging infections (mostly zoonoses) (Lederberg et al. 1992; Will et al. 1996), rising levels of nosocomial infections such as multiresistant *Staphylococcal aureus* (MRSA) and unrealised potential for health gain for many of these topics (Duckworth and Charlett 2005). These combined to make a convincing case for a concerted health-protection strategy.

Box 30.7 The need for health protection – continuing and chronic threats

Resurgence and rising levels of infection

- Sexually transmitted infections – gonorrhoea and syphilis.
- Tuberculosis.
- HIV.
- Rising levels of type C meningococcal disease in European countries.
- The next influenza pandemic.
- International and national gastrointestinal disease.

Emergence of new infections

- Viral haemorrhagic infections (lassa, ebola, etc.).
- New zoonoses (BSE, hendra and nipah viruses).

Exposure to exotic infections abroad and in the UK

- Malaria.
- Dengue fever.
- Other arboviral infections.

Threats associated with healthcare

- Healthcare-associated infections.
- Antibiotic-resistant organisms.
- Xenotransplantation.
- New blood-borne infections.

Novel threats to health

- Chemical, radiological and toxic challenges.
- Bioterrorism.
- Chemical and hormone residues in foods.

Unrealised health gain

- Undiagnosed infections (genital chlamydia and infertility).
- 'Silent' water infections (cryptosporidiosis).
- New and underutilised vaccines (pneumococcal and influenza vaccines).

Definition and limits of health protection

Health protection has been defined as those elements of the public health function which protect the population against communicable diseases and non-communicable environmental hazards (such as chemical fires and radiation threats) (*see* Box 30.1). It includes the public health aspects of the emergency response but is more than 'blue-light' public health. Routine public health tasks such as ensuring good immunisation coverage, tuberculosis control, infection control in healthcare settings and assessing environmental hazards are also within the health-protection repertoire (*see* Box 30.7). Health protection can also be defined by the threats it manages and this provides an audit tool. Any proposed local, national or international health-protection arrangements can be assessed for their likely safety by considering whether they would and do cope well with a series of threats – so-called *'acid tests'* – and these provide a ready list for exercises and contingency plans (*see* Box 30.7) (Health Protection Agency 2004; Lightfoot *et al.* 2001).

Broader roles for the health services

Severe acute respiratory syndrome (SARS), the events of September 11th 2001 and the threat and reality of bioterrorism (specifically the domestic anthrax attacks in the USA) radically changed the appreciation of governments of the role of public health, health protection and the health services in emergencies. Previously the role had essentially been to deal with the consequences of the event and casualties. Responding to casualties remains an important role as has been seen in events like the Indian Ocean tsunamis (WHO 2005) and the evacuation of New Orleans. However, with SARS and anthrax releases it became apparent that there was also potentially a role in early detection, investigation, containment and the delivery of counter-measures. For example, during SARS the best defence was how initial cases were managed when they appeared in hospitals (Tambyah 2004). It was astute clinicians and microbiologists (alerted by public health officials) that detected the release of weaponised anthrax in the USA in the autumn of 2001 (US Public Health Service Centers 2001). During the white-powder releases in Europe in 2001–2 ('copycat' releases of the American attacks) public health investigators worked jointly with the police and security services (www.hpa.org.uk). This was also to an extent true after the natural disaster of the tsunamis around the Indian Ocean in 2004–5 and after the failure of New Orleans levees with the role of public health services being detecting and intervening against potential outbreaks of infectious disease (www.hpa.org.uk; US Public Health Services, www.bt.cdc.gov/disasters/hurricanes/infectiousdisease.asp).

Health protection and environmental health in combination

Though the core roles of health protection are well defined it is less clear where health protection stops. The inclusion, for example, of low-level chemical and radiation threats in the environment can logically be extended to include physical threats (habitat alteration and safety hazards) and accident prevention (Gordon 1993; Kotchian 1997). Indeed there is considerable overlap between the concepts of health protection and environmental health and many arguments for combining the two (*see* Table 30.2).

Table 30.2 Health protection and environmental public health – a comparison in relation to human health

Component	Health protection	Environmental public health
Prevention and control of infectious disease	Yes	No
Controlling infectious disease threats in the non-human environment	Yes	Yes

Table 30.2 (Continued)

Component	Health protection	Environmental public health
Controlling chemical threats	Yes	Yes
Controlling radiation threats	Yes	Yes
Public health surveillance	Yes but only as relates	No
Hazard reduction	Limited	Yes
Environmental design and health	No	Yes
Accident prevention	No	Yes
Health aspects of the responses to emergencies	Yes	Yes

International developments, health and civil protection – responding to emergencies

The English Chief Medical Officer's initiative was in tune with increasing international interest in health protection centring around the ability of societal institutions, including public health structures, to deliver civil protection. Recent events, bioterrorism (real and hoax threats), large and international infection outbreaks, emerging infections, chemical spills and floods and other natural disasters have provided international '*acid tests*', frequently revealing gaps in civil protection in many countries. A number of these have found their arrangements lacked resilience, especially at the local level (Anon 2000, 2001; MacLehose *et al.* 2001; US Department of Health and Human Services 2002).

In the United States the Centers for Disease Control and Prevention (CDC) was able to mobilise and focus its national staff and trainees to respond to the terrorist attacks of 11 September 2001, and domestic deliberate releases of anthrax that followed (CDC 2001). This left it well positioned to respond to subsequent disasters – for example, being able to mobilise the whole organisation to respond to the New Orleans flooding disaster. However, it was recognised that American local public health epidemiological and microbiological capacity was highly variable and often weak. Consequently the federal government directed emergency funding of over $1 billion in 2002–3, much of it to strengthen state and county structures though a problem has been that this has been so related to responding to bioterrorism that it has not necessarily led to a general and sustained increase of capacity (www.hpa.org.uk). The Canadian response to SARS in Ontario suffered from poor coordination at the local level and an inability to readily provide 'surge capacity' where it was needed. Following a critical report this led to the creation of a Public Health Agency for Canada (Health Canada 2003). The response to SARS was stronger in Hong Kong but still it has created a Centre for Health Protection (Hong Kong SARS Expert Committee 2003). Building on its successful response to a number of outbreaks of infection the World Health Organization has a developing capacity for advising on health protection, including biological and chemical threats (WHO-CSR 2001). This has been focused especially at the Geneva headquarters but there is now an attempt to partially distribute this capacity to WHO's six regional offices. With the experience of SARS, avian influenza and other zoonoses the most progress has been made in the Western Pacific

Region which covers China and much of South-East Asia. This has been facilitated by substantial investment from the Asian Development Bank. Investment is much less in other WHO regions and hence, above the national level, the preparedness for an influenza pandemic is weak in Africa and the Americas.

European developments

Europe has possessed administrative arrangements for dealing with infectious disease threats since 1998 when a European Union Decision (Decision 2119) created a network to coordinate surveillance and control of infectious diseases (European Commission: http://europa.eu.int/comm/health/ph_threats/com/comm_diseases_en.htm).

A problem for this approach was that it had no competent coordinating body for the network and its small disease surveillance networks (EUROHIV, EUROTb, etc.). In 2001 the European Commission created a European Centre for Disease Prevention and Control (www.ecdc.eu.int) from a central capacity under an urgent civil protection directive adopted in October 2001 (European Commission 2001). This Centre was established in Stockholm in 2005 and in its first period of work (2005–8) will rapidly expand to about 300 staff. It is intended to coordinate rather than replace the substantial capacity of some European countries. It is hoped that it will be able to work with the European Commission to stimulate other established EU countries to develop their capacity along with the accession countries like Romania, Bulgaria and Turkey. There are other European level agencies and institutions that the new Centre has to work with if health protection is to be delivered in Europe. These include the European Food Safety Authority, the European Medicines Agency and agencies dealing with injecting drug use, occupational health, etc., as well as the diverse parts of the European Commission.

Some individual European countries have strengthened their capacity of late. In France following September 11th additional staff were added to the complement of the central Institute of Veille Sanitaire (INVS) for bioterrorism along with some additional roles following the perceived failure to respond to the heatwave of the summer of 2004. Germany has recently modernised its public health law and overcome years of resistance to federal reporting by its *Landers* (regions). However, Spain and Italy have given more powers of late to their regions and to an extent weakened their national health-protection capacity. Both countries still do not have national reporting of HIV infection. In the UK there has been no major additional sustained investment in health protection with the formation of its Agency and the emphasis has instead been on intensive planning, exercises and acquiring specialised equipment and supplies. Surprisingly few other European countries have reinforced their public health infrastructures in response to the recent developments and threats (*see* Box 30.4). This is despite the important role that public health will play in delivering health protection against terrorism and deliberate release and the fact that there are already major differences, and obvious deficiencies, among European countries in their current ability to deliver health protection.

The legal basis of health protection

Neither microbes nor chemicals respect political or administrative boundaries and in view of globalisation and interconnectivity health-protection functions have to operate within UK, European and other international frameworks and networks. Many threats (*see* Box 30.6) have extended across European boundaries and the borders of Europe with the rest of the world – the most classic recent example being SARS and the most tangible future threat being pandemic influenza.

New international health regulations

Until 2005 the legal basis for detection of control of infections at the international level, the International Health Regulations, could be considered antiquated. They only required the reporting of three infectious diseases (cholera, plague and yellow fever), did not allow WHO to take account of non-official information sources, could not respond to new and emerging infections and worked with the outdated notion that infection could be stopped at national boundaries by strict border controls. SARS showed their inadequacies. As it was a new disease and certainly not one of the three reportable infections, China, the source of human infection, did not have to report the first outbreaks of severe respiratory disease in Guangdong in November 2002. WHO was hampered in its efforts to pursue unofficial reports of outbreaks of serious respiratory disease once China had erroneously declared they had identified a known pathogen among the cases and efforts to control its entry into other countries by exit and entry screening were only partially successful because of SARS's long incubation period. A country could not protect itself against SARS by what it did at its borders (short of stopping all incoming people). What was crucial was how it managed cases that came into emergency rooms and hospital wards.

Spurred on by the SARS experience almost all member states of WHO adopted new modern International Health Regulations at the World Health Assembly in 2005 which among many provisions included an obligation on *all* countries to strengthen internal disease surveillance and control and to report any incident that potentially represented a public health emergency of international concern (World Health Organization, *International Health Regulations*). In addition WHO is now officially able to use informal reports such as those that come through Promed and non-government agencies. A drawback however is that the implementation date for the seeming more onerous obligations (e.g. strengthening surveillance) is more than 2 years away. It is also unclear whether in poorly resourced countries either governments or donor agencies will be willing to fund the unglamorous field of general strengthening of public health structures (WHO-CSR 2001).

Europe, the Fifth Freedom and training in field epidemiology

Europe gives a good example of the importance of the new Regulations. The European Union (EU) and its internal market deliver four freedoms of movement of people, services, goods and capital. Though the freedoms are not complete they are considerably greater than for movements into the EU from other countries (Summary of Legislation – Internal Market: http://europa.eu.int/scadplus/leg/en/s70000.htm). Those responsible for public health and health protection in Europe therefore sometimes talk about the *Fifth Freedom*, the freedom of movement of infections as a consequence of the easy movement of goods and people. In May 2004 the EU expanded to 25 countries and a total population of around 470 million. The range, prevalence and incidence of infections to be found within the EU borders are wide and the ease of movement results in frequent transfer of infection, disease and threats between countries. Some recent examples published in the weekly electronic European journal *Eurosurveillance* are shown in Box 30.8. Partly to counter this the EU-supported European Programme for Intervention Epidemiology Training (EPIET) programme produces trained staff used to moving rapidly between countries to respond to infection threats (Henderson, Handford and Ramsay 2000; Lieftucht and Reader 1999). This is building on the successful model of trainees in the American Centers for Disease Control and Prevention's Epidemiology Intelligence Service (www.cdc.gov/eis/) and other national and regional Field Epidemiology Training Programmes (Australia, Germany, etc.). Increasingly these training schemes are providing field personnel for when WHO is asked to provide for field teams under its Global Outbreak and Response Network. Unfortunately European states have not always recognised the value of such trainees and only a few countries have created the posts to retain EPIET graduates in senior national positions.

Box 30.8 Recent examples of human infections consequent on free movement of goods or people in Europe

Salmonella from Southern Europe into The Netherlands, Norway, Sweden and the UK in salads and eggs 2003–4:

- www.eurosurveillance.org/ew/2004/041216.asp
- www.eurosurveillance.org/ew/2004/040219.asp
- www.eurosurveillance.org/ew/2004/041216.asp#2.

LGV (lymphogranuloma venereum, an STI) to and fro between London and Amsterdam 2004:

- www.eurosurveillance.org/ew/2004/040122.asp.

West Nile Virus from Portugal into Ireland 2004:

- www.eurosurveillance.org/ew/2004/040805.asp.

Norovirus in travellers from Ireland to Andorra 2003:

- www.eurosurveillance.org/em/v08n01/0801-221.asp.

Rabies from North Africa through Spain into France 2004 in a 'decoy' dog:

- www.eurosurveillance.org/ew/2004/040902.asp.

Intersectoral resilience at the international level

Responding to major health-protection threats requires responses that extend beyond the health sector. This is not confined and over a decade ago the United Nations family created UNAIDS (United Nations Joint Programme on AIDS) to pull together the response of bodies like WHO, UNICEF, UNDP, etc. (www.unaids.org/en/default.asp). It has been recognised that natural disasters and complex health emergencies (emergencies where security is threatened) produce special threats to health particularly involving infectious diseases (Connolly *et al.* 2004). This led to the creation of sections in bodies like WHO and the UK Department for International Development that quickly deliver responses when there are international disasters such as the South Asian earthquake and tsunamis in 2005. The most recent development has been the creation of small coordination offices in the United Nations family to prepare multisectoral responses to influenza.

The UK and the Health Protection Agency

The UK's new Agency provides an opportunity to develop multiple roles and functions for the benefits of the public's health (*see* Boxes 30.4 and 30.5). In England the groups who deliver health protection at regional and national levels are diverse, and their activities have not always been well co-ordinated (Phillips, Bridgeman and Ferguson-Smith 2000). The Agency gives a co-ordinating capacity to other groups essential to health protection but outside the HPA (*see* Box 30.3). From its inception in addition to dealing with infections the Agency also deals with radiation and chemicals and poisons. The field of radiation has been well served at the national level with the UK wide National Radiation Protection Board which is now the Radiation Division of the HPA. Investment in protection against chemicals and poisons has previously been inadequate with a series of *ad hoc* local arrangements. The Agency by having a national Division can now take a more systematic approach. However difficulties remain because of the HPA needing to be cost neutral and it being hard therefore without considerable reorganisation for its local staff to extend their work to encompass the considerable needs of chemical protection. However that is now being achieved by the formation of local teams with specialisation among team members, including for chemical and environmental work.

Opportunities for strengthening public health protection

Below are some examples of the opportunities the Strategy (Nicoll and Murray 2002) and the Agency provide to develop the tools, workforce and organisation for the delivery of health protection, and also the challenges and issues that arise.

Reviewing and strengthening surveillance

The Strategy prescribes strengthening surveillance through a number of mechanisms. These include broadening the number of clinical staff required to report the occurrence of infectious diseases and further developing case definitions for reporting (Nicoll and Murray 2002). It is proposed that a duty of care be placed on all microbiology laboratories to report for public health purposes. New elements of surveillance are to be introduced to cover important infectious disease problems which are not well described currently and that there be greater use made by those responsible for chemical and radiation hazards in creating a single point – the Centre for Infections, taking over the previous function of the Communicable Disease Surveillance Centre (DHSS 1980) – for coordination, analysis and reporting on all the different systems of infectious disease surveillance. The Strategy envisages better use being made of diverse local data provided through public health observatories. It should then be possible to integrate other systems of data which are relevant to the prevention and control of human infectious diseases and providing better protection against chemicals – for example, from veterinary surveillance – working with those devising a new veterinary surveillance strategy (DEFRA 2003) – environmental monitoring, antimicrobial prescribing patterns and trends in patient care data. Modern technology should make a number of improvements possible – for example, to achieve greater and more accurate knowledge about infectious disease problems in the population, more effective analysis and more rapid feedback to frontline staff and improve interfaces with international surveillance systems.

To an extent this assumes that monies are made available for relevant information technology in the HPA. The HPA was established with 'flat funding' (no more funding than the parts from which it was made) but was expected to also deal with new areas of work, such as responding to chemical threats (environmental public health). It was also made subject to some recurrent financial constraints following the 2005 Arms Length Bodies Review. Hence it is not likely to have monies for all the major internal investments in service IT that it would wish. Initially it has had to concentrate on meeting its own considerable internal needs. That might not matter given the considerable investment in IT in the NHS. However, it is unclear how much priority will be given to links with bodies outside the NHS family and use of data for public health purposes for what is sometimes regarded as 'secondary purposes' and therefore of less importance.

Improving communications and information flows

Closely related to strengthening surveillance is improving communications for health protection. Currently the Centre for Infections is able to communicate electronically with all consultants in communicable disease control and HPA laboratories. For example, it acts as the broadcaster of information received on new threats received through the European Early Warning and Response System (EWRS) and the WHO's Global Outbreak Alert and Response Network (GOARN) (European Commission DG Health and Consumer Protection, Public Health European Early Warning and Response System). As the focal point for GOARN and (with the Department of Health) for the EWRS system, the Centre cascades information to the technical leads in the UK's devolved administrations in Northern Ireland, Scotland and Wales (Communicable Disease Surveillance Centre (CDSC) Northern Ireland, Health Protection Scotland and the National Public Health Service Wales).

These networks and connections need to be extended to all microbiology units and key clinical groups (e.g. lead consultants in accident and emergency, intensive care and infectious disease units) and should also be available to those responsible for control of chemical and radiological threats. A prototype HPA system exists, the *Health Protection Alerting System* modelled on an American system, but this needs to be formally recognised and supported.

An issue that emerges at intervals is whether considerations of patient privacy and confidentiality should constrain such communications. For example, if a patient is diagnosed as unexpectedly having anthrax, e.g. following a deliberate release, can the anonymised information be communicated without patient consent? Such legitimate considerations have to be balanced against the expectations of the public to be protected against health threats (Verity and Nicoll 2002).

Surge capacity and risk assessment

Many of the acute threats that require a response from health protection come from events outside the health sector (*see* Box 30.9) and the potential impacts on human health must be speedily considered for any major activity or accident.

Classic UK examples are the accidental release of aluminium in Camelford in Cornwall in 1988 (Rowland *et al.* 1990) and the disposal of millions of cow and sheep carcasses in England and Wales in 2001 (Department of Health 2001a).

The HPA and public health services will therefore need to have access to risk assessment and modelling capacity that is rapid and effective. Estimating a risk is only the first step to delivering health protection. One initial problem during foot and mouth disease control was that local public health and veterinary networks did not assume an executive role, or provide emergency liaison (notwithstanding the recommendations of the Phillips report). If a risk is identified there needs to be robust management structures that can immediately identify, organise and re-deploy appropriately skilled staff to areas of need.

Box 30.9 Drivers for the acute and chronic threats

Increasing overseas travel:

- exposure to exotic infections
- importation of exotic infections.

International trade in foods and animals:

- importation of exotic infections
- international outbreaks of food poisoning.

Clearance of new areas from virgin forest:

- emerging infections.

Global warming:

- changes in distribution of vectors and associated illnesses
- threats to safe water supplies.

Developments in food processing:

- emergence of new food pathogens (variant Creutzfeldt-Jakob disease -- vCJD).

Industrialised animal husbandry:

- emerging zoonoses
- explosive outbreaks of zoonoses.

Technological advances in medicine:

- more transplantation and use of blood products
- greater scope for nosocomial infections.

Aging populations and a rising prevalence of people living with chronic illnesses:

- greater scope for nosocomial infections.

More use of antimicrobial agents in human and animal sectors:

- antimicrobial resistance.

Changing social behaviours:

- rising sexually transmitted infections
- greater potential for infection in children (greater use of day care).

Industrialisation and interdependence:

- development and use of novel agents (chemicals and genetic engineering).

Rising public expectations:

- issues around safety of vaccine, medicines, food and from low levels of radiation and chemicals.

War and emergencies – complex public health emergencies:

- difficulties in controlling conventional infections
- spread of infections by troops, associated persons (journalists and relief agencies) and refugees
- exposure to CBRN (chemical, biological, radiological or nuclear) agents.

Partnership with local government

Local authorities, key players in delivering health protection, have, outside of classical emergencies, not formally been included in health-protection planning – while of course in reality they have often played major roles in the local *acid tests* (*see* Box 30.9) and have indeed developed some of their own health-protection plans. Since Regional Directors of Public Health have moved into Government Regional Offices that has changed; they are now able to pick up some of the powerful local levers that were lost to public health when Medical Officers of Heaith posts were abolished in 1974 (Galbraith 1980). The creation and expansion of public health observatories provides useful foci for local information assembly as do attempts to align local authority and health authority structures.

Recognising the contribution to public health and health protection of all practitioners

Health protection cannot be delivered by the new Agency, or even public health on its own. The contributions of others outside the public health families are essential (*see* Boxes 30.2 and 30.5) (Chief Medical Officer 2001; Secretary of State for Health 1998). Currently professional rules for doctors' work do not satisfactorily encompass communications for protecting the health of the public. While there are publications from the General Medical Council on good medical practice and the duties of doctors to individual patients, confidentiality and research there is no cohesive statement on the public health responsibilities of doctors. Certainly the contributions of all doctors and nurses outside formal public health posts need to be more formally acknowledged by regulatory bodies as there can be times when the duties to the patient and the duties to others come into conflict.

At the individual level this can be when a doctor is aware that their patient has an infection such as infectious hepatitis B or HIV that puts at risk a sexual partner but that the patient refuses to tell the partner or take precautions. More collectively there is a debate as to whether health personnel should contribute important patient data to population surveillance systems without seeking explicit individual consent.

Modernising public health law and port health

The UK's public health law requires modernisation to meet the challenge of health protection and this is promised in *Getting Ahead of the Curve* (Department of Health 2002a). For example, it needs to be clear who locally will bear responsibility for communicable disease control. Currently local authorities have responsibility for this, though they are rarely factored into current health service thinking as much as they should be and the relevant field operatives, environmental health officers, are some of the least recognised and underfunded personnel in local authorities (SOLACE Health Panel 2001).

After the revision of the International Health Regulations the challenge now for the UK and the Health Protection Agency is to modernise its regulations and structures in the light of this. A particular candidate are port health services which currently often operate on the basis of ineffectively screening a few people perceived as being sick on entry to the UK. An interesting case study is that of screening or personal surveillance for tuberculosis in migrants and visitors to the UK. A common misconception is that this could all be picked up at ports of entry. However, the majority of those coming to the UK who will later develop tuberculosis would be screened negative by any port health service. Control of tuberculosis in those coming to live in the UK is about integrated services in the community, not screening at entry.

Providing emergency preparedness and response

One of the rationales of the Agency was improving the response to emergencies and to effect this a new group concerned with emergencies was created. Initially there was some confusion in that it was imagined by some that this group would lead, coordinate or deliver the response to emergencies, sometimes to the exclusion of the subject specialists in the area affected. This issue has beset a number of national and international bodies when creating emergency sections or departments. When one of the *acid tests* becomes an emergency the whole organisation has to adapt to support and use the relevant subject specialists while at the same time not letting drop other core and essential services. Leadership usually passes to the Chief Executive of the national/international body or to a head of operations and shift working put into place as 24/7 patterns take over. In the biggest emergencies government departments or politicians assume overall leadership. Not all organisations manage this successfully. A criticism of WHO in Geneva as an organisation during SARS was that it relied on and could not adequately support its Director General and a small group of subject specialists who almost burnt out between March and August 2003. In the HPA and other bodies the emergency group's function has become clarified as the focus for insuring that emergency preparedness is present throughout the system through the production and testing of plans in frequent and diverse field exercises. When emergencies occur they support but do not lead. Beyond the level of individual bodies there are occasional times, usually during national emergencies, when government has to act in a concerted way to deliver coordinated action across sectors. Examples of this would include the response to an influenza pandemic and terrorist action. The UK has a robust mechanism for doing this through the

Cabinet Office system where there is a Civil Contingencies Secretariat which prepares for a variety of threats including those that affect or threaten health. These national arrangements are mirrored in the devolved administrations and at regional levels with Regional Resilience Teams.

Developing public health pathology

With a constantly changing National Health Service and much detail to be worked out in the health-protection strategy there are dangers that opportunities are missed or that functions are lost in the transition. The strategy *Getting Ahead of the Curve* intended that reference services be better managed while much of the non-reference diagnostic work previously undertaken by the Public Health Laboratory Service in England (PHLS) would move into the NHS. This leaves the role of the HPA as prime provider of specialist and reference microbiology and a body for determining standards. It was considered important that the personal specialist and expert contribution to the public health of the PHLS microbiologists (medical and non-medical) should be retained even though they have moved over to the NHS. Equally the NHS undertakes much public health microbiology work, reporting infections to the Centre for Infections and supporting outbreak investigations where there are now no public health laboratories. These strengths need to be encouraged and developed with it being clear for hospital managers that these are essential roles for their laboratories with a public health contribution to be written into every microbiologist's job description.

Pathology services have been being modernised for a number of years and the concept of public health microbiology should be extended to other aspects of pathology services (Department of Health 2002b). Laboratories undertaking work relating to chemicals and toxins should be reporting to the chemicals equivalent of the Centre for Infections which has been created within the Agency at its Chiltern site building on the strengths of the National Radiation Protection Board (NRPB).

Health Protection UK

In 2005 the Health Protection Agency Bill was passed by Parliament and the scope of the Agency extended from England to also encompass the devolved administrations of Northern Ireland, Scotland and Wales. There are a number of good working patterns already. Radiological protection has been on a UK-wide basis for many years under the National Radiological Protection Board (now part of the HPA) and the so-called *Five Nations Group* (the four UK countries plus Ireland) of public health specialists from what is now the Centre for Infections (England), CDSC (Northern Ireland), Health Protection Scotland and the National Public Health Service Wales have been working together for a number of years running a successful annual conference for field workers. However, coordination will not necessarily be easy especially when it comes to getting the non-specialist services to work together as, although there are national foci in each country, the field arrangements are significantly different in England, Wales and Scotland with a re-organisation pending in Northern Ireland (*see* Table 30.1). In England health protection and general public health are in separate organisations with national and local tiers (the HPA and NHS); in Scotland there is no local Health Protection Scotland services with the NHS providing both general and specialist public health services; while in Wales both general and specialist public health are combined at national and local levels in the National Public Health Service Wales.

A stronger workforce for health protection

A number of important steps needs to be taken in the UK to develop the health protection workforce.

Health protection and general public health

Health protection is an integral specialty of general public health, and basic public health skills are essential to its delivery. Indeed with its emphasis on environmental threats health protection is taking public health back to its roots in the sanitation movements of the 19th century. However, health-protection practitioners have to address mainstream public health priorities such as inequalities and the determinants of ill health. Differentials in levels of communicable diseases across communities in the UK are as least as great as the social differentials seen for the chronic illnesses; cancers and cardiovascular disease. Parts of East London have a higher notification rate for tuberculosis than Romania, while prosperous areas of England can rival the low levels of Scandinavia. Also poorer communities are more likely to experience exposure to environmental hazards from chemical sites (Arden). Equally, general public health practitioners will need to include health protection in their portfolio of basic skills if they are to comprehensively address inequalities and the determinants of ill health. They will still be expected to contribute to on-call arrangements, though supported by specialists in the HPA.

Developing surge capacity

A dedicated core workforce is essential to health protection on an ongoing basis as it is not just responding to events. However, health protection against substantial outbreaks of infection or chemical releases often require the rapid mobilisation of trained staff who have to be deflected in short order from their usual tasks, so-called 'surge capacity'. This need to secure surge capacity for health protection has been recognised by Parliament and is an issue for all the countries in the UK (House of Commons Select Committee on Health 2001). Public health teams will be based in each of England's PCTs which will support health protection (Department of Health 2001b). However, that point is yet to be made to most PCTs and their minimum staffing for health protection has not been made clear. The situation is likely to be confused by further structural change in the NHS since the 2005 UK election. It is unclear that the advantages of the changes in public health arrangements justify the disruption that will follow.

Strengthening local public health workforces

At the local level in England and Wales health protection is delivered by common staff groupings built around Consultants in Communicable Disease Control (CsCDC), infection control nurses, public health scientists and their support staff. Numbers of CsCDC were determined by the 1988 Acheson report at roughly one per local health authority. However, the expectations on these teams have increased greatly since the 1980s as they have been required to take on antimicrobial resistance, hospital-associated infection, sexually transmitted infections as well as threats from non-communicable disorders and responding to potential bioterrorism. Consequently even 5 years ago a survey undertaken for Regional

Directors of Public Health (RDsPH) found workforce deficiencies in England in medical, non-medical and nursing staff (Public Health Laboratory Service 1997). A similar survey in 2001 found the deficiencies were still great at the local level where staffing was surprisingly variable (CDSC unpublished data). Therefore with limited development funds available the local level would seem an initial priority for investment. In accordance with general trends in the NHS greater use will be made of the non-medical groups and it is wholly welcome that the Faculty of Public Health has opened up full membership by examination to non-medical specialists.

Training programmes and career structures

Training will be key to successful implementation of the strategy. Some local workforces will need training in areas that are new to them (e.g. for some CsCDC dealing with non-communicable environmental threats). More training for emergencies is needed now that initial planning is completed. There are training programmes for medical public health specialists but they can be inadequate for health protection, which should be recognised as a formal specialty of public health. However, there are hardly any training programmes for public health nurses and scientists. There are opportunities now for imaginative approaches and continuing professional education sufficient to ensure an adequate workforce for health protection. Strong training programmes are also essential for 'surge capacity'. Trainees, if well supported, gain immensely from being assigned to surge requirements. Here the UK is vulnerable. Specialised health-protection training is not often undertaken and a doctor can still become a CCDC after less than 6 months of communicable disease control training and even less training in the chemical response. Workforce planning for public health promised in the 1999 white paper *Saving Lives* is underway but it is unclear if health protection will feature in this.

Responses to chemical and radiation hazards

As it stands at present national chemical hazards protection is relatively weak, in part because the structures for health service support are more poorly developed compared to infection control or radiation control. There are few national reference laboratories and no body equivalent in capacity to the Centre for Infection or the National Radiological Protection Board. These organisations have been developed for over 20 years and have trained and experienced staff. Chemical support is more patchy and has only been recognised over the last 4–6 years following the development of chemical incident provider units in 1996 and the National Focus in 1997 (National Focus for Chemical Incidents: www.natfocus.uwic.ac.uk/). Few medical toxicologists have been trained in the UK in recent years and most have a clinical rather than an environmental public health focus.

Organisation for health protection

Constant changes in the National Health Service poses problems for health protection. In accordance with the philosophy of *Shifting the Balance of Power* (Centre for Health Protection, Hong Kong: www.chp.gov.hk/index)the function should generally not be centrally directed, except in a strategic sense – for example, setting targets and standards and monitoring performance. Health protection should be based on appropriately trained and accredited professionals, operating through managed local networks to agreed, national evidence-based policies and guidelines. It should be accountable in two directions, upwards eventually to the Chief Medical Officers, and to the populations it serves. However, it should rely on local professionalism that will be judged against explicit standards, not on central direction. A series of routine and priority programmes needs to be in place, and delivering on a routine basis. Policies for dealing with the public health aspects of case management will need to be standard and be available locally and applied at all times.

However, it cannot be the case that local health-protection practitioners can work in isolation. Good, almost instant communications will be key and there will need to be regional or national direction and coordination when local events have broader, national or international implications – for example, when there is an outbreak stretching across the country (Killalea *et al.* 1996), or a rare event with major implications (e.g. the appearance of vCJD in humans). This is why CDSC (now within the HPA's Centre for Infections) was established in 1977 following a series of poorly coordinated incidents. There needs to be designated responsibility, authority, capacity and expertise at national and regional levels to draw together rapidly and coordinate the multi-agency working required for tackling outbreaks and incidents (*see* Box 30.7). As ever the key to the success of the new arrangements in the emergency situation will be good team-working, strong infrastructure and speed of response; essential public health skills (Trotter and Edmunds 2002).

Managed health-protection networks

PCTs will contribute to health protection through their public health teams (Centre for Health Protection, Hong Kong: www.chp.gov.hk/index). However, even the larger PCTs will not justify having the specialist staff needed for health protection, and staff numbers and complement will depend on local need (e.g. more dedicated tuberculosis nurses in high incidence areas). Consultants in communicable disease control (CsCDC) will be in the Agency and have joined together within managed health-protection networks to offer flexible arrangements and some degree of specialisation to serve geographically defined populations. Quite often these arrangements represent the evolution of progressive pre-existing arrangements in a number of parts of the country. The networks will have to be managed because of the need for rapid resource management when threats occur (*see* Box 30.9) (Trotter and Edmunds 2002). They will not be rigidly blueprinted but will comprise medical and nursing consultants (e.g. CsCDC) and non-medical public health specialists, a range of specialist and non-specialist support staff such as an information officer, public health/infection control nurse, lead immunisation nurse, etc. Hopefully they will also encompass public health microbiology and chemical incident response capacity. Health protection is the personal responsibility of RDsPH. With regional populations of millions they cannot achieve this single-handed. They will need some protection themselves. Hence there are regional and sub-regional posts in the

Agency equivalent to the regional epidemiologists and advising and delivering for them the public health microbiology from the NHS and agency laboratories, IPPC in full services, chemical incident responses, etc. These networks will also provide career structures, for example for CsCDC who previously had usually been kept single-handed and had to leave their jobs if they wished to progress professionally.

Challenges and opportunities

Producing the Strategy (*see* Box 30.3) has been the first step to delivering effective health protection but the next steps were also essential. There are a series of organisational challenges (*see* Box 30.10). There is a danger from creating this Agency that people imagine will alone deal with all aspects of health protection – the '*silo phenomenon*' of everyone retreating into their own area of defined responsibility. The same could happen between the centres in the Agency and its local services. It would be a tragedy if current good working (for example, between public health and reference microbiology) was lost. If either those inside or outside the Agency imagine it alone will deliver health protection it will fail. Therefore an exciting partnership development with all relevant organisations and agencies provides the best prospects for the future. The NHS's constant organisational churn produces unhelpful challenges as the HPA constantly has to seek new arrangements with new bodies and people at every level. Doing this while responding to the ever-present threats to health (*see* Box 30.11) can be likened to unravelling, redesigning and re-knitting a complex sweater while still wearing it (and undertaking vigorous outdoor exercise). However, there is a strategic vision for the future and it is up to all the stakeholders to constructively determine the important 'knitting patterns' that will deliver the exciting promise of the strategy. With goodwill and workforce support and adequate funding even more effective arrangements can be created.

Box 30.10 Six organisational challenges for public health and health protection services from the *acid tests*

1 Are there the specialist expertises for the technical response and can they be drawn upon efficiently when they are needed?
2 Can smaller local services be made to co-operate to deliver a coordinated response?
3 Can large organisations be made flexible enough to be entirely refocused onto a single task for a sustained period?
4 Can naturally competitive national bodies be made to co-operate in times of stress?
5 Are command and control systems adequate?
6 Can services across a range of sectors (health, education, transport, security, etc.) act together to give a concerted response to major threats such as pandemic influenza and natural disasters?

Box 30.11 Scenarios which health protection has to deliver against – the *'acid tests'*

- A major community outbreak of a gastrointestinal disease, Legionnaires' disease, etc.
- An urgent need to reduce incidence of a specific infection, e.g. tuberculosis, genital chlamydia, meningococcal disease, etc.
- An outbreak of a unknown illness – could be biological or result of a chemical or radiological exposure.
- A breakdown of infection screening quality.
- A large fire in a plastics factory.
- The appearance of an unrecognised pathogen in the national blood supply.
- Uncontrolled serious infection contracted in hospitals.
- Chemical, biological or radiological contamination of a water supply.
- A lost radiation source.
- A major flood or another disaster requiring evacuation of a large community.
- A local, national or international vaccine scare.
- A hepatitis virus-infected healthcare worker who has practised in many areas.
- A serious imported infection affecting a number of hospitals.
- The emergence of a new STI or the re-emergence of a previously recognised STI.
- The next influenza pandemic.
- A suspected deliberate or accidental release of a biological agent attack.
- A major national or local animal epidemic with implications for human health.

References and further reading

Anonymous (2000) *An Evaluation of the Arrangements for Managing an Epidemiological Emergency Involving More Than One EU Member State*. Bielefeld: Institute of Public Health.

Anonymous (2001) New York City Department of Health response to terrorist attack, September 11. *Mortality and Morbidity Weekly Report*. 28 September. **50**(38): 821–2.

Arden K (ed.) *Report on Cancer Cases in North Liverpool. Possible links with incinerator*. www.nwpho.org.uk/reports/livfaz.pdf.

Baxter PJ (1990) Review of major chemical incidents and their medical management. In: V Murray (ed.) *Major Chemical Disasters: medical aspects of management*. London: Royal Society of Medicine, pp.7–20.

Brown P (2000) A view from the media on vaccine safety. *Bulletin of the World Health Organization*. **78**: 216–17.

CDC (2001) Update: investigation of bioterrorism-related anthrax and interim guidelines for clinical evaluation of persons with possible anthrax. *Morb Mortal Wkly Rep*. **50**(42): 909–19. www.cdc.gov/mmwr/preview/mmwrhtml/mm5042a1.htm.

Civil Contingencies Secretariat, Cabinet Office UK: www.ukresilience.info/home.htm.

Chief Medical Officer (2001) *CMO Update. Emergency preparedness*. Chief Medical Officer, England. www.doh.gov.uk/cmo/cmo_32.htm#1.

Connolly MA, Gayer M, Ryan MJ *et al.* (2004) Communicable diseases in complex emergencies: impact and challenges. *Lancet.* **364**: 1974–83.

Department for the Environment, Food and Rural Affairs (DEFRA) (2003) *UK Veterinary Surveillance Strategy.* London: DEFRA. www.defra.gov.uk/animalh/diseases/veterinary/strategydoc.pdf.

Department of Health (2001a) *A Rapid Qualitative Assessment of Possible Risks to Public Health from Current Foot and Mouth Disposal Options.* June. www.doh.gov.uk/fmdguidance/disposalriskassessment.htm.

Department of Health (2001b) *Shifting the Balance of Power – securing delivery.* www.doh.gov.uk/shiftingthebalance/initialconsult.htm.

Department of Health (2001c) *The Report of the Chief Medical Officer's Project to Strengthen the Public Health Function.* London: Department of Health. www.doh.gov.uk/cmo/phfunction.htm.

Department of Health (2002a) *Getting Ahead of the Curve: a strategy for combating infectious diseases (including other aspects of health protection).* January. London: Department of Health. www.doh.gov.uk/cmo/idstrategy/idstrategy2002.pdf.

Department of Health (2002b) *Pathology Modernisation.* February. London: Department of Health. www.doh.gov.uk/pathologymodernisation/index.htm.

Department of Health and Social Security (DHSS) (1980) *Health Service Development. Co-ordination of epidemiological services for communicable diseases and food poisoning: Communicable Disease Surveillance Centre.* Health Circular HC(80)2, LAC (80)1. February. London: DHSS.

Donnelly CA, Fisher MC, Fraser C *et al.* (2004) Epidemiological and genetic analysis of severe acute respiratory syndrome. *Lancet Infectious Diseases.* **4**: 672–83.

Duckworth G and Charlett A (2005) Improving surveillance of MRSA bacteraemia. *BMJ.* **331**: 976–7.

European Commission (2001) *European Commission Council Decision of 23 October 2001 Establishing a Community Mechanism to Facilitate Reinforced Cooperation in Civil Protection Assistance Interventions.* 2001/792/EC. Euratom.

European Commission DG Health and Consumer Protection. *Public Health. European Early Warning and Response System*: http://europa.eu.int/comm/health/ph_threats/com/early_warning_en.htm.

Fleming D (2005) Influenza pandemics and avian flu. *BMJ.* November. **331**: 1066–9.

Galbraith S (1980) The impact of the 1974 reforms. *Journal of the Royal Society of Medicine.* **35**.

Gordon LJ (1993) The future of environmental health (Part 1). *J Environ Health.* **55**: 28–32.

Harling R, Twisselmann B, Asgari-Jirhandeh N *et al.* for the Deliberate Release Teams (2001) Deliberate release of biological agents: initial lessons for Europe from events in the United States. *Eurosurveillance.* **6**: 166–71.

Health Canada (2003) *Learning from SARS. Renewal of public health in Canada. A report of the National Advisory Committee on SARS and Public Health.* October. www.hc-sc.gc.ca/english/pdf/sars/sars-e.pdf.

Health Protection Agency (2004): www.hpa.org.uk.

Health Protection Agency Chemical Hazards and Poisons Division: www.hpa.org.uk/chemicals/default.htm.

Henderson B, Handford S and Ramsay M (2000) Rapid reporting system for meningitis W135: 2a: P1.2, 5 prompted by haj outbreak. *Eurosurveillance Weekly.* 16 November. **46**. www.eurosurv.org/update/.

Hong Kong SARS Expert Committee Report (2003) *From Experience to Action.* September. Government of Hong Kong. www.sars-expertcom.com.gov.hk/english/reports/reports_fullrpt.html.

House of Commons Select Committee on Health (2001) *Report on Public Health.* Para 218.

Killalea D, Ward L, de Louvois J *et al.* (1996) International epidemiological and microbiological study of *Salmonella agona* infection from a ready to eat savoury snack. I. England and Wales and the United States. *BMJ.* **313**: 1105–7.

Kotchian S (1997) Perspectives on the place of environmental health and protection in public health and public health agencies. *Ann Rev Publ Health.* **18**: 245–59.

Lederberg J, Shope R and Oaks SC Jr (1992) *Emerging Infections: microbial threats to health in the United States.* Washington, DC: National Academy Press.

Lieftucht A and Reacher M (1999) Case control study of Salmonella paratyphi B infection associated with travel to Alanya, Turkey. *Eurosurveillance Weekly.* 28 October. **44**. www.eurosurv.org/update/.

Lightfoot N, Wale M, Spencer R, Nicoll A (2001) Appropriate responses to bioterrorist threats. *BMJ.* **323**: 877–8. www.bmj.com/cgi/content/full/323/7318/877.

MacLehose L, Brand H, Camaroni I *et al.* (2001) Communicable disease outbreaks involving more than one country: systems approach to evaluating the response. *BMJ.* **323**: 861–3. http://bmj.com/cgi/reprint/323/7317/861.pdf.

Morita H, Yanagisawa N, Nakajima T *et al.* (1995) Sarin poisoning in Matsumoto, Japan. *Lancet.* **346**: 290–3.

Mort M, Convery I, Baxter J and Bailey C (2005) Psychosocial effects of the 2001 UK foot and mouth disease epidemic in a rural population: qualitative diary based study. *BMJ* doi:10.1136/bmj.38603.375856.68.

National Radiation Protection Board (2004) *Mobile Phones and Health.* www.hpa.org.uk/radiation/publications/documents_of_nrpb/pdfs/doc_15_5.pdf.

Nicoll A, Calvert N, Wilson D and Borriello P (2001) Managing major public health crises. *BMJ.* **323**: 1321–2. http://bmj.com/cgi/reprint/323/7325/1321.pdf.

Nicoll A and Hamers F (2002) Are trends in HIV, gonorrhoea, and syphilis worsening in western Europe? *BMJ.* **324**: 1324–7.

Nicoll A and Murray V (2002) Health protection – a strategy and a national agency. *Public Health.* **116**: 129–37.

Okumura T, Suzuki K, Fukuda A *et al.* (1998) The Tokyo subway sarin attack: disaster management, Part 1: Community emergency response. *Academic Emergency Medicine.* **5**(6): 613–17.

Phillips Lord, Bridgeman J and Ferguson-Smith M (2000) *The BSE Enquiry.* London: HMSO.

Public Health Agency for Canada: www.phac-aspc.ca.

Public Health Laboratory Service (1997) *CDSC Communicable Disease Control Survey.* PHLS.

Regan M (1999) Health protection in the next millennium from tactics to strategy. *J Epidemiol Community Health.* **53**: 517–18.

Rowland A, Grainger R, Smith RS *et al.* (1990) Water contamination in North Cornwall: a retrospective cohort study into the acute and short term effects of the aluminium sulphate incident in July 1988. *J R Soc Health.* **110**(5): 166–72.

Secretary of State for Health (1998) *Saving Lives: our healthier nation.* London: HMSO. www.archive.official-documents.co.uk/document/cm43/4386/4386.htm.

Simms I, Macdonald N, Ison C *et al.* (2004) Enhanced surveillance of lymphogranuloma venereum (LGV) begins in England. *Eurosurveillance.* **8**. www.eurosurveillance.org/ew/2004/041007.asp#4.

SOLACE Health Panel (2001) *The Role of Modern Local Authorities in Creating Health Communities.* June. Society of Local Authority Chief Executives.

Tambyah PA (2004) Severe acute respiratory syndrome from the trenches, at a Singapore university hospital. *Lancet Infectious Diseases.* **4**: 690–6.

Trotter CL and Edmunds WJ (2002) Modelling cost effectiveness of meningococcal serogroup C conjugate vaccination campaign in England and Wales. *BMJ.* **324**: 809.

US Department of Health and Human Services (2002) *Presentation of the President's Fiscal Year 2003 Budget for the US Department of Health and Human Services*. Press release, 4 February. www.hhs.gov/news/press/2002pres/20020204b.html.

US Public Health Service (2001) Centers for Disease Control and Prevention update: investigation of bioterrorism-related anthrax and interim guidelines for clinical evaluation of persons with possible anthrax. *MMWR*. 2 November. **50**(43): 941–8.

United States Public Health Services, Centres for Disease Control and Prevention. *After a Hurricane: infectious diseases. Hurricane Katrina*. www.bt.cdc.gov/disasters/hurricanes/infectiousdisease.asp.

Verity C and Nicoll A (2002) Consent, confidentiality and the threat to public health surveillance. *BMJ*.

WHO-CSR (2001) *Public Health Response to Biological and Chemical Weapons*. www.who.int/emc/deliberate_epi.html.

Will RG, Ironside JW, Zeidler M *et al.* (1996) A new variant of Creutzfeldt-Jakob disease in the UK. *Lancet*. **347**: 921–2.

World Health Organization (2001) *Communicable Disease Surveillance and Response: Global Outbreak and Response Network (GOARN)*. www.who.int/emc/global_outbreak_network.htm.

World Health Organization. *International Health Regulations; renewing the health regulations*. www.who.int/emc/IHR/int_regs.html.

World Health Organization (2005) *South East Asian Earthquake and Tsunami: moving beyond the Tsunami. The WHO Story*. WHO South East Asian Office.

Chapter 31

Academic public health

Selena Gray

Academic public health is an essential part of the public health endeavour. Without an academic base, how will the public health professionals of the future be trained and educated? How will they know what the key public health problems are, how they can tackle them most effectively, and whether they are making a difference?

Defining the public health sciences

Public health has been defined as *'the science and art of preventing disease, prolonging life and promoting health through the organised efforts of society'* (Acheson 1998). A helpful description of the public health sciences is given in Box 31.1.

Box 31.1 Description of the public sciences

Traditionally, the basic sciences of public health have been considered to be epidemiology and biostatistics, but increasingly, there is an awareness that multidisciplinary perspectives are needed to understand a range of influences on behaviour and to develop effective strategies to improve health. This requires contributions from the biological, physical and social sciences including disciplines such as economics, sociology, anthropology, demography, nutrition, psychology and policy analysis. (The Wellcome Trust 2004)

In his influential report, *Securing Good Health for the Whole Population*, Wanless (2004) recognised the wide-ranging nature of public health research, and highlighted a particular need for synthesis of existing evidence and new research that *'designs, tests and evaluates interventions and policy initiatives'*. Similar concerns about research capacity in public health have been identified in other developed countries. *The Future of Public Health* report in the USA (Institute of Medicine 1998) highlighted the disarray of the public health system and the need for investment in surveillance and research. In Canada, in response to the SARS outbreak in 2003, there has been a substantial investment in the public health infrastructure, which includes the establishment of six National Collaborating Centres for Public Health, each drawing together research expertise in different areas (Health Canada 2005). There are also concerns that, at a global level, public health research in developing countries needs strengthening (WHO 2004).

Research capacity in the UK

The diverse nature of disciplines involved in public health can lead to challenges in identifying capacity in public health research. For example, economics is a critical part of a public health research base, but unless the talents and energies of an economics department are applied to a public health problem, they are not *per se* contributing to the public health research endeavour, although they may represent a latent capacity to do so. An example of how different disciplines may be applied to a public health problem is shown in Table 31.1.

Table 31.1 Applying different scientific disciplines to public health research: illustrative case study using tobacco control

Discipline	Application
Epidemiology	Eliciting and quantifying the association between tobacco consumption and illness.
Bio-statistics	Trials of individual and community-based interventions. Modelling likely future impact on health of current tobacco use.
Biological sciences	Understanding mechanisms of damage from tobacco use. Developing therapeutic approaches to nicotine dependency. Measuring exposure to tobacco.
Social sciences	Surveys to establish trends in consumption and attitudes to tobacco use by age and social class.
Economics	Modelling to determine the impact of price rises/taxation on consumption.
Sociology and anthropology	Understanding the social context of tobacco use; developing contextually appropriate interventions.
Psychology	Developing and testing interventions to support cessation.
Marketing	Analysis of advertising strategies and their effects. Examining relationship of exposure to tobacco advertising and uptake of smoking.
Policy analysis	Developing effective means of tobacco control at national and global level.
Evidence synthesis	Underpins the effective use of research evidence in a variety of fields. Informs guideline development and policy action.

A study undertaken in England in 2000 (Milner 2004) attempted to map public health research capacity in both named and 'non-named public health' departments in university and in non-university settings such as government and health authorities. They identified 26 named public health departments, and a further 31 departments which, although not described as public health, such were undertaking public health work. Over three quarters of the 864 staff identified were based in the named departments; many were on short-term contracts. The most common discipline in named departments was epidemiology (42%) and in non-named departments behavioural or social sciences (24%). In terms of performance in the 2001 Research Assessment Exercise (a UK exercise which aims to assess the quality of research undertaken by universities), only three named and six non-named departments were ranked as 5 or 5*; three and seven as a 4 rating; and eleven and seven respectively a 3a or 3b. (Ratings were on a scale from 1 to 5 dependent on how much of the work is judged to reach national or international levels of excellence and directly affect income to universities.)

More recently, a worrying decline in the number of medically qualified public health academics employed by medical schools in the UK has been reported. Between 2001 and 2003 the number of whole-time equivalents fell from 215 to 146 (Silke 2004), despite an increase of 29% of medical student numbers since 2000. Less than half of all posts are funded by the universities and a similar number by the NHS.

Concerns about capacity in the public health sciences were reiterated in the Wellcome Trust Report on the Public Health Sciences (2004), and in *Securing Good Health for the Whole Population* (Wanless 2004). The latter identified gaps in the capacity to undertake applied or secondary research, particularly in evidence synthesis, health economics and modelling. However, without an adequate primary research base, the contribution of applied and secondary techniques will be limited.

Encouraging signs

The developments in evidence synthesis and dissemination that have characterised the evidence-based medicine movement – with substantial input from public health academics – are now being more systematically applied to public health. There are increasing numbers of systematic reviews available of direct relevance to public health practice available within the international Cochrane Collaboration. The establishment of the Health Development Agency in 2002 and its incorporation in the National Institute for Health and Clinical Excellence (NICE) in 2005 in England and Wales should provide increasing expertise in the development and synthesis of a robust evidence base to support public health practice. NICE will aim to provide national guidance on the promotion of good health and the prevention and treatment of ill health. Work has begun to develop a framework for deriving grades of recommendations for public health interventions based on a synthesis of all relevant research, which will be piloted on obesity in the first instance.

The establishment of the Health Protection Agency in the UK, which has as one of its key goals building and improving the evidence base through a comprehensive programme of research and development, offers significant opportunities to develop and consolidate research capacity in the field of health protection. Similar opportunities exist with the establishment of the Food Standards Agency, an important funder of nutrition-related public health research.

Within all four countries of the UK, there has been welcome investment in public health surveillance and expertise with the establishment of public health observatories in England (*Saving Lives: our healthier nation*, DH 1999) and similar developments in Wales and Scotland.

Funding for public health research

For many researchers, the type of work undertaken is highly dependent on access to research funding; dedicated funding in key areas will mobilise research talents in different directions. For example, the investment by the Economic and Social

Research Council in their Variations in Health programme (1996–2001), which focused on the social determinants of health inequalities, enabled social science researchers to explicitly address the issues of health inequalities. One of the reasons for the relative dearth of public health intervention, as opposed to descriptive or epidemiological research (Millward *et al.* 2003), has been lack of funding for this type of work, with funding from public and private sources geared towards biological and medical sciences and interventions (Wanless 2004).

Despite the publication of a public health strategy in 2001 by the Department of Health in England (DH 2001a,b), the UK has lacked a parallel and *sustained* investment in the public health sciences. This is in contrast to health services research, where development has been heavily supported by investment and funding by the NHS Health Technology Assessment Programme (NHS HTA 2005). There are some signs that this may be changing. The English white paper *Choosing Health* (Secretary of State for Health 2004) has made several very positive statements about the need to prioritise and fund public health research. One early outcome is the launch of the National Prevention Research Initiative (NPRI 2005), a broad consortium of public funding and charity sectors mobilised under the umbrella of the National Cancer Research Institute to support research in the field of prevention. It is imperative that such investment is not seen as 'one off' but is sustained over time. Another is the arrival of the Public Health Research Consortium trailed in *Choosing Health*. The Department of Health has also published a new health research strategy, *Best Health, Best Research* (Department of Health 2006). This has been criticised for its clinical dominance and its restricted focus on public health.

However, we must be also be wary of an over-simplistic paradigm of 'intervention research' based predominantly on individual behavioural interventions aimed at changing lifestyles as the solution to all public health problems. Experience demonstrates the need to consider wider socio-economic, environmental and political factors in addressing public health problems.

Methodological developments in academic public health

Recent advances in public health research have included the developments in systematic approaches to evidence synthesis and guideline development already referred to above. While not by any means a comprehensive list, other emerging areas include:

- the application of economics and modelling to public health issues as in the Global Burden of Disease Report (Murray and Lopez 1994) and the Wanless report (Wanless 2004)
- complex modelling of infectious disease outbreaks and the effects of different control strategies
- life-course approaches that recognise the cumulative effect of disadvantage at different stages of the life course and offer new insights as to how and when to intervene (Kuh and Ben-Shlomo 1997)
- the application of social marketing techniques to public health issues
- public health genetics: the rapid developments in genetics provide opportunities to greater understanding of mechanisms of disease, and through the use of techniques such as 'Mendelian randomisation' (Davey Smith and Ebrahim 2003)

offer potentially powerful ways of using genetics and epidemiology to elucidate causal associations of risk factor exposure and disease. While welcome, there is some concern that developments in genetics offer the potential for an enormous diversion of research funding from less glamorous areas of public health practice.

Areas of concern

The implementation of the Data Protection Act and its impact on the use of personal data is a serious threat to public health research. Although mechanisms have been developed in England, under the Health and Social Care Act (Section 60) 2001, to allow access to personal data without explicit consent, this provides an additional bureaucratic hurdle both for public health surveillance and for research. Some research may become literally impossible if informed consent has to be obtained – or the ensuing biases may render the results difficult to interpret. More worryingly, the cumulative effects of such barriers may deter researchers from undertaking research requiring access to such data. While it is entirely appropriate that proper protection should be put in place for personal data, including consent where appropriate, and anonymisation techniques, the overzealous application of such principles may jeopardise the collation of data that most would see as being in the public interest. An appropriate balance must be struck between individual confidentiality and public health research. Evidence from a survey of academic departments in the UK undertaken under the auspices of the UK Faculty of Public Health in 2004 (Smith 2004) suggests that meeting the current interpretations of these requirements is adversely affecting the validity, feasibility and costs of public health research.

A further area of concern is the fragmentation between academic departments and service public health, where the creation of many small public health bodies in England, and to some extent in Wales, has led to the disruption and loss of existing strong relationships and support between academic and service public health colleagues. There is a strong sense that, despite shared values and common interests, the differing external pressures are serving to drive the two groups apart rather together to work on their common agendas. Thus while those working in public health in the NHS setting face a plethora of short-term targets, those in academic settings face enormous pressure to deliver research that fulfils the criteria of national or international excellence to meet the expectations imposed upon them by their universities under the Research Assessment Exercise. For each party, failure to secure these goals will jeopardise their short- and medium-term security, thus generating little incentive and practical difficulties for both in finding mutually beneficial ways of working together. Yet this engagement between the two is essential if we are to sustain a strong public health community in the long term. Given the degree to which the NHS has historically supported posts in academic public health departments, lack of engagement may yet further jeopardise capacity.

There has been particular concern that the UK Research Assessment Exercise (RAE), with its perceived lack of weighting given to applied research, has been damaging to clinical academic medicine, and in particular to community-based subjects such as public health (Banatvala *et al.* 2005). The next RAE in 2008 will use a similar peer-review methodology, but panel chairs are advised that it is intended to ensure that *'appropriate measures of excellence are developed which are suf-*

ficiently wide as to capture all types of research, including practice-based research, applied research, basic/strategic research, interdisciplinary research' (RAE 2005). Detailed guidance on the process has not yet been issued, but it is essential that appropriate weighting and consideration is seen to be given to a wider range of applied research if capacity is not to be further damaged.

Education and training

Alongside research, another fundamental role of academic public health is to teach and train the public health practitioners and specialists of tomorrow, and also to inculcate a basic understanding of public health in a much wider group. While dedicated Master's level courses in Public Health are essential for training the specialists and leaders of tomorrow, there are many other professionals and groups who require an understanding of public health principles as a part of their basic training. This includes those wishing to work specifically in a public health role such as community public health nurses (health visitors and school nurses) and environmental health officers, as well as new roles such as 'health trainers' as outlined in the white paper *Choosing Health* (Secretary of State for Health 2004). Accreditation requirements for registration for specialist community public health nursing, the new third part of the Nursing and Midwifery Council Register (which currently contains existing health visitors but in due course will include school and occupational health nurses), now contain explicit statements about public health skills and competencies (Nursing and Midwifery Council 2004). The important and projected growth of the role environmental health officers play in improving the public's health and reducing health inequalities over the next 10 years was highlighted in a pivotal report (Burke *et al.* 2002), and public health skills are increasingly prominent in the core curriculum for environmental health officers. These changes may provide new opportunities for interprofessional learning between key groups such as school nurses and environmental health officers, which may be pivotal in creating a workforce that can work together effectively in future.

Other key groups requiring a basic grounding in public health are doctors, other health professionals and many managers in the statutory and voluntary sector in both health and local authorities and the voluntary sector.

While universities are of paramount importance in delivering this substantial educational agenda, it must be delivered in partnership with those working in the public health service and the NHS. There is a need for public health teaching at both undergraduate level, as part of vocational degrees such as nursing, medicine, environmental health, at postgraduate level and as part of continuing professional education. Following the Acheson report (Acheson 1988), a number of universities established Master's level courses in public health (usually attached to medical schools) for the first time. Over the last few years, there has been a further substantial expansion in the number of institutions providing Master's level courses, including the 'new' universities, many of whom are already active in the field of nursing education and environmental science. It is estimated that there are now of the order of 90–100 Master's level courses in public health or related subjects now running in the UK, some of which were initially more orientated to health education and promotion at their inception (personal communication, Dr S George). Although there is undoubtedly variability in the content and approach taken by these courses, they are nonetheless catering for a wider and more diverse audience than in previous years and are widening access to public health skills.

Concerns exist about the capacity to deliver these substantial educational needs; for example, despite a 29% increase in medical students since 2000 there has been a substantial decline in the number of clinical public health academics to teach them (Silke 2004). However, if public health is not entirely to be a 'values-led' discipline, it is essential that public health practitioners gain some understanding of the science and evidence base that informs their practice.

In conclusion, the need for a strong and vibrant academic base in public health has never been greater. However, academic public health may struggle to deliver all that is expected of it now and in future if it is not adequately resourced and supported (*see* Box 31.2). Sustained investment and support from all key players is essential if academic health is to thrive. It is too important to be left to universities alone.

Box 31.2

To address the almost complete absence of an evidence base on the cost-effectiveness of public health interventions, substantial investment will be necessary, backed up by building the capacity of the public health research sector in England, establishing clear priorities and ensuring that responsibility to collate what evidence does exist is assigned. (Derek Wanless)

References

Acheson D (1988) *Public Health in England. Report of the Committee of Inquiry into the Future Development of the Public Health Function.* London: HMSO.

Banatvala J, Bell P and Symonds M (2005) The Research Assessment Exercise is bad for UK medicine. *Lancet.* **365**: 458–60.

Burke S, Gray I and Paterson K *et al.* (2002) *Environmental Health 2012: a key partner in delivering the public health agenda.* London: Health Development Agency.

Davey Smith G and Ebrahim S (2003) 'Mendelian randomization': can genetic epidemiology contribute to understanding environmental determinants of disease? *Int J Epidemiol.* **32**: 1–22.

Department of Health (1999) *Saving Lives: our healthier nation.* London: Department of Health.

Department of Health (2001a) *A Research and Development Strategy for Public Health.* London: Department of Health.

Department of Health (2001b) *Health and Social Care Act.* London: Department of Health.

Department of Health (2006) *Best Health, Best Research.* London: Department of Health.

Health Canada (2005) www.hc-sc.gc.ca/english/ (accessed 2 May 2005).

Institute of Medicine (1988) *The Future of Public Health.* Washington DC: IOM.

Kuh D and Ben-Shlomo Y (eds) (1997) *A Life Course Approach to Chronic Disease Epidemiology: tracing the origins of ill-health from early to adult life.* Oxford: Oxford Medical Publications.

Millward LM, Kelly MP and Nutbeam D (2003) *Public Health Intervention Research. The evidence.* London: Health Development Agency.

Milner P, Mistral M and Brown L *et al.* (2004) Academic public health research capacity and development in England 2000–1: capacity, capability and concerns. *Critical Public Health.* **14**: 251–60.

Murray CJL and Lopez AD (1994) *Global Comparative Assessments in the Health Sector. Disease burden, expenditures and intervention packages.* Geneva: World Health Organization.

National Prevention Research Initiative (2005) www.mrc.ac.uk/index/funding/fundingspecific_schemes/funding-calls_for_proposals/funding-npri.htm (accessed 2 May 2005).

NHS Health Technology Assessment Programme (2005) www.ncchta.org/ (accessed 2 May 2005).

Nursing and Midwifery Council (2004) *Standards of Proficiency for Specialist Community Public Health Nurses*. London: NMC.

Research Assessment Exercise (RAE) (2005) *Guidance to Panels*. RAE 01/2005. Bristol: Higher Education Funding Council for England.

Secretary of State for Health (2004) *Choosing Health*. London: The Stationery Office.

Silke A (2004) *Clinical Academic Staffing Levels in UK Medical and Dental Schools*. May. London: Council of Heads of Medical Schools.

Smith WC (2004) *Impact of Data Protection on Public Health Research. Responses to a survey of academic departments of public health in the UK*. London: Faculty of Public Health.

Wanless D (2004) *Securing Good Health for the Whole Population*. London: HM Treasury.

The Wellcome Trust (2004) *Public Health Sciences: challenges and opportunities*. London: The Wellcome Trust.

World Health Organization (2004) *The Mexico Statement on Health Research*. Geneva: WHO.

Chapter 32

Public health systems and performance management

Tony Jewell

Introduction

The UK public health system has a good international reputation for the surveillance and epidemiological analysis of population-based data, which has its roots with the public health pioneers of the 19th century. Modern landmark reports such as the 1980 Black Report (Black *et al.* 1980) and the Acheson report on *Inequalities in Health* (Independent Inquiry into Inequalities in Health 1998) in 1998 have rigorously identified public health inequalities and the fact that in many cases they stubbornly persist or the gap is widening in the UK between socio-economic, cultural or ethnic groups. Despite huge advances in the state of the public's health, as assessed by measures such as the decline in infant mortality rates and rising life expectancy, there is concern that we are not effectively developing the public health workforce, moulding it into a public health system or performance managing those organisations and professionals with statutory accountability for the public's health.

This chapter describes the current arrangements in place in England as an example of how monitoring performance can be used for development and active management of public health programmes and the public health system.

The structure: statutory responsibilities and population levels

Choosing Health (Department of Health 2004a), the most recent English public health white paper, is the government's response to the final Wanless report, *Securing Good Health for the Whole Population* (HM Treasury 2004).

The Wanless report was critical of the public health delivery system:

> The major drivers of public health have been recognised since the 1970s, with numerous 'upstream' and 'downstream' public health strategies having been proposed. However, 30 years on, despite some successes, implementation has been partial at best. To achieve the 'fully engaged' scenario will require a step change in effort and achievement. The fundamental challenge is now to 'make it happen', particularly focussing on incentives, levers and delivery. (HM Treasury 2004, p.23)

An example of not making it happen, according to the Wanless report, is the tobacco programme and particularly the process for target setting and review of the smoking cessation programme in the NHS. He asks basic questions such as: who had estimated the population impact expected from smoking cessation targets? Was this the most cost-effective intervention to make? Inability to answer such questions reflects the lack of evidence and economic analysis in policy making. Equally, there is a lack of rigour in setting targets for performance management of the NHS. Comparison between processes (e.g. smoking cessation services) and outcomes (fewer people smoking the rest of their lifetimes) are not sufficiently taken into account in determining the priority for action.

The priorities in *Choosing Health* include reducing health inequalities, tackling tobacco-related harm, controlling alcohol use, improving sexual health, reducing obesity, increasing physical activity and reducing accidents and injuries. These are typical priorities which increasingly focus on modern behavioural and lifestyle factors (*see* Chapter 2) and can only be tackled effectively through partnership working.

Choosing Health does, however, have policies and plans for their monitoring and delivery at national, regional and local levels. Their relevance is underlined by the emphasis placed on public service agreements (PSA targets), performance measures which monitor actions and accountabilities at each of these three levels.

At a central level, statutory accountability rests with the Cabinet Office and with individual government departments. Regionally it lies with regional government or regional 'offices' and at a local level with local government or PCT (NHS) levels. At a national level the PSA targets, such as life expectancy and infant mortality targets, are agreed by Cabinet, and the Cabinet Committee chaired by the Deputy Prime Minister oversees the performance nationally. Individual government departments have their specific targets and lead responsibilities, e.g. Department of Health for cancer and heart disease targets or Department for Education and Science for Health Promoting Schools standards.

The Office of the Deputy Prime Minister (ODPM) is the common pathway for the targets that are specific for local government. The review processes for local authorities involve the Audit Commission as a regulator and the Comprehensive Performance Assessment (CPA) as the process through which best value is ensured and progress toward local PSA targets is monitored. This process increases the central overview of the local government system, perhaps at odds with emphasis on local democratic accountability, and is exemplified by the introduction in 2004 of local area agreements (LAAs), local contracts which need to be signed between local partners, including the NHS, in upper-tier authorities (counties and unitary local authorities). These contain local 'stretch targets' which accelerate the achievement of local PSA targets by building in financial incentives to reward achievement on agreed performance measures over a 3-year period. The LAAs have a public health focus, highlighting economic development, safe and secure communities, a healthy start for children, and health and wellbeing of older people. Despite the fact that politically the move toward democratically elected regional government has faltered (apart from the Greater London Authority) the regional government offices in England are the place where these LAAs are coordinated and agreed for signing off by ODPM (*see* Figure 32.1).

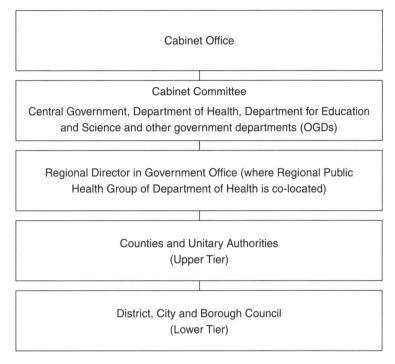

Figure 32.1 Levels within local government.

The Department of Health now oversees, through its Permanent Secretary, both health and social care. The NHS with its £60 billion budget and 1.3 million staff is an important part of the Department of Health delivery arm for health and not just concerned with health services. It is the source of national policies both for health and the health service – for example, the *NHS Improvement Plan* (Department of Health 2004b), *Commissioning a Patient-led NHS* (Department of Health 2005), the National Service Frameworks and *Choosing Health* (Department of Health 2004a). Possibly because of this relationship, and the need to deliver new policies as they emerge from the political system, the NHS therefore finds itself subject to frequent structural reforms.

As we write we know that the structure we have in 2005 in England is changing. Current organisation has three levels of governance – Department of Health in central government, the strategic health authorities which cover populations of between 1.5 and 2.5 million, and primary care trusts with populations of between 100,000 and 300,000. PCTs both provide primary care services and commission care from acute hospitals, mental health and ambulance provider trusts. In addition to NHS providers there are independent sector providers, NGOs, charities and voluntary carers. In the future there will be fewer PCTs and they will become commissioning bodies, not providers. The local primary care system will include practice-based commissioners and a plurality of providers. Strategic health authorities will become regional with strategic performance and market management functions (*see* Figure 32.2).

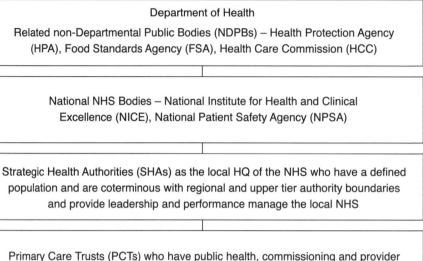

Department of Health

Related non-Departmental Public Bodies (NDPBs) – Health Protection Agency (HPA), Food Standards Agency (FSA), Health Care Commission (HCC)

National NHS Bodies – National Institute for Health and Clinical Excellence (NICE), National Patient Safety Agency (NPSA)

Strategic Health Authorities (SHAs) as the local HQ of the NHS who have a defined population and are coterminous with regional and upper tier authority boundaries and provide leadership and performance manage the local NHS

Primary Care Trusts (PCTs) who have public health, commissioning and provider functions for registered populations of between 100–300,000 people

Hospital Provider Trusts (including Foundation Trusts) in Acute Care, Mental Health and Ambulance Trusts

Figure 32.2 Levels within the NHS.

Thus there are two arms of the accountability machinery engaged in performance managing public health. The wider determinants of health are monitored through the Cabinet Committee which sets the overarching public service agreement (PSA) targets (half of which have a public health component). The delivery systems broadly work through the regional government to local organisations. The health service contribution is monitored through the strategic health authority rather than the regional government office. As shown in Figure 32.2, public health governance is through the regional public health groups and the SHAs as the intermediate tier.

An important player in the public health delivery system is the Health Protection Agency (HPA), a comparatively new non-departmental public body (*see* Chapter 30). Its remit covers an important domain of public health and the HPA has a parallel but complementary national, regional and local team structure.

The Audit Commission is part of the regulatory structure for local government and related public services while the Healthcare Commission and the Social Care Inspectorate are the regulatory bodies for health and social care (*see* Chapter 9). The small number of foundation hospital trusts is currently regulated by a comparatively new organisation called Monitor which has a predominantly financial scrutiny remit and does not contribute at present to public health governance.

With this complexity it is not difficult to see why development of a public health system is not a simple task, and performance management of such a system requires collaboration and communication between all the different players.

Three domains of public health

Since public health policy and practice is as complex as the determinants of health, one useful framework which assists the performance development and performance management of public health is the identification of three distinct and inter-related domains of practice – health improvement, health protection, and health and social care services (Griffiths *et al.* 2005). Constructing frameworks at each level to scope public health responsibilities and accountabilities usefully holds together the complexities of the public health system. These can be shown diagrammatically as in Figure 32.3.

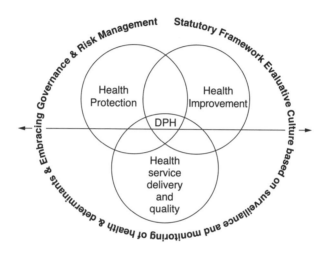

Figure 32.3 Three domains of public health.

Health protection incorporates the infectious diseases, biological, chemical, and radiological factors. While the HPA is a national agency for health protection, policy is determined at DH level and health-protection accountabilities are exercised through PCT Directors of Public Health. Immunisation programmes and local infection control measures will be overseen by the PCT and local NHS provider trusts.

The health-improvement domain covers health promotion and tackling health inequalities through the modification of material and structural factors, e.g. child poverty and poor housing. Partnership working through the local strategic partnerships is a crucial part of the process in identifying the health needs and inequalities and agreeing a multi-agency programme to address them.

Health and social care services represent direct clinical services for people, including advice on healthy lifestyles, preventive measures and treatment services. Many conditions in modern developed societies are long term and the close working relationships between health and social services, including carers and the voluntary sector, are vital.

In Figure 32.3, the three domains are deliberately shown as overlapping zones requiring a performance-management system which covers all elements. Effective accountability is most easily achieved by primary health and social care services, coterminous with environmental health and housing, education and transport functions in upper-tier local authorities, understanding and reporting on these relationships. The role of the Director of Public Health, with joint public health accountabilities (*see* Chapter 25), facilitates greater clarity for statutory organisations charged with oversight of the social, economic and environmental determinants of health and the wellbeing of the defined population (Association of Directors of Public Health 2004). Public health specialists, trained in each of the three domains, are in an ideal position to provide Chief Officer level input into the local authorities and NHS in this role.

Performance managing public health: performance reviews

Reviewing the performance of public health contribution by the different organisations in the NHS and local government takes place at different levels with a variable level of detail and rigor. Locally PCT DsPH and CEOs are subject to accountability reviews through the local strategic health authority and nationally via the Healthcare Commission (*see* Chapter 9); these reviews are changing but assessments will typically look at structure, process and outcomes.

An example of the framework for public health reviews includes questions about the areas in Box 32.1.

Box 32.1 Framework for public health reviews

Structure:

- DPH as Executive Director of PCT.
- Joint appointment with local authority (LA).
- Staffing levels and who is in the team.
- Public health networking arrangements between PCTs.
- Other resources – training, library services and management support.

Process:

- DPH annual report recommendations to PCT and LA.
- Local strategic partnership (LSP) working.
- Health equity audits and actions taken to reduce inequalities.
- Engagement with local area agreement processes.
- Sure Start.
- Health Promoting Schools.
- Sexual Health Strategy.
- Obesity/physical activity strategies.
- Relationships with and use of public health observatory.
- Working with the local Health Protection Unit (HPA).

Outcomes (in relation to PSA and other PH targets):

- Smoking prevalence and cessation targets.
- Childhood obesity prevalence.
- Teenage pregnancy rates.
- Life expectancy and infant mortality rates.
- Reducing inequalities.
- Cancer mortality rates and breast and cervical screening uptake.

- CHD mortality rates, CHD service indicators such as thrombolysis/revascularisation rates.
- Suicide rates.
- Accident and injury rates.

Locally the strategic health authorities hold PCTs to account for public health performance; local authorities use the Comprehensive Performance Assessment process and increasingly are subject to LAAs. These are scrutinised at regional office level with inputs from the regional public health groups. At present the different performance-assessment review systems are not sufficiently joined up.

At national level the Department of Health through the CMO monitors Regional Public Health Directors through a limited range of public health performance measures at regional level. The national inspection and regulation bodies such as the Healthcare Commission, Audit Commission and Social Care Inspectorate report to national government on star ratings and thematic reviews and include commentary on public health.

Conclusions

Public health and the public health system are of vital importance to all countries, including the developed world. The Wanless reports identified the risk to modern societies if some of the lifestyle determinants, such as food, exercise and obesity, are not tackled effectively and individuals and communities engaged in the endeavour. We have many strengths in the UK public health system, notably good surveillance and public health clinical indicator sets collected locally, regionally and nationally. However, the complex relationships described above reflect the difficulty many people have in determining who is accountable for health gain. Moves in recent years to ensure that public health is part of the performance assessment of both the NHS and local government are welcome but would be strengthened by clarification of public health accountabilities at all population levels. This would ensure that the system becomes more joined up and the public health performance review processes can be clearer. Recent developments such as the *Choosing Health* delivery plan give cause for optimism, using national PSA targets to create a framework which clearly designates organisations and their accountabilities within the framework.

Other contributions include the National Service Frameworks which take a broad view and build public health programmes through promoting health, preventing disease, enhancing the quality of treatment and care services in a way which does not just concentrate on sickness but includes a wider social perspective. The NSFs help communicate the public health narrative, identifying who needs to do what at different parts of the programme.

Key players at all levels of the public health system are the Directors of Public Health (DsPH) (*see* Chapter 25). With DsPH increasingly appointed jointly across PCTs and upper-tier local authorities we will see greater congruence and the possibility of healing the 1974 rift when Medical Officers of Health were moved from local authorities to the NHS (*see* Chapter 15). The DPH role as an accredited public health specialist, appointed at executive director or chief officer level to a statutory organisation with public health accountabilities, holds the key to ensuring that with all the continuing organisational changes the public health needs of defined populations will be assessed and addressed. However, performance development and management arrangements will need to be more clearly described and integrated into performance activities at the intermediate and national levels to enhance performance and meet ambitious public health targets.

References

Association of Directors of Public Health (2004) *The Role of the Director of Public Health*. London: Faculty of Public Health.

Black D, Morris J, Smith C *et al.* (1980) *Inequalities in Health: The Black Report*. London: Penguin.

Department of Health (2004a) *Choosing Health: making healthy choices easier*. London: Department of Health.

Department of Health (2004b) *NHS Improvement Plan*. London: Department of Health.

Department of Health (2005) *Commissioning a Patient-led NHS*. London: Department of Health.

Griffiths S, Jewell T and Donnelly P (2005) Public health in practice: the three domains of public health. *Journal of Public Health*. **119**(10): 907–13.

HM Treasury (2004) *Securing Good Health for the Whole Population*. London: HM Treasury.

Independent Inquiry into Inequalities in Health (1988) *Independent Inquiry into Inequalities in Health Report*. London: The Stationery Office.

Part 5

Tools

Introduction

Having described the context, issues, priorities and practice in the earlier part of this book the contributions in this section provide some perspectives from those engaged in areas of work which have emerged as important to the public health agenda over the last few years.

Trailed as an idea in the 1999 English white paper, *Saving Lives: our healthier nation*, Public Health Observatories (PHOs) have become an essential part of the public health system. Based as they are at regional level they have the potential to act as the hub for population surveillance not only across the NHS but across all sectors of the population. John Wilkinson provides a description of their development, current role and future potential as well the problems they face. The opportunity afforded by the NHS Information Strategy, the growing awareness of the need to work closely with the Health Protection Agency and the issues around confidentiality and registration provide challenges to be faced. However, hopefully, PHOs look set to survive.

One of the organisations promoted in *Saving Lives* which has had a short-lived existence is the Health Development Agency (HDA). During its lifetime the HDA, as one of its roles, reviewed evidence of effective practice in public health. In April 2005, it was integrated with the National Institute for Clinical Excellence, now known as the National Institute for Health and Clinical Excellence while retaining the NICE acronym. In his chapter on evidence-based public health Michael Kelly describes how the principles which Archie Cochrane, the guru of evidence and effectiveness, outlined in 1972 have finally come to pass in 2005 in public health. The task of the Centre for Public Health Excellence, the transfigured HDA within NICE, is to take an evidence-based approach to effectiveness for public health combined with a concern for the cost-effectiveness of interventions. Recommendations will be not only for the NHS but all sectors, and will include not only personal behaviour change but societal interventions. As Kelly says:

> There is a considerable task ahead for NICE. The problem of inequalities in health remains stubbornly resistant to change, and the burden of disease and premature mortality caused by technically preventable diseases remains a problem for the population as a whole, and is disproportionately concentrated among the most disadvantaged. The best ways to change the health of the population will be subject to evidence-based scrutiny. Guidance development is, at least on this scale, a genuinely new departure for public health. Although it will be hard, the possibilities of this evidence-based approach to health improvement offer one of the most exciting opportunities in several generations in public health. The aspirations are high, the task difficult, but the prize potentially considerable.

Linked to this ambitious development to promote evidence-based guidance to the population is the whole question of how we manage knowledge in a world of exponentially and readily available information. Daragh Fahey and Muir Gray describe the basics of a knowledge management framework and system for public health practice, ending by reminding us that the public and professionals need clean clear knowledge just as they need clean clear water:

> *Ignorance is like cholera; it cannot be tackled by the individual alone and requires the organised efforts of society. It is thus a public health responsibility.*

Another developing theme in public health over the last few years is the need for networks. Allison Thorpe describes the emergence of public health networks and their utility, particularly at times of change. She reminds us that at its most fundamental, a network is a way of 'joining up' people with, or

> *around, a common interest. The connections may be simple – for example, a face-to-face, person-to-person connection – or a more complex and fluid matrix, involving multiple layers. Physically, there may be little connection between the layers, but in practice, it functions like a spider's web, as it is made stronger by the ability to be flexible in the direction travelled and nodes pulled into play. The different people sitting at each of the nodes where the web joins may have different skills and areas of expertise and different methods of communication may be used.*

This concept of linking, sharing and supporting public health delivery through organised networks has received support in all four UK countries, but has been implemented with varying success, often dependent on the people and resources available. Their success, in turn, is often dependent on their leadership and management.

The theme of networks and public health leadership is picked up by Neil Goodwin, who describes leadership as '*a process played out between leaders and followers, without whom leadership cannot exist*'. In his exploration of leadership he highlights that it is a dynamic, relationship-based process that uses a twofold approach of creating an agenda for change using a strong vision; and

> *building a strong implementation network to get things done through other people.*

> *Good leaders sense an environment, absorbing and interpreting hard and soft data without having it spelt out for them.*

Reminiscent of the definitional phrase of 'the science and the art', we are reminded once again of the balance between personal characteristics and positional power. The characteristics of public health practitioners able to deliver the future policy agenda are the subject of the last chapter. Steve Feast *et al.*'s vision of what things could be like, the new roles and ways of working that could emerge, gives us all food for thought.

Chapter 33

Public health intelligence and public health observatories

John Wilkinson

Introduction

Public Health Observatories (PHOs) were set up in England in 1999, having been announced in the *Saving Lives: our healthier nation* white paper (Department of Health 1999). Previously strong health intelligence functions had existed in the former regional health authorities (RHAs). These were abolished in 1994. The size of some of these regional information departments had been quite impressive, in some cases with staff of 100 people.

Origins of observatories

The first PHO in England was set up in Liverpool in 1990. The Liverpool Observatory described the term 'public health observatory' as a location and a responsibility for the public health surveillance and intelligence function within a defined administrative jurisdiction.

Its stated objectives were to *'stand back from phenomena and events, providing objective description and analysis, and forecasting patterns, interrelationships, processes and outcomes'* (Liverpool Public Health Observatory 2004).

However, the term 'observatory', for other than astronomy, has become widely used within the countries of the European Union. The use of the term 'observatory' in this new context appears to derive from France where the term is widely used to describe institutions, networks and organisations that have a responsibility for a sector or problem.

In France, there are observatories for most domains of knowledge and expertise. These include 'observatories' in the field of economics, law, health, environment, by specific area of knowledge, e.g. legislation, and for particular issues, e.g. rural (Le Petit Observatoire d'AdminNet 2004). 'Observatories' can operate at a national and regional level.

It has been said that *'souvent, en France, devant un probleme, on crée une observatoire'* (trans. 'Often in France, confronting a problem, an observatory is created') (Le Petit Observatoire d'AdminNet 2004).

PHOs were first established in the Ile de France surrounding Paris in 1974. Eventually, health observatories were set up in all regions of France including the overseas departments. France has a well-established national network of public health observatories – FNORS (Federation National Observatoires Regionaux de Sante) (Fédération national observatoires régionaux de la santé 2004). Equivalent terms have been utilised in other European countries, in Italy 'Osservatore' (Osservatorio – nazionale sulla salute nelle regioni italiane 2004), 'observatorium'

(Schweizerisches Gesundheitsobservatorium 2004) and other European countries. There are plans to establish health observatories in other parts of Europe, e.g. Hungary, Switzerland.

In the UK the term 'public health observatory' has become synonymous with the development of the public health surveillance and intelligence function. The UK is not noted for integrating European approaches within its health sector, least of all from France. However, in public health there is a precedent, as 'surveillance', the predominant function for public health observatories, is a French term.

Role of public health observatories

On being established in 1999, PHOs in England were given a number of explicit roles. These were as follows:

- monitoring health and disease trends and highlighting areas for action
- identifying gaps in health information
- advising on methods for health and health inequality impact assessments
- drawing together information from different sources in new ways to improve health
- evaluating progress by local agencies in improving health and cutting inequality
- looking ahead to give early warning of future public health problems.

They were also given a list of organisations with whom they were expected to work. These were:

- NHS bodies
- NHS Executive Regional Offices
- Government Offices
- Regional Development Agencies
- Health Development Agency.

This list provided an important clue about the direction that PHOs were expected to take and how they were to be distinguished from public health information departments in the former regional health authorities – the main difference being the focus on the determinants of health, rather than on the running of the health service.

Initially, eight PHOs were created in England, one in each of the NHS regions. When public health groups were aligned with Government Office regional boundaries, an additional public health observatory was created bringing their number up to nine.

Since their creation, PHOs have taken on a number of additional functions. Shortly after their arrival, PHOs took on the development of regional safe havens for hospital episode statistics (HES). In the 1990s the Department of Health had established a number of pilots to encourage the greater use of hospital data. As a result of the pilots, it was decided to establish regional safe havens in PHOs. The remit was for PHOs to encourage better use of this important data source at regional level.

Recognising the developing role of PHOs, the National Treatment Agency (NTA) asked PHOs to establish Regional Drug Treatment Monitoring Services (NDTMS). The initial priority of this development was to obtain good national data on the efficacy of treatment for drug misuse. Not all PHOs took on this responsibility. In later years the NTA agreed to fund analytic staff which enables regional PHOs to make much more effective use of this data source.

There has also been closer working between cancer registries and PHOs. This came about because of a request from the Chief Medical Officer for England. With the devolution of responsibility for the funding of cancer registries to primary care trusts (PCTs), it became apparent that these organisations had a varying understanding of the importance of the national surveillance function for cancer. Some PCTs refused to fund their local cancer registries. This led to considerable difficulties and a threat to the ongoing, very effective system of national cancer surveillance. In 2004, the responsibility for the funding of cancer registries was returned to the Regional Directors of Public Health (RDsPH). Some RDsPH took the opportunity in some cases to merge the PHOs and the cancer registries. However, this has not happened universally, in a number of cases because of the lack of coterminosity in some parts of England.

What do observatories do?

Hemmings and Wilkinson (2003) described the key components of an observatory. They suggested that an observatory, in this context, has a number of features, namely: it serves to combine a number of qualities of academic departments and state-based public health departments by providing high-quality, relevant regional intelligence for those who need it. The observatories do this to a short timetable, enabling them to respond to new, rapidly developing situations. They noted that observatories were often small organisations with a degree of autonomy. Observatories often hold very little data themselves and are not normally involved in its collection, but are able to access data readily and, using a range of skills and expertise, assemble it in a way that can influence policy makers.

PHOs have a number of activities

The activities of PHOs include:

1 The production of reports on selected topics. All PHOs have now published a wide range of reports on various public health topics, set according to either national or local priorities.
2 Website developments. All PHOs have websites on which a wide range of material of use to public health practitioners and the wider public can be found. The Association of Public Health Observatories has its own website which produces rapid access to all the PHO websites and material.
3 Capacity development and training. All PHOs are involved in training, be that at undergraduate or postgraduate level. Most PHOs are a core resource within their region for training and many have trainees attached. Some PHOs run courses and are involved in training in many diverse ways. Dissemination of the work of PHOs is crucial through conferences, workshops and seminars.
4 Support to the local public health community. PHOs provide a range of help and support to local public health intelligence specialists working in a range of organisations e.g. local authorities, PCTs and SHAs.

Wanless report

PHOs predated both Wanless reports (Wanless 2002, 2004). The second report was commissioned by the UK government *'to focus on prevention and wider determinants of health in England and on the cost of effectiveness of action … to reduce inequalities in health'*. In essence the review was asked to assess the state of readiness of the public health system to deliver the 'fully engaged scenario' described in the first Wanless report.

Wanless commented on the paucity of information of the current wellbeing of the population, particularly at local authority or PCT level. He went on to suggest the strengthening of the role of PHOs and suggested that there needed to be a better coordination of 'information activities at local level'.

Public health white paper: *Choosing Health*

The English white paper *Choosing Health* (Department of Health 2004) consolidated the recommendations of Wanless and produced a wide-ranging list of recommendations and conclusions. In terms of public health intelligence, the following key recommendations were made:

- The need to create a modern public health information and intelligence strategy was identified.
- The creation of a public health intelligence task force was signalled.
- There should be a framework for health surveillance at regional level.
- There should be development of skills, e.g. in equity audits and HIA.
- Information for PCT reports should be produced in an accessible style.
- Reports for local communities should be produced at local authority level.
- Real-time information at local level across the NHS and in the local community should be developed.

Additional resources for PHOs and the public health intelligence function were identified (£5 million in 2005 and £10 million in 2006).

The subsequent delivery plan, *Delivering Choosing Health* (Department of Health 2005), consolidated these recommendations for developing public health intelligence in the following four key areas:

- developing a regional health intelligence strategy in support of the RDPH and his or her team
- developing training (on both national and regional scales) and building capacity in public health intelligence
- producing reports/community profiles for local authorities
- supporting areas of national policy importance.

Each of these areas is considered below.

Developing a regional health intelligence strategy in support of the RDPH and his or her team

The development of regional health intelligence strategies is now crucial to make best use of the limited resource available in the regions, in health and social care organisations and in local authorities. These need to be connected together much more effectively. In recent years public health intelligence capacity in England has been fragmented across many organisations. This has hampered the ability to provide a good information base for the delivery of public health in England.

Developing training (on both national and regional scales) and building capacity in public health intelligence

The need to develop public health intelligence capacity has been highlighted as a priority for a considerable time. Working closely with others, implementing the voluntary register observatories will need to play a full part in rolling out expertise and assisting to create an appropriate career structure for those working in public health intelligence.

Producing reports/community profiles for local authorities

The very specific task of producing local health reports for local authorities has been taken forward as quickly as possible, with the development of the first set of proposals completed in mid-2006. PHOs are gaining new skills in this area as more material is targeted directly to the public.

Supporting areas of national policy importance

There is much that PHOs can do to support the national agenda and we will continue to do this along with our partners. PHOs will be expected to be more closely involved in broader NHS policy such as the National Service Frameworks (e.g. in diabetes, heart disease). The changes following NICE's incorporation of the former HDA provide another opportunity to review the relationship between evidence and information.

The development of observatories in other parts of the United Kingdom and Ireland

In other parts of the UK, following devolution in 1998, there have been different approaches taken to the organisation of health services, in which at the present time public health inevitably becomes embroiled. In Wales, the public health function has become much more centralised and at the same time has attempted to maintain local contact. It has done this by appointing all its senior public health personnel to the Wales Centre for Health, and then outposting staff to local primary care groups. There are now 22 of these organisations covering the whole of Wales and two regional health authorities, north and south. Wales has also created its own PHO as part of the Wales Centre for Health. This has very similar functions to the PHOs in England, with the notable additional task of providing health information to the general public, a role which is not explicitly part of the PHOs' responsibilities in England.

   In Scotland, where there has been for many years a much greater emphasis on the importance of information, and indeed less structural change, the position is very different. Boundaries of health boards in Scotland have been unchanged since the mid-1970s. More recently, following a brief excursion into separating the purchaser and provider function, the Scots have created single integrated health organisations. This has meant that the health boards have always had for many years fairly stable intelligence functions as part of these organisations. However, some of the health boards are quite small (such as Orkney and the Western Isles). Nationally Scotland has had a very strong public health intelligence function, as part of its Information and Statistics Division (ISD), and now as part of NHS Health Scotland, which was formed in 2004 as a result of the merger of the Public Health Institute for Scotland and the Health Education Board for Scotland.

In Northern Ireland, boards have had responsibility for combined health and social care for many years and have operated for a population of around 1.7 million. In the future, it is likely that the number of health boards will be reduced, as a health reorganisation is currently underway in the province.

Lead areas

When PHOs were established, it was agreed that each PHO should develop expertise in a key area of policy, in order to avoid duplication between the PHOs and to provide leadership and input into national decisions. The lead areas of PHOs have recently been revised, and are at the time of writing as shown in Table 33.1.

Table 33.1 Lead areas of PHOs

Region/country	Website address	Lead area
North East	www.nepho.org.uk	Mental health, prisons, Europe and international
North West	www.nwpho.org.uk	Drug misuse, crime and violence, alcohol
West Midlands	www.wmpho.org.uk	Older people, cancer
East Midlands	www.empho.org.uk	Food and nutrition, renal disease, teenage pregnancy
South West	www.swpho.org.uk	Accidents and injuries, sexual health
London	www.lho.org.uk	Black and ethnic minorities, tobacco, inequalities in health
South East	www.sepho.org.uk	Physical activity, obesity, transport, coronary heart disease, stroke
Eastern	www.erpho.org.uk	Rural health, primary care
Wales	www.wch.wales.nhs.uk	Environment and sustainable development
Yorkshire and the Humber	www.yhpho.org.uk	Children and young people, diabetes

In addition, PHOs have individually taken on the responsibility to link with key departments of government, agencies and other organisations. The links are as shown in Table 33.2.

Association of Public Health Observatories

The Association of Public Health Observatories (APHO) was created at the outset of PHO development in England. The roles and responsibilities of the APHO were agreed to be as follows: a learning network for members and participants, a single point of contact for external partners, an advocate for users

Table 33.2 PHOs' links with other organisations

PHO	Linked organisations
North East	Department of Health, National Patient Safety Agency
North West	Health Protection Agency
West Midlands	UK Association of Cancer Registries
East Midlands	Health and Social Care Information Centre
South West	Office of the Deputy Prime Minister
London	National Institute for Health and Clinical Excellence
South East	Office for National Statistics
Eastern	Healthcare Commission
Yorkshire and the Humber	Department for Education and Skills

of public health information, and a coordinator of work across the network of PHOs.

The real strengths of PHOs have been those of a managed national network. In summary these have been in the pooling of a wide range of skills (information technology, web development and analytic skills). The development of lead areas has enabled skills to be pooled and developed providing a national resource. PHOs have been able to be flexible and the APHO has facilitated rapid transference of skills and techniques across the dispersed network. The APHO is playing a critical place in the development of public health intelligence capacity both regionally and nationally. Finally, the threats to public health intelligence through legitimate concerns about data protection are being dealt with through continuing dialogue with the Office for National Statistics (ONS), the National Treatment Agency (NTA) and Neighbourhood Statistics (NeSS). In short PHOs have been able to build on a critical mass of IT, web development and analytic skills, a system of lead areas. Flexibility and the ability to learn from different models has been a strength. A core role has been in training and development, and finally PHOs have been able to develop a collective advocacy for public health intelligence.

PHOs have concluded that with the strengthening of PHOs the APHO will also need to be strengthened and to develop more national capacity.

Current challenges and the future

There are a number of challenges to the future stability of the public health function within England. The major challenge is the need to expand the availability and capacity of the public health intelligence workforce. With the fragmentation of the public health intelligence function as a result of *Shifting the Balance of Power* (Department of Health 2002), this scarce resource has been scattered through a variety of poorly connected public health organisations. This means that, very often, public health intelligence specialists have been working in isolation and unsupported. There are a number of exceptions – where, for example, effective public health networks have been established – but unfortunately these are not effective universally. The Faculty of Public Health is now attempting to strengthen the public health intelligence function with the creation of a voluntary register which will include public health intelligence specialists as a 'defined group'. It is expected that this will improve the recognition and the career prospects of this group of skilled staff.

Disclosure and confidentiality issues are a serious threat to the effective utilisation of public health intelligence. People clearly have a right to preserve confidentiality over their personal medical details. However, society needs to recognise the value of data on health about the whole population. Cancer registries are a very good example of how data has been collected over many years and is now being put to good effect to target the improvement of cancer services and to monitor their effectiveness. Unfortunately named data has been required to enable individual histories to be followed and to avoid duplication. Although this has required the collection of named data, the use of the name has only been essential for these purposes. In the future various techniques are likely to be developed to allow such functions to be carried out without the need to collect named data. However, these schemes remain in their infancy. Other concerns relate to the unintended identification of individual circumstances through the publication of data on very small populations. The Department of Health has announced a review of this issue.

A third challenge is the need for organisational stability. The history of the NHS in the UK, and especially in England, is not good in this regard with the plethora of reorganisations in recent years. This leads to a particular set of problems where health intelligence is concerned. Not only are the personal lives of the staff concerned disrupted, but public health intelligence needs long-term stability to monitor disease trends. Numerous organisational boundary changes add an additional burden to this process, when for example it may be necessary to track disease patterns in a particular geographical location over a period of 10–20 years.

New developments in information systems present new opportunities

The massive investment currently taking place as the National Programme for IT, newly renamed *Connecting for Health*, presents huge opportunities for gaining a better understanding of the population's health in England. This project, which is estimated to be costing £6 billion, originated out of a combination of activities – the development of the NHS Care Records Service, together with huge political impetus in establishing a system which would allow patients sitting with their general practitioner a choice of hospitals in which to be treated and at the same time setting a date for treatment. Effectively creating a database of the whole population in England, including all health records, presents huge opportunities for understanding health in our society. In time it could replace the need for such systems as cancer registration and at the same time provide equivalent 'registries' in all other areas of morbidity. However, the public health benefits of such a system have only latterly been recognised. Nonetheless, this potential is now being taken into account. It will be the 'Secondary Users Service' (SUS) which will be the way in which population information data is transmitted and interpreted.

The SUS will protect patient confidentiality and provide data and information for other purposes than direct clinical care and includes:

- planning
- commissioning
- public health
- clinical audit
- benchmarking
- performance improvement
- research
- clinical governance.

In time, SUS will take data from other sources including cancer waiting times, clinical audit, and later data from non-health sources such as ONS, workforce data.

Regional role of PHOs with non-NHS partners

From the outset PHOs have had a remit to work with non-NHS partners. Initially these were included in the list in *Saving Lives: our healthier nation*:

- NHS Executive Regional Offices
- Government Offices
- Regional Development Agencies
- Health Development Agency.

In all regions, PHOs are working closely with their respective Regional Development Agencies (RDAs), Regional Assemblies and Government Offices. PHOs are supporting the process of local area agreements which are tools being used by Government Offices to manage significant changes at local authority level including health and wellbeing. All regions of England have generic observatory functions, concentrating on the wider information needs in the region. Generally, these are funded by the RDAs, but work closely with PHOs. PHOs have also worked to produce reports on crime (e.g. from South West PHO) and a range of other topics.

PHOs are also working closely in a number of cases with Local Authority Overview and Scrutiny Committees whose remit now includes a health dimension.

Impact/fate of PHO reports

Assessing the impact of PHOs is difficult. It is easy to look at website hits and volume of reports downloaded, and where this has been done, this has been informative but clearly limited. An evaluation of PHOs was carried out in 2003 by the West Midlands PHO and individual observatories have undertaken small evaluations of their own local activities. These have all yielded useful insights and all PHOs can point to examples where reports have been used.

Relationship with the Health Protection Agency (HPA)

PHOs are developing links with the HPA at both regional and national levels. At regional level, some regional epidemiology units are co-located with the public health observatory and a number of regional teams and PHOs have produced joint reports (North East: www.nepho.org.uk/index.php?c=206, South West: www.swpho.nhs.uk/resource/browse.aspx?RID=5). A memorandum of agreement was signed between APHO and the former Centre for Disease Control (CDSC), this is now being updated. Clearly there are many skills which PHOs have which are of value to the HPA; these include expertise in geographical mapping techniques, novel statistical approaches, demographic data, and data on inequalities.

Regional indications

A major piece of work has been undertaken by the Association of Public Health Observatories at the request of the Chief Medical Officer for England. Observatories were commissioned to produces a series of reports which were aimed to highlight various aspects of public health performance and to focus on inter-regional comparisons. A series of 'traffic-lighted' indicators were produced for 46 (check) indicators under five headings. These headings are:

- population health status
- priority public health interventions
- effectiveness in partnerships
- wider determinants and risk factors
- public health capacity.

In addition to the regional reports, themed reports have also been published. The topics covered by these themed reports are:

- lifestyles
- ethnicity and health
- sexual health
- mental health
- child health.

On average three reports are published each year with extensive use being made of control chart methodology. Originally taken from industry, control chart methodology aims to identify outliers where remedial action may be called for. This technique is more fully described by Mohammed *et al.* (2001). Its advantage is that it provides a credible alternative to more standard methods of presentation (e.g. bar charts, league tables) and has the advantage that it identifies points (in this case local authorities) which lie outside the expected predefined range, rather than a simple ranking.

This Regional Indications series of reports has been aimed to stimulate action at both national and regional level and provides some 'hard' data on which public health activities can be performance managed which it can be argued is more likely to focus managers' attention on public health issues in the same way as attention is focused on such data as waiting lists in the healthcare setting.

Conclusions

PHOs have now been in existence for over 5 years and look to continue for at least the foreseeable future. Their development emphasises the increasing importance of making best use of intelligence to improve the health of the population. Some important progress has been made, but there is still a long way to go.

References

Department of Health (1999) *Saving Lives: our healthier nation.* Cm 4386. London: The Stationery Office.

Department of Health (2002) *Shifting the Balance of Power.* London: Department of Health.

Department of Health (2004) *Choosing Health: making healthier choices easier.* Cm 6374. 16 November. London: The Stationery Office.

Department of Health (2005) *Delivering Choosing Health.* London: Department of Health.

Fédération national observatoires régionaux de la santé (FNORS) (2004). www.fnors.org.

Hemmings J and Wilkinson JR (2003) What is a Public Health Observatory? *Journal of Epidemiology and Community Health.* **57**: 324–6.

Le Petit Observatoire d'AdminNet (2004) Adminet. http://adminet.com/obs.

Liverpool Public Health Observatory (2004) www.liv.ac.uk/PublicHealth/obs/root/liverpool%20public%20health%20observatory/index.htm.

Mohammed MA, Cheng KK, Rouse AA *et al.* (2001) Bristol, Shipman, and clinical governance: Shewhart's forgotten lessons. *Lancet.* **357**: 463–7.

Osservatorio – nazionale sulla salute nelle regioni italiane (2004) Istituto di igiene, Rome. 5 December. http://www.osservasalute.it/.

Swiss Public Health Observatory (2004) www.obsan.ch/e/index.htm.

Wanless D (2002) *Securing Our Future Health: taking a long term view.* www.hm-treasury.gov.uk/Consultations and Legislation/wanless/consult wanless final.cfm (accessed 22 July 2002).

Wanless D (2004) *Securing Good Health for the Whole Population: final report.* 25 February. London: HM Treasury.

Chapter 34

Evidence-based public health

Michael P Kelly

Introduction: the emergence of the evidence-based approach

The use of evidence is not new in public health. Public health as an academic discipline, and as a form of practice, has used evidence from its very beginning. When John Snow in 1850s' London, in perhaps the most famous of all public health interventions, identified the possibility that cholera was a water-borne disease, he was using observation and evidence in a logical and rational way. Although the understanding was rudimentary by today's standards, it neverthe-less led to effective preventive strategies and the Broad Street pump in Soho had found its infamous place in the annals of public health (Chave 1958). When the first Medical Officers of Health plotted epidemic prevalence and linked it to poor housing (Checkland and Lamb 1982), and when Victorian social reformers tracked the relationship between poverty and poor physical health (Briggs 1959), they were following a route prescribed by the evidence. Some of the most important breakthroughs in prevention of non-communicable diseases have been made using epidemiological evidence. The evidence which demon-strated the relationship between smoking and lung cancer (Doll and Hill 1952), the lack of exercise and heart attack (Morris *et al.* 1953), and exposure to asbestos and lung cancer (Doll 1955) are striking examples of the powerful use of evidence. More recently the very many investigations which have shown the relationship between cardiovascular disease and various lifestyle factors (Batty *et al.* 2003; Marmot and Elliott 1992; Unal *et al.* 2004), and the relationship between the wider determinants of health and health inequalities (Davey Smith *et al.* 2002; Lynch *et al.* 2000; Marmot and Wilkinson 1999), have been grounded in very advanced uses of evidence.

However, taking an evidence-based approach contemporarily has come to mean more than simply *using* evidence or doing well-conducted scientific studies. The evidence-based approach refers to taking a scientific approach to the accumulation and understanding of the evidence itself (Chalmers *et al.* 2002; Egger *et al.* 2001)! A major impetus in this has been the development of evidence-based medicine (Greenhalgh 2001).

Evidence-based medicine

Evidence-based medicine has evolved in the last 40 years or so for a variety of reasons. First, there has been a dramatic escalation in the amount of available medical evidence. The sheer volume of scientific information has become too vast for even the most conscientious scientist or doctor to keep pace with. Ways of making the large volume of evidence easily accessible became a necessity and this in turn led to more systematic ways of organising databases of evidence than had conventionally been the case (Greenhalgh 2001).

Second, as ways of synthesising and reviewing the vast amounts of information generated by medical and other scientists became an urgent priority, this was greatly assisted by the development of new technologies. Computer databases, and powerful search engines to access the databases quickly, allowed much more comprehensive ways of finding information than was ever possible by manual methods. The existence of the new technologies has meant that it was technically possible to gather large amounts of information, on a scale congruent with the volume of new evidence appearing, and then search it comprehensively and rapidly.

Third, bias has been identified as a critical problem in science (Egger *et al.* 2001). There are two different aspects to the problem of bias. Initially there are those biases that arise as a consequence of the types of method used. Methodologists had written for decades about the problems of bias, of the fact that subjects involved in scientific investigations often behave differently to how they would behave normally, of placebo effects, and of failures to observe and record things accurately, and of the process of recording information to reflect the prejudices of the researchers. The evidence-based approach seeks to minimise these kinds of bias. The other issue is more social in origin. It has been argued that scientists have tended to be much less systematic towards the *accumulated* scientific evidence than they have been to the process of gathering evidence in the first place. And, worse, they have tended to be very selective in their approach to their favoured evidence. The history of science is full of many examples of scientists preferring their own pet theories and models, in spite of accumulated evidence which contradicted them (Kuhn 1970). Bias, intentional or accidental, is an endemic hazard of scientific and medical activity (Greenhalgh 2001).

Fourth, in spite of the great successes of medicine stretching back to the early 19th century and the undoubted benefits to the overall health of populations of these advances, especially in developed countries (Bunker 2001) – aseptic surgery, control of infectious disease, antibiotics, immunisation, hip and knee replacement surgery, dramatic declines in the rate of infant mortality, and increasing life expectancy – by the 1950s and 1960s medicine found itself under mounting criticisms from a variety of directions. Some dismissed the claims that medical technologies had actually produced health benefits. They argued instead that general improvements in social conditions were responsible for the majority of health gain (McKeown 1976). Others argued that medicine did more harm than good and encouraged a tendency to medicalise ordinary everyday life (Illich 1977). Still others saw medicine as a conspiracy to exert power and control over docile populations (Freidson 1970). Catastrophic medical disasters like the thalidomide affair, worries over organ transplantation, and in the end an apparent impotence in the face of the modern scourges of cancer and heart disease, all contributed to this state of unease within medicine and to criticisms from the outside.

Fifth, originally in the United States, but more recently elsewhere, a penchant for patients to sue their doctors added to the unhappy state which medicine found itself in the second half of the 20th century. The rise of consumerism with patients vocally demanding the best and most appropriate treatments were parts of the same trend. And finally the sheer costs of modern healthcare led to pressures from the funders of medical services to determine whether what was being done in the name of medicine was in fact cost-effective.

The evidence-based approach in clinical medicine emerges not so much in direct response to these criticisms and to these developments, so much as taken together these different things created a fertile ground in which evidence-based medicine could develop. One of the most influential British texts in the history of the evidence-based approach originally appeared in 1972. This was Archie Cochrane's essay, *Effectiveness and Efficiency: random reflections on health services*. Cochrane, himself an eminent physician, was part of the chorus of criticism. He argued that health services have a tendency towards inefficiency, mostly because of organisational, institutional, demographic, and technical factors and a variety of other things including human failure. His principal concerns were that there was no agreed way to determine what worked or did not work, and therefore it was not possible to tell whether interventions did more harm than good, or had neutral effects. He also complained that no one could tell how much anything cost, so there was no way of telling what was good value for money and what was not. His solution was to advocate the use of the clinical trial and to argue that economic appraisal must be undertaken of medical interventions.

The randomised controlled trial (RCT) is the most precise way to determine effectiveness of an intervention. With subjects properly randomised and with investigators blind to which is the experimental group and which is the control group, it provides the best way to determine whether or not something works and allows bias of various kinds to be to a large extent controlled. The use of the RCT as the means of determining effectiveness became the gold standard, and indeed the best available way of determining effectiveness. In spite of certain philosophical and medical discussions around points of detail, this method remains the most reliable as far as determining effectiveness is concerned (Davies *et al.* 2000). Cochrane's demands for a science of health economics led in Britain to the development of very sophisticated tools to compare different treatments on a cost–benefit and cost-effectiveness basis. Alan Williams, an economics professor at the University of York and collaborator with Cochrane, was a particularly influential figure in this regard.

Despite Cochrane's arguments and the development of health economics it was not until the House of Lords Select Committee on Science and Technology in 1988 identified the fact that too little research was being carried out that was relevant to practitioners, managers and policy makers that a significant shift towards the evidence-based approach actually took place (Davies *et al.* 2000). This in turn led to the formulation of the NHS *Research and Development Strategy* in 1991 and was a major impetus to the development of both the Cochrane Collaboration itself and the establishment of the NHS Centre for Reviews and Dissemination at the University of York, both of which act to review primary evidence in systematic, transparent and auditable and replicable ways (Davies *et al.* 2000). These organisations were and are engaged in the systematic searching for evidence, its critical appraisal and its synthesis. They have become world leaders in the evidence-based approach.

The principles of building the evidence base are straightforward enough. It starts from the idea of the accumulation of evidence. Accumulated evidence is aggregated. The idea of cumulation of findings is simple. Rather than generalise from one particular study to the world as a whole, the idea is to increase representativeness of findings by putting together many studies which will provide a closer approximation to what is really going on. By increasing representativeness by pooling observations and results, the idea is that bias may be reduced (Egger *et al.* 2001). So in the evidence-based approach the assumption is made that the more often a finding occurs in different studies the more likely it is to be an accurate representation of reality. To rely on a single result from a single study and to generalise to a broader reality is unwise because any single result may in a statistical sense be an outlier, and/or the result of random chance. The greater the number of cases the greater the likelihood that statistical aberrations will be nullified and the real effect will be found.

The process of building the evidence base involves therefore finding and then gathering together as many examples of studies of a particular type as possible. Then the best studies methodologically are identified and poor studies eliminated. After deciding which studies have met the methodological rigour in terms of design, sampling, control of bias, the results are summed in some way, either to detect the general direction that the evidence points, or by trying to accumulate the results from multiple studies into one statistical calculation in what is called meta-analysis. The results of the best studies are synthesised. The elimination of poor studies is important. Studies which do not reach predefined standards of methodological rigour need to be excluded from the evidence base because if they are methodologically unreliable so too will be their results. This was in principle what Archie Cochrane had argued for.

The development of powerful computer search engines to interrogate properly compiled and indexed databases, on a scale that scholars who used to have to work by hand and index card could never have imagined, makes systematic discovery of relevant papers much more straightforward than it once was. The development of the tools of systematic review and of meta-analysis make synthesis, as opposed to traditional literature reviewing, a much more auditable, transparent and exhaustive process. Not all that many years ago it was simply not feasible even to suggest that a literature search would cover the entire scientific output in the world on a particular topic. Instead the scholar would begin with one or two key articles or textbooks and then search on the basis of what was in the bibliographies and work outwards. Personal communication, gossip, attendance at conferences and meetings all were sources to help the researcher add to their literature. When the author came to write their review or to assemble their evidence, it was not usual to indicate why certain material was included, why some was excluded, and what kind of process had been used to search library catalogues and so on. Obviously this kind of approach was inherently subject to bias and there was little or no way for others to check the degree of bias. The systematic review, as the name implies, tries to be open and transparent, and can claim greater representativeness by virtue of the ability researchers now have to synthesise large volumes of data using the available computer technology. It is of course not perfect, but it is a lot less likely to be subject to the biases mentioned above.

The development of a public health evidence base

In the UK the move to developing an evidence-based approach in public health was slower than in clinical medicine. The real impetus occurred with the publication of the *Saving Lives: our healthier nation* white paper (Secretary of State for Health 1999) and in the Department of Health's *Research and Development Strategy* (Department of Health 2001). The Health Development Agency (HDA) was established as a special health authority in 2000, following the publication of that white paper. One of the Agency's core functions was to build the evidence base in public health and health improvement, particularly with regard to the reduction of health inequalities. The *Research and Development Strategy* indicated that the HDA's work on the evidence base should provide high-quality evidence to reduce inequalities in health, bring various knowledge bases together, identify gaps in the evidence and be accessible.

From 2000 to 2005 the Agency reviewed the evidence on health inequalities and on the effectiveness of public health interventions. Reviews were undertaken of the evidence dealing with the prevention of low birth weight (Bull *et al.* 2003), social support in pregnancy (Bull *et al.* 2004), the prevention of drug misuse (Canning *et al.* 2004) , sexually transmitted infections and HIV (Ellis *et al.* 2003; Ellis and Grey 2004), the promotion of physical activity (Hillsdon *et al.* 2005), accidental injury prevention (Millward *et al.* 2003), the management of obesity and overweight (Mulvihill and Quigley 2003), the prevention of alcohol misuse (Mulvihill *et al.* 2005) and smoking (Naidoo *et al.* 2004), the promotion of breastfeeding (Prothero *et al.* 2003), and the prevention of teenage pregnancy (Swann *et al.* 2003).

The work of the Health Development Agency in building the evidence base was taken over by the National Institute for Health and Clinical Excellence (new NICE) in April 2005. The role of new NICE was signalled in the 2004 white paper, *Choosing Health* (Department of Health 2004). The Centre for Public Health Excellence in new NICE will develop public health guidance based on the best available evidence. The work will not be confined to particular populations or settings, and very importantly the focus on health inequalities and the wider determinants of health, which were such a feature of the work of the Health Development Agency, will be retained. The guidance will relate to public health activities that are direct (for example, providing a particular service, such as family planning or smoking cessation) or indirect (for example, the creation of safe open spaces for physical activity as part of general environmental upgrading). The guidance will concern both explicit and traditional public health topics (for example, the welfare of nursing and expectant mothers) and more implicit issues associated with wider determinants of health, such as the control of the number of fast-food and alcohol outlets in inner-city regeneration schemes.

The evidence-based public health guidance of NICE will make recommendations at population, community, organisational, group, family or individual level. It will recognise the wide spectrum of determinants of population and individual health. This spectrum includes factors from the social structure, economy and environment, through access to services, to individual choices and behaviours. The guidance will embrace and involve the appraisal of a variety of approaches including traditional health education and public campaigns as well as community development.

In the course of developing guidance the evidence of effectiveness and cost-effectiveness will be evaluated in order to make recommendations. The methods of economic appraisal will build upon existing NICE methods, with appropriate modifications to reflect the evidence available in public health. The starting point for the economic analysis will be cost per QALY (quality-adjusted life year – a method pioneered by Alan Williams) supplemented where necessary and appropriate by cost consequence analysis. The area of public health economics will present particular challenges and doubtless will evolve from this starting point. In particular the fact that there is very little good quality cost data in much of public health, and that some of the assumptions which have worked in clinical models will need to be reviewed, poses an interesting set of problems. The time periods over which appraisal can most appropriately be done also raises difficult challenges.

The implications for health inequalities will be considered in the new guidance, because the assumption that health improvement in the population as a whole reduces health inequalities is not borne out by the evidence. So special attention will need to be paid to the precise way interventions and policies impact on the different component parts of the population.

Before April 2005, NICE's remit was to develop guidance only for the NHS. From April 2005, the audiences for the guidance products will explicitly be extended beyond the NHS. The audiences for the guidance developed by the Centre for Public Health Excellence will include the NHS, local government and education, the utilities, and the private and voluntary sectors as well as a range of central government departments and their delivery arms that are responsible for taxation, benefits, roads, transport, housing, criminal justice and other aspects of services that determine the health of the public. Therefore the targets for NICE public health guidance will include chief executives and senior managers in the NHS and local government, public health specialists, medical and dental general practitioners, nurses, community practitioners (such as health visitors), other NHS staff, local authority managers, officers and employees, local politicians, managers and employees of the utilities, teachers and people working in certain parts of the private and voluntary sectors. The audience will also include policy makers and planners in all these areas.

Conclusion

So the principles which Archie Cochrane outlined in 1972 have finally come to pass in 2005 in public health – an evidence-based approach to effectiveness combined with a concern to make clear what the cost-effectiveness of interventions is. There is a considerable task ahead for NICE. The problem of inequalities in health remains stubbornly resistant to change, and the burden of disease and premature mortality caused by technically preventable diseases remains a problem for the population as a whole, and is disproportionately concentrated among the most disadvantaged. The best ways to change the health of the population will be subject to evidence-based scrutiny. Guidance development is, at least on this scale, a genuinely new departure for public health. Although it will be hard, the possibilities of this evidence-based approach to health improvement offer one of the most exciting opportunities in several generations in public health. The aspirations are high, the task difficult, but the prize potentially considerable.

References

Batty GD, Shipley MJ and Marmot M *et al.* (2003) Leisure time physical activity and coronary heart disease mortality in men symptomatic or asymptomatic for ischemia: evidence from the Whitehall study. *Journal of Public Health Medicine.* **25**: 190–6.

Briggs A (1959) *The Age of Improvement.* London: Longmans.

Bull J, McCormick G, Swann C et al. (2004) *Ante and Post Natal Home Visiting Programmes: a review of reviews.* London: Health Development Agency.

Bull J, Mulvihill C and Quigley R (2003) *Prevention of Low Birth Weight: assessing effectiveness of smoking cessation and nutritional intervention: evidence briefing.* London: Health Development Agency.

Bunker J (2001) *Medicine Matters After All: measuring the benefits of medical care, a healthy lifestyle, and a just social environment.* London: The Stationery Office/The Nuffield Trust.

Canning U, Millward LM, Raj T et al. (2004) *Drug Use Prevention: a review of reviews.* London: Health Development Agency.

Chalmers I, Hedges L and Cooper H (2002) A brief history of research synthesis. *Evaluation and the Healthcare Professions.* **25**: 12–37.

Chave SWP (1958) John Snow, the Broad Street pump and after. *The Medical Officer.* 13 June. **99**: 347–9.

Checkland O and Lamb M (eds) (1982) *Health Care as Social History: the Glasgow case.* Aberdeen: Aberdeen University Press.

Cochrane AL (1972) *Effectiveness and Efficiency: random reflections on health services.* London: British Medical Journal/Nuffield Provincial Hospitals Trust.

Davey Smith G, Dorling D, Mitchell R et al. (2002) Health inequalities in Britain: continuing increases up to the end of the twentieth century. *Journal of Epidemiology and Community Health.* **56**: 434–5.

Davies HTO, Nutley SM and Smith PC (2000) *What Works? Evidence based policy and practices in public services.* Bristol: Policy Press.

Department of Health (2001) *A Research and Development Strategy for Public Health.* London: Department of Health.

Department of Health (2004) *Choosing Health: making healthier choices easier.* London: Department of Health.

Doll R (1955) Mortality from lung cancer in asbestos workers. *British Journal of Industrial Medicine.* **12**: 81–6.

Doll R and Hill AB (1952) Smoking and carcinoma of the lung. *British Medical Journal.* **2**: 84–92.

Egger M, Davey Smith G and Altman BG (2001) *Systematic Reviews in Health Care: meta-analysis in context.* London: BMJ Books.

Ellis S, Barnett-Page E, Morgan A et al. (2003) *HIV Prevention: a review of reviews assessing the effectiveness of interventions to reduce the risk of sexual transmission: evidence briefing.* London: Health Development Agency.

Ellis S and Grey A (2004) *Prevention of Sexually Transmitted Infections (STIs): a review of reviews into the effectiveness of non-clinical intervention: evidence briefing.* London: Health Development Agency.

Freidson E (1970) *Profession of Medicine.* Chicago: Chicago University Press.

Greenhalgh T (2001) *How to Read a Paper: the basics of evidence based medicine.* London: BMJ Books.

Hillsdon M, Foster C, Cavill N et al. (2005) *The Effectiveness of Public Health Interventions for Increasing Physical Activity Among Adults: a review of reviews* (2e). London: Health Development Agency.

Illich I (1977) *The Limits to Medicine.* Harmondsworth: Penguin.

Kuhn TS (1970) *The Structure of Scientific Revolutions* (2e). Chicago: Chicago University Press.

Lynch JW, Davey Smith G, Kaplan G et al. (2000) Income inequality and mortality: importance to health of individual income, psychosocial environment or material conditions. *British Medical Journal.* **320**: 1200–4.

Marmot M and Elliott P (eds) (1992) *Coronary Heart Disease Epidemiology: from aetiology to public health.* Oxford: Oxford University Press.

Marmot M and Wilkinson R (eds) (1999) *Social Determinants of Health.* Oxford: Oxford University Press.

McKeown T (1976) *The Role of Medicine: dream, mirage or nemesis?* London: Nuffield Provincial Hospitals Trust.

Millward LM, Morgan A and Kelly MP (2003) *Prevention and Reduction of Accidental Injury in Children and Older People: evidence briefing.* London: Health Development Agency.

Morris J, Heady JA, Raffle PAB *et al.* (1953) Coronary heart disease and physical activity at work. *Lancet.* **ii**: 1053–7, 1111–20.

Mulvihill C and Quigley R (2003) *The Management of Obesity and Overweight: an analysis of reviews of diet, physical activity and behavioural approaches: evidence briefing.* London: Health Development Agency.

Mulvihill C, Taylor L and Waller S (2005) *Prevention and Reduction of Alcohol Misuse. Evidence briefing* (2e). London: Health Development Agency.

Naidoo B, Quigley R, Taylor L *et al.* (2004) *Public Health Interventions to Reduce Smoking Initiation and/or Further Uptake of Smoking, and to Increase Smoking Cessation: a review of reviews; evidence briefing.* London: Health Development Agency.

Protheroe L, Dyson L, Renfrew MJ *et al.* (2003) *The Effectiveness of Public Health Interventions to Promote the Initiation of Breastfeeding.* London: Health Development Agency.

Secretary of State for Health (1999) *Saving Lives: our healthier nation.* London: Stationery Office.

Swann C, Bowe K, McCormick G *et al.* (2003) *Teenage Pregnancy and Parenthood: a review of reviews: evidence briefing.* London: Health Development Agency.

Unal B, Critchley JA and Capewell S (2004) Explaining the decline in coronary heart disease mortality in England and Wales between 1981 and 2000. *Circulation.* **109**: 1101–7.

Chapter 35

Managing knowledge

Daragh Fahey and Muir Gray

Introduction/background

- Historical perspective.
- Definition of knowledge and knowledge management (KM).
- Knowledge vs data/information.
- Contextual perspective of KM (including policy drivers).

Why is knowledge management important?

> *There is no knowledge that is not power.* (Ralph Waldo Emerson)

> *... by getting what we know into practice we will have a bigger impact on health and disease than any drug or technology likely to be developed in the next decade.* (Muir Gray)

Why do large commercial organisations know much more about their customers than most public sector organisations? They know what food they like, where they eat, what transport they use, what paper they read and what type of people they are. Their wealth of knowledge contrasts sharply with that of primary care trusts (PCTs) who struggle to know basic health statistics such as what percentage of children and teenagers in their catchment area are obese. The explanation behind this contrast lies in the different priorities and values which the organisations place on knowledge and information. Commercial organisations recognise knowledge management (KM) as a vital ingredient in providing an efficient user-orientated service. They see the cost-effectiveness of investing resources to manage their knowledge in order to remain competitive and stay in business. They recognise that poor KM leads to duplication of efforts, spread of bad practice and the inappropriate targeting of resources. It is difficult to know why PCTs are not prepared to invest as much resource in KM. Possible reasons include the following.

- They do not appreciate the cost-effectiveness of KM.
- They rely on central government to manage their knowledge.
- They are overwhelmed by the quantity of targets and service requirements leaving neither time nor money to invest in the knowledge infrastructure, which ultimately would make their work easy.
- Lack of foresightedness.
- Not sufficiently incentivised centrally to better manage their knowledge locally.

These factors highlight the need to publicise the value of KM and its benefits. Knowledge management is not a particularly exciting concept but it is a critical component of evidence-based practice and efficiency. Health professionals are drowning in a river of guidelines, reports and recommendations while crying out for better information to help them to do their work. We need to better manage how we provide, communicate and present the knowledge we already have to improve its relevance, accessibility, timeliness and usefulness. In a desperate effort to be seen as innovative and to push the boundaries of what we can do there is an inappropriate focus on providing the latest and most innovative technologies without considering what we can do to better utilise and spread what is already known. This nearsightedness is leading to chronic under-investment in one of the critical ingredients of a successful health service – knowledge management.

Types of knowledge

- Research.
- Data.
- Experience.

What are we trying to achieve?

> Not everything that can be counted counts, and not everything that counts can be counted. (Albert Einstein)

If you were to ask the board of a PCT to define what it means to have a good KM system there would be a wide range of views varying from those who see KM as a fancy term to describe what the librarians have traditionally done to those who would see it as an organisational wide document management and/or information technology system. Very few would recognise a good KM system as being an organisational (and possibly community) wide system and way of working which captures, collates, analyses and shares data and information with a view to providing accessible, useful, timely and relevant information to those who want it at the times they need it to support the actions they need to take.

In a PCT with good KM, health professionals should have, at the touch of a button, a user-friendly, detailed profile of the demography, consumer profiles and health of their population (or an individual within that population). This should be contextualised by the evidence base on how ill health within that individual/population might be managed, a toolkit on the practicalities of providing such a service, grey literature on how the same problem was managed before in similar populations, details on how such a service could be evaluated appropriately, readily available outcome measures to monitor such a service and contact details of a local expert to provide advice.

For example, in response to a request from the board to tackle the rising prevalence of childhood obesity locally, a Director of Public Health should have sub-ward-level details of where obesity in their population is a particular problem and in what sub-groups. They would have information on their population's consumer profiles in order to target health-promotion campaigns appropriately. They would have the latest summarised evidence base on tackling obesity in childhood along with toolkits on providing an obesity service, which would outline the resource implications and the practical steps required to deliver and evaluate such a service. Similarly they would be given information on what indicators to monitor and how they can record the information to populate these indicators. To support local implementation they would have contact details for the nearest obesity expert and grey literature on how this problem was tackled in this area or similar areas before. Having started the project they should have ready access to all the relevant documentation, correspondence and progress reports. This might seem like utopia but the information is there; we just need to manage it appropriately.

How can we improve KM within our organisation?

He is wise who knows the sources of knowledge – who knows who has written and where it is to be found. (A Hodge)

Improving KM within an organisation is not a task to be undertaken lightly. It needs careful planning, senior level engagement and support and a strategy, which is likely to take at least 2 years to fully implement. Box 35.1 outlines the features of a good KM system and strategy.

Box 35.1 Key features of a good KM system/strategy

- Aligned with organisational culture.
- Senior management and broad organisational support and engagement.
- Championed through good leadership.
- Well-resourced KM staff.
- Supportive and comprehensive IT infrastructure.
- Well linked to the organisational business strategy and individual user requirements.
- Good communication of the need and benefits of KM.
- Training and support for the organisation.
- Proof of the effectiveness of KM.

Good KM should affect the whole organisation; therefore all employees within the organisation should both support and participate in a strategy to improve KM. Senior managers are particularly inclined to see KM as something they can pass onto someone else with the hope that they will provide them with the timely, relevant KM system they desire. However, the goal of KM is to provide a system which satisfies both individual user requirements and the business strategy and objectives of an organisation. Therefore it is essential that everyone within the organisation is involved in defining what knowledge is required and when and how they want it. One useful exercise is to ask individuals to describe the common decisions they make, identify what information they need to make that decision, how they want it presented and how they want to access it.

Success of the KM depends on good leadership from the knowledge manager him/herself and that of sponsors within the organisation. There needs to be a senior director level sponsor such as the Director of Public Health to work with the knowledge manager to champion the strategy. The sponsor has a critical role in selling the vision to the organisation and ensuring sufficient resources are made available.

The KM strategy needs to be aligned with the organisational culture. The culture can be defined as 'the way we do things around here' and its importance and potential as a showstopper should not be underestimated. For example, a strategy which proposes that all correspondence is done electronically is likely to be vehemently opposed in an organisation where traditionally all meetings are face to face. It is not easy to change the culture of an organisation so it is best to align the strategy within the current culture.

Having identified what is needed and having achieved appropriate support there are some key practical issues which need to be addressed. First, who is going to develop and implement the strategy and where should they be based? This question depends on the size of the strategy but a typical PCT should have a chief knowledge officer (CKO) who would be supported (probably part-time) by other knowledge officers who would report to a steering committee of key stakeholders. The knowledge officers would typically be based within the information technology division of the trust but they are often found within human resources or dispersed throughout the organisation.

It is advisable that rather than initially trying to tackle the whole KM problem within an organisation the CKO should pilot a small KM initiative within a high-profile area that is very likely to be successful. For example, they could set up communities of practice which would be supported by document management systems and virtual meeting rooms and discussion boards. This would provide the CKO and his or her sponsor with a high-profile, successful early deliverable which would provide the basis to achieve organisation-wide engagement and to argue for more resources.

As the KM strategy is being implemented it is essential that it is monitored and progress is reported and communicated widely. Training should be provided to employees within the organisation who will need support to adapt to a new way of working. There is a tendency for data holders to initially hoard their information for data protection reasons so a knowledge officer may be given the responsibility to ensure that data has not been inappropriately protected. Often, the data holders only need reassurance that for public health purposes it is entirely reasonable to provide the information even if it is personally identifiable information.

The strategy itself should endeavour to eventually provide a comprehensive KM service, although this could be done in stages and will probably include a number of pilots. It is bad practice to attempt to correct one aspect of KM without considering the implications for the whole service. For example, one might introduce an excellent tagging system for PCT documents but then subsequently realise that this is unsuitable for documents from key partner organisations such as local authorities.

Two types of knowledge

If we define knowledge as information in action, it can be divided into two main types: generalisable knowledge and particular knowledge.

Generalisable knowledge is that which can be used by a public health professional in any setting in any country. There are three types of generalisable knowledge:

- knowledge derived from research, sometimes called evidence
- knowledge derived from the analysis of routinely collected or audit data, sometimes called statistics
- knowledge derived from experience.

These types of generalisable knowledge have to be blended with particular knowledge, namely knowledge that is relevant principally to:

- the population being served and
- the social and economic context in which the public health professional is working.

It is also recognised that there is another very important type of knowledge, namely ignorance. We have to be explicit when it is clear that there is uncertainty about a particular issue or course of action. There are two types of uncertainty – certain uncertainty and uncertain uncertainty. In uncertain uncertainty the public health professional does not know if anyone knows. After completing an effective literature search the public health professional will either find a piece of knowledge or will be certain that nobody knows – certain uncertainty.

The James Lind Library is developing a Database of Uncertainties about the Effectiveness of Treatments, and a similar database is needed for uncertainties about public health interventions. To do this, however, requires that public health knowledge be well organised, and the development of a National Library for Public Health in England is one attempt to organise knowledge.

Communities of practice

Knowledge from experience can be stored either in the form of a casebook or through a community of practice, and there is now an extensive literature on communities of practice. The use of Groupware offers the opportunity of managing a community of practice effectively and efficiently, and all public health professionals should work within a community of practice as well as working within the bureaucratic organisation that employs them.

Websites, search engines and databases

> *Whatever is worth doing at all, is worth doing well.* (Chesterfield)

In general, good KM depends on good technology but one of the big mistakes in KM is to set up a website or a database as a means of managing information/knowledge without thinking about the data vocabulary, cataloguing or standards required. This is the reason why internet/intranet users frequently experience frustration at the lack of meaningful results when they look for a resource using search engines. They know that the data or documents are there, so why can they not find them? The simple answer is that entering data or documents onto an electronic database is the easy part of managing knowledge; the key to providing a good search engine is to set up a good database behind the engine, which can easily identify the items to which the search terms relate. This requires that the IT specialist work closely with those who create, use and enter the data.

The typical organisational scenario in developing these search engines is for a senior manager within an organisation to employ an IT consultancy to come in and set up a website for him or her to manage their knowledge. Typically the IT consultants will receive their brief from the manager and then proceed to hide themselves in a room for months before coming out with the 'solution'. Nine times out of ten this solution will be close to useless and abandoned after a year or two. There are two key reasons for this:

1 Setting up IT systems to support KM must be done in conjunction with frequent input from the users of the system and those inputting the data to ensure the solution is delivering what it is supposed to.
2 Every piece of information on the database needs to be associated with a label and/or a code and inputted according to predefined standards and definitions.

The second point relates to the issues with language; the same word can mean different things to different people or it may be contextually specific. For example, 'sensitivity' could be used to mean 'compassion' or used to describe the validity of a test. Similarly we can have two words describing the same entity or concept (e.g. 'myocardial infarction' or 'heart attack'). Therefore we need to set up a system whereby each piece of data is given a label or a code to identify what it means. Those entering the data should have data dictionaries to define what each of these codes/labels means. Those setting up the databases should have systems, which map commonly used search terms to the appropriate labels to improve the relevance of their search results. For example, if we searched the database for the words 'heart attack', the cross-mapping might identify the appropriate label as 'myocardial infarction' (which might have its own code defining the concept where an individual has chest pain, abnormal ECG and abnormal cardiac enzymes) and thus retrieve all the resources with this label. In the case where 'sensitivity' is inputted, the website/database could be set up where the user is asked to indicate which 'sensitivity' they mean or the user may find that in order to find sensitivity as it relates to the concept of interest they need to drill down through the labelling systems (e.g. MeSH headings in Medline).

If these standards, data dictionaries, labels and codes are set up and agreed across different databases and websites then we can have interoperability where a search on one site can automatically search a partner database or website to produce a more comprehensive result. Such a system has been set up in England where certain public health networks have set up their electronic networks using the same common public health language and tagging system used by the public health observatories. Therefore, if, for example, when a local public health professional retrieved no resources to match a search on their local database for 'fuel poverty' they could easily extend this search to check the databases in other interoperable local public health networks or observatories.

These examples illustrate the importance of having data dictionaries, standards, labelling systems and appropriate coding of data when inputting the data and meaningful mappings when building search engines to search databases. Although this might seem somewhat dictatorial and stifling it is seen as very worthwhile when one considers the added functionality and meaningful search results it brings.

How do we know we have got it right?

Each public health team needs to develop an evaluation framework. The traditional framework of structure, process and outcome is appropriate.

- Criteria relating to structure include items such as whether or not the public health professional has access to the internet at work and home and whether they have access to the Campbell Collaboration database.
- Process criteria would include measures about the use made of knowledge – for example, does an audit of the Public Health Department's papers show that the papers are based on a systematic review of the literature, e.g. how many papers are produced that have no references? How many papers are produced that do not have a summary of the methods used to search and retrieve information?
- Outcome measures are, as always, the most difficult, but it is possible to identify policies that have brought about change which have been based on evidence or interventions by the public health team which has changed the policies and practices of the organisations in which they work because of effective knowledge mobilisation.

Just do it

The public and professionals need clean clear knowledge just as they need clean clear water. Ignorance is like cholera; it cannot be tackled by the individual alone and requires the organised efforts of society. It is thus a public health responsibility.

The most important step for public health to take is the first step – just do it. There is a large amount of free software available, for example on www.freedomsoftware.net. Much of the debate about free software relates to debates about office software but there are other types of software even more helpful for knowledge management.

Every public health professional should have a blog, a web log, www.blogadoc.com. Every department should put together and manage its website, receiving RSS feeds from other sources, and offering a knowledge service to its local population. Free software is also available to run discussion groups, for example www.hphbb.com.

Protecting the public from tainted knowledge

The Director of Public Health (DPH) has a responsibility to ensure that the population they serve has universal and equal access to clean clear knowledge. The DPH should identify populations with unmet knowledge needs, and be assured that the quality of knowledge procured and provided, including that provided by their own department, is based on good evidence and is readable.

In doing this work the DPH and all public health professionals practise knowledge management. It is, however, essential to remember the changes brought about not only by words but also by tools. A historical text of great power and importance is a short book called *Medieval Technology and Social Change* by Lyn White Jr (1962). In this book Lyn White demonstrates, with evidence, that although they could not write, the people who invented the stirrup or the heavy plough had an impact on society at least as great as those who sought to achieve change by words and ideas.

The public health professional of the 19th century was responsible for the infrastructure of their cities, for food and housing and water and sewerage. The public health professional of the 21st century is also responsible for infrastructure and should get their hands on the tools that are available to organise, mobilise and deliver knowledge to those in need.

Reference

White L Jr (1962) *Medieval Technology and Social Change*. Oxford: Oxford University Press.

Chapter 36

Leadership in public health

Neil Goodwin

Introduction

Although there are hundreds of definitions of leadership the principles and practice apply equally to most organisations. It is principally local context that largely determines the leadership approach to be adopted, meaning local challenges, the history and relative strength of local relationships, local resource issues and local ways of doing things. This is why a wholly national approach to implementing change is not realistic and why one approach will work in one place but not in another. For public health in particular, local context also means the local impact of national government policies and strategies, and the strength of local partnerships and inter-organisational working. Partnership and inter-agency working have always been a feature of delivery in public health but they are given strong emphasis in *Choosing Health* (Secretary of State for Health 2004) along with public service agreement targets, transformational change and the incorporation of public health in a new performance framework for all health and social care organisations. All of this will require greater leadership from public health not only within the NHS but, equally importantly, across NHS boundaries to other organisations, particularly local government.

Leadership is not a characteristic of one person: it is a process played out between leaders and followers, without whom leadership cannot exist. Leadership also is not always synonymous with hierarchical position because there can be numerous leaders across organisations or systems, each leading on different issues. Management is different from leadership. Managers are concerned with stability and keeping the service or system turning over primarily using analytical and decision-making processes designed to be used in similar ways across most situations. Managers will propose change but mainly by changing structures and reorganising work processes, which often results in short-, rather than longer-term, success. Managers also will use authority based on their formal position using transactional tactics such as negotiation, bargaining, rewards and coercion.

Leaders are different from managers because they view people from an emotional perspective, seeing them as individuals. They will pursue change by developing influential and empathetic interpersonal relationships, which will often include influencing other people beyond organisational boundaries. Given the delivery agenda now facing public health this is particularly important. In summary, leadership is a dynamic, relationship-based process that uses a twofold approach:

- creating an agenda for change using a strong vision and
- building a strong implementation network to get things done through other people.

Finally, leadership and management are not mutually exclusive. Managers' plans do not have to be visionary and budgets do not necessarily have strategies. In relatively stable working environments, limited leadership coupled with strong management works well, but in times of major change or chaos, strong leadership with some limited management may be what is required (Kotter 1990).

The importance of context

The leader is potentially the biggest influence on their immediate working environment. However, there has been much more research on the consequences of leader behaviour than on its determinants such as the impact of external forces on the effects of leadership (Lieberson and O'Connor 1972; Yukl 1994). This is probably because of the view to see leaders as players who shape events rather than being shaped by them. Although there is a strong view that leadership is critical to organisational success, this underplays the significant environmental, macro-economic, and national and local political influences that potentially impact on organisational or system performance. Most people are often only dimly aware of wider contextual issues both within and beyond their organisation. Consequently, distilling the wider context, such as national government policy, into local understanding and management of the potential implementation implications, is a powerful leadership skill. For public health practitioners wishing to develop their leadership role across health and local government, which they will now need to do much more so for personal and organisational success, distilling national context into local understanding is essential.

It is not always realised that leaders in high-level positions, such as chief executives and directors, actually have unilateral control over fewer resources and policies than might be assumed. Significant investment and change decisions will require the approval of other senior colleagues, the board and, increasingly for public health directors, other organisations and stakeholders. What this means is that people within organisations will often constrain the behaviour of leaders. This is particularly so when dealing with other organisations but time taken with key individuals to understand their agendas and corporate culture can help overcome any potential inter-organisational friction. What all people in leadership roles will need to accept is that their impact on organisational outcomes will sometimes be small and their influence is often a product of the internal and external constraints on their relative ability. However, strong evidence for a definitive view of leadership is difficult to establish because of the research challenge of gaining access to observe top management in action in organisations.

Context is important to leaders because they rely extensively on their ability to read situations both local and national. Good leaders sense an environment, absorbing and interpreting hard and soft data without having it spelt out for them. Is this a natural instinct or can it be learnt? It is probably both and it is certainly true that some individuals seem to have an intuitive ability to read situations. The ability to do this is helped by developing informal networks of contacts for exchanging information and gossip; or by improving their emotional intelligence and systematic training in interpersonal skills. In the NHS there are many opportunities available for interpersonal skills training with advice available from employer organisations and from the leadership centre based in the new NHS Institute for Innovation and Improvement. The importance of context is also underscored by a study of leadership development in 30 public and private sector organisations where evidence was found of a contextual model of leadership with successful leadership contingent on factors such as culture, interpersonal working and the development of co-operative inter-organisational networks (Alimo-Metcalfe and Lawler 2001; Pettigrew *et al.* 1994). Understanding context, and recognising and seizing opportunities is also referred to as adaptive capacity, which is seen as the single quality that determines success rather than other personal variables such as IQ (intelligence quotient), educational attainment, ethnicity, race or gender (Bennis and Thomas 2002).

Vision and passion

Vision is an agreement and positive image about future direction. It is the essence of leadership and the prerequisite to providing inspiration and momentum. This is important because people are not led by written polices, strategies and quantitative analysis: people actually do business with other people. To create effective visioning through team-working, leaders must develop a culture built on trust that also rewards creativity and diversity. Effective visioning requires a willingness to explore all options and commitment to a plan of action even if this results in unwelcome changes. The process is more time consuming and harder to achieve when working on inter-organisational issues, which may present problems when action is required over a shorter timescale. Clear, frequent and, above all, personal communication is crucial if the vision is to be accepted and people inspired. Paper and email cannot distribute visions but they can reinforce them. Finally, in today's complex world, heroic leadership is no longer appropriate: one person cannot know everything and do it all. Consequently, leadership teams are essential.

Passion is an essential personal characteristic if followers are to be motivated and inspired. People who are motivated produce their best and the best way to motivate others is to be passionate and motivated yourself. Facts and quantitative analyses abound in public health and they are important in generating support for change but so are emotions. However, passion also can be dangerous because history is littered with examples where it has deceived, clouded judgement and destroyed. For these reasons passion needs to be underpinned by trust, clear values and a willingness to assess risk. Achieving that requires the leader to surround themselves with a strong and trusted team capable of complementing the leader's opinions and skills with their own. For public health leaders the use of organisational development practitioners and team coaching can help here.

Emotional intelligence and failure

Because leadership is an interpersonal dynamic process, leaders will fail if they cannot drive emotions in the right direction, both their own and those of people around them. As such, leadership is subject to the human foibles that we all possess. Leadership demands respect for people's need for direction, protection and order and it requires compassion and support at times when change is distressing. This is often difficult to fulfil and, consequently, leaders are always failing somebody and sometimes themselves. Knowing how hard to push others and ourselves, when to pause and when to stop are important leadership judgements.

Emotional intelligence is concerned with how leaders manage themselves and their relationships with others. It is argued that certain human competencies –

such as self-awareness, self-discipline, persistence and empathy – are of greater significance and importance than traditional intelligence in much of life (Goleman *et al.* 2002). When IQ scores are compared with career achievement, intelligence counts for only a quarter of the difference between high and low achievers. The concept of emotional intelligence focuses on being intelligent about emotions but it is not about being emotional. Leaders need to be able to manage distressing emotions, whether in themselves or others, so they do not get in the way of their work.

Good leadership demands more than putting on a good face every day. It requires a leader to determine, through personal reflection, how emotions drive the moods and actions of others and to adapt personal behaviour accordingly. Emotions can be useful; for example, aggression can be focused onto being the best; passion will drive the visionary leader; and service-based healthcare organisations will need emotion to understand the consumer perspective. Leaders fail if they cannot drive emotions in the right direction and nothing will work as well as it could or should. This is why emotional intelligence is crucial to leadership success.

There are links between leadership failure, self-esteem and emotional intelligence. It is no surprise that self-esteem increases with success and decreases temporarily at times of failure. However, good leaders are unlikely to be emotionally destabilised when failure occurs: and the very best leaders are those with a fine-tuned intuition to which they listen. These people have an ability to understand and work positively with their own feelings and those of others. Such skills are rare, however – the more so in men. Women tend to be much more attuned to their feelings and those of others. Intuition and feelings are important personal characteristics at times of failure because if failed leaders have developed self-awareness, they will look dispassionately at what went wrong and extract the learning for the future. They will recognise when personal support is needed from a colleague, mentor or coach, perhaps to help understand personal strengths and weaknesses and issues that are likely to precipitate personal stress. It is crucial for all leaders to think through, perhaps with the help of a mentor or coach, how to manage failure when it occurs.

Leadership teams and networks

Recent research on leadership in the UK NHS has produced two important conclusions (Goodwin 2002). First, it is the successful management of significant local issues seen as important to local stakeholders, such as service change and financial strategies, that for leaders and their teams creates a local leadership culture. This then forms a basis for pursuing further, successful implementation of major change such as that flowing from government policy. Second, the extent to which a leadership culture can be successfully created is determined by the ability to manage and explain the interaction between national and local objectives; and the extent to which the leader is influenced by or personally influences the following variables:

- the quality of the leader's team as seen by external players
- the impact of local relationships and other leaders in local networks on the team

- the creation and use of interpersonal and inter-organisational networks by the team
- the extent networks are used to create inter-organisational power sharing, alliances and partnerships.

For public health leaders, the research emphasises that pursuing successful leadership is built on a process and relationship-based approach requiring a high-quality team that can operate successfully across organisational boundaries. The specific actions and approach that public health leaders need to take to pursue successful leadership are fivefold:

1 Give high importance to developing and maintaining interpersonal relationships within and beyond organisational boundaries.
2 Develop and maintain extensive inter-organisational networks.
3 Clarify for all players the agenda for change.
4 Recognise the importance of creating and developing a high-quality leadership team.
5 Build personal leadership credibility by successfully tackling issues viewed as important to local stakeholders.

An organisation-based system can be viewed as a network of other organisations within which the system consists of a field of relationships binding the organisations together. For public health leaders, therefore, networks not only set the context for the actions they wish to take, thereby providing resources and constraints, but they are also there to be manipulated in order to provide more resources and fewer constraints. Studies show that senior managers will often call on their entire network of work-based relationships to pursue change, using tactics such as simply asking people to take action, using resources to negotiate, exerting influence through intermediaries, and occasionally using intimidation and coercion (Kotter 1999).

Networks are continually shaped and reshaped by the actions of individuals and it is those occupying central positions exercising control over the flow of information who are most likely to emerge as leaders (Bass 1990; Brass and Burkhardt 1992; Kotter 1982; Yukl 1994). Also, individuals who establish links with other powerful people will increase their power although not on every occasion. While other powerful people may provide useful information in a communications network, negotiating with other powerful people in a bargaining network may produce negative results. Reflecting on the importance of interpersonal relationships in leadership, networks are an important source of soft data, complementing the use of hard information (Goddard *et al.* 1999). A simplistic distinction is that soft data is subjective and qualitative, while hard data is objective and quantitative. This generates the tendency to view hard data as being more valid or reliable than soft data, which can be seen as subject to bias and distortion. However, when hard information is used in isolation it can be inadequate and sometimes misleading. There are drawbacks with placing too much emphasis on the use of soft information such as the potential for obtaining distorted views, largely because much soft information is collected in discussion with individuals who may be pursuing their own agenda. For public health leaders to obtain and make increasing use of soft information requires much greater emphasis on interpersonal and network-based styles of management.

Network studies in the health sector are hard to find but two are useful in exploring the implications of developing network-based healthcare organisations. First, a study of UK health authorities identified the following key networking attributes and skills as important to success:

- strong interpersonal communications and listening skills
- an ability to persuade
- an ability to construct long-term relationships (Ferlie and Pettigrew 1996).

Second, key lessons for healthcare from networks across three other major industries identified a number of challenges (Goodwin *et al.* 2003). The first challenge for managers of networks is to understand the scope to which they are able to change their own position within it to secure or retain a central position from which to exert influence. This is important because from that position the leader has more ability to access resources from others in the network and provide a base from which to manipulate and/or steer the objectives of the network. Leaders matter in networks because they are necessary to promote the network to their peers. Importantly, in health networks it was found that leaders ideally should come from a professional or clinical background with a level of charisma. This reflects the findings that professionals within broader networks are distinct groups that respond best to charismatic leadership from one of their own.

Partnership and collaboration

Networking is rarely explained in the context of systems and partnership working. The reality is that networking is a simple and low-risk activity with little or no commitment required. Networks can also absorb rather than unlock resources in the short and medium term, and become too preoccupied with discussion and process rather than with problem solving and outputs. It is only when networking moves on to more formal working, coupled with a commitment to reach joint agreements, that organisational and personal risk increases.

The term collaborative advantage emerged from research work with large public sector organisations (Huxham 1996). It is concerned with the creation of synergy between collaborating organisations and their management teams. Collaboration means focusing on outputs that could not have been achieved in other ways, which is important because it emphasises the need for each organisation to achieve its own objectives better than it could alone. Collaboration also implies a positive, purposeful relationship between organisations that retains autonomy, integrity and distinct identity, and thus the potential to withdraw from the relationship (Cropper 1996). The implications are that networking is only one level of activity along a developmental continuum of inter-organisational working (*see* Table 36.1). To pursue network leadership across systems requires a twofold approach: first, a facilitative style because of the multi-organisational basis of systems; and, second, a focus on team-working with a commitment to understand each organisation's culture and to work in genuine partnership.

Table 36.1   From networking to collaboration

Level	Category	Definition
1	Networking	The most informal level and therefore can be used most easily. Defined as exchanging information for mutual benefit. Involves little or no risk.
2	Coordination	This requires more organisational involvement than networking. Defined as exchanging information and altering activities for mutual benefit and to achieve a common purpose.
3	Co-operation	This too requires even greater organisational commitments and may involve legal arrangements. Defined as exchanging information, altering activities and sharing resources for mutual benefit and to achieve a common purpose.
4	Collaboration	Defined as exchanging information, altering activities, sharing resources and enhancing the capacity of another for mutual benefit and to achieve a common purpose. To do this requires sharing risks, responsibilities, resources and rewards, all of which can increase the potential of collaboration beyond other ways of working together. Collaboration is a relationship in which each person or organisation wants to help their partners become better at what they do.

Developing leadership

Since leadership is a dynamic, relationship-based process based on creating an agenda for change and building a strong, people-based implementation network, developing public health capability and capacity needs to focus on developing sustainable, effective interpersonal skills of individuals and teams. This will then facilitate the development and achievement of inter-organisational, system-based strategies and objectives. However, attending formal training away from the workplace is unlikely to result in long-term benefit because only a fraction of new knowledge is used and retained. This is because when leaders return to work, the realities of their day-to-day lives, work pressures and lack of personal time result in the learning not being thought through and applied in the local context. Consequently, greater emphasis on experiential learning, reflecting on real local challenges, is needed to facilitate sustained change in personal behaviour and leadership practice (Mintzberg 2004). Against the backdrop of how public health delivery will need to be undertaken in the future, experiential learning needs to be carried out with individuals and teams who work also across health and local government systems. Processes such as inter-organisational team building, local strategy development and partnership and individual team coaching can help on the understanding that, above all else, time and personal commitment from public health and local government leaders are essential for a successful outcome.

References

Alimo-Metcalfe B and Lawler J (2001) Leadership development in UK companies at the beginning of the twenty-first century. Lessons for the NHS? *Journal of Management in Medicine.* **15**(5): 387–404.

Bass BM (1990) *Bass and Stogdill's Handbook of Leadership Theory, Research and Managerial Applications.* New York: The Free Press.

Bennis W and Thomas R (2002) *Geeks and Geezers.* Boston: Harvard Business School Press.

Brass DJ and Burkhardt ME (1992) Centrality and power in organisations. In: N Nohria and RG Eccles (eds) *Networks and Organisations: structure, form, and action.* Boston: Harvard Business School Press.

Cropper S (1996) Collaborative working and the issue of sustainability. In: C Huxham (ed.) *Creating Collaborative Advantage.* London: Sage.

Ferlie E and Pettigrew A (1996) Managing through networks: some issues and implications for the NHS. *British Academy of Management.* **7**: S81–S99.

Goddard M, Mannion R and Smith PC (1999) Assessing the performance of NHS hospital trusts: the role of 'hard' and 'soft' information. *Health Policy.* **48**: 119–34.

Goleman R, Boyatzis R and McKee A (2002) *Primal Leadership. Realizing the power of emotional intelligence.* Boston: Harvard Business School Publishing.

Goodwin N (2002) *The Leadership Role of Chief Executives in the English NHS.* PhD thesis, University of Manchester.

Goodwin N, Perri 6, Peck E *et al.* (2003) *Managing Across Diverse Networks of Care: lessons from other sectors. Policy report.* Birmingham: Health Services Management Centre.

Huxham C (ed.) (1996) *Creating Collaborative Advantage.* London: Sage.

Kotter JP (1982) *The General Managers.* New York: The Free Press.

Kotter JP (1990) What leaders really do. *Harvard Business Review.* May–June: 103–11.

Kotter JP (1999) What effective general managers really do. *Harvard Business Review.* Reprint 99208. March–April.

Lieberson S and O'Connor J (1972) Leadership and organisational performance: a study of large corporations. *American Sociological Review.* **37**: 117–30.

Mintzberg H (2004) *Managers Not MBAs.* Harlow: Pearson Education Limited.

Pettigrew A, Ferlie E and McKee L (1994) *Shaping Strategic Change, Making Change in Large Organisations: the case of the National Health Service.* London: Sage.

Secretary of State for Health (2004) *Choosing Health: making healthy choices easier.* London: HMSO.

Yukl G (1994) *Leadership in Organisations.* New Jersey: Prentice-Hall.

Chapter 37

Networks: supporting public health

Allison Thorpe

> *Networking is about community, not hierarchy.* (Agre 2003, p.2)

Networks are not a new concept. We all have experience of the process of networking, be it personal, functional, social, or more recently web-based interactions. At its most fundamental, a network is a way of 'joining up' people with, or around, a common interest. The connections may be simple – for example, a face-to-face, person-to-person connection – or a more complex and fluid matrix, involving multiple layers. Physically, there may be little connection between the layers, but in practice, it functions like a spider's web, as it is made stronger by the ability to be flexible in the direction travelled and nodes pulled into play. The different people sitting at each of the nodes where the web joins may have different skills and areas of expertise and different methods of communication may be used. Thus, the successful network is characterised by its ability to respond quickly and flexibly to changing and challenging agendas.

This chapter will focus on a specific use for the networking concept – the public health network in England – drawing on a study of the specialist workforce carried out by the Faculty of Public Health in 2004 as part of the *Choosing Health* English white paper consultation process (Griffiths *et al.* 2006).

Looking backwards: the policy context

From the structural changes announced in *The New NHS* (Department of Health 1997), via a redefinition of the key roles, and a mass workforce relocation and re-organisation, public health has been through a period of intense change, as other chapters have described (*see* Box 37.1).

Box 37.1 Networks: the policy incubation period

1997: *The New NHS: modern, dependable* (Department of Health 1997)

- Structural changes announced: creation of PCG/Ts and reduction in number of health authorities.
- CMO to review public health.

1998: CMO's report (Department of Health 2001c)

- Focus on public health capacity and capability to deliver the agenda.
- Partnership working as delivery mechanism.
- Defining the public health workforce.

1999: *Saving Lives: our healthier nation* (Department of Health 1999)

- Primary care mandate for public health.
- Developing multidisciplinary working – sharing good practice.

1999: *Clinical Governance: quality in the new NHS* (HSC 1999)

- Critical mass as key to good clinical governance of health authority functions.

2000: FPH guidance on networks
2001: Hunt speech (Department of Health 2001b)

- New local focus for public health services within PCT.
- Public health networks as delivery mechanism.
- Board level DPH in each PCT.

2001: *Shifting the Balance of Power: securing delivery* (Department of Health 2001a)

- Dates set for dissolution of existing health authorities.
- Strengthen PCT public health function.
- Pool resources and talent.
- Managed public health networks – geographical – SHA focus and performance management role.

2002: *Getting Ahead of the Curve* (Department of Health 2002)

- Changes in organisation of health protection.

2004: Department of Health white paper: *Choosing Health: making healthy choices easier* (Department of Health 2004a)

- Partnership working.
- Engaging all staff in health improvement.

2005: *Commissioning a Patient Led NHS* (Department of Health 2005)

- Structural changes: improve coordination with social services through greater congruence of PCT and local government boundaries.
- Practice-based commissioning.
- Strengthened public health delivery system as key outcome measure.

Thus the composition of the public health workforce has been realigned over recent years to reflect multidisciplinary working, and with many DPH posts going to non-medical qualified specialists for the first time,[1] mobility of the workforce has increased exponentially with recurrent reorganisations (Connelly *et al.* 2003). It is within this context that the concept of public health networks has evolved as a way to address concerns about professional isolation, the changing structures of delivery,

---

[1] Reflected in the removal of the word 'Medicine' from the title of 'Faculty of Public Health' (FPH) in 2003. To avoid confusion, FPH will be used throughout this chapter at all times to refer to this professional organisation.

professional accountability and the need to coordinate a fragmented public health system (Connelly and Emmel 2003; Scottish Partnership Agency 2000). Public health is not alone in going down the networking pathway. Clinical networks have become a common feature in many specialties, not least in cancer care. Work in Scotland has demonstrated that the most successful networks share a common core of characteristics (*see* Box 37.2).

Box 37.2 Common core principles of a network (Scottish Partnership Agency 2000)

- Clarity and unity of purpose.
- Coverage, structure and management – with clear management arrangements and designated leadership with dedicated time and adequate staffing support determined by the size, population coverage, geographical area and structure of the network.
- Membership.
- Clinical governance.
- Education and training.
- Value for money.

These characteristics are reflected in the definition of networks proposed by the Faculty of Public Health:

> *linked groups of public health professionals working in a* co-ordinated *manner across organisations and structural boundaries who will have a common agenda to promote health improvement and reduce inequalities.* (Faculty of Public Health *et al.* 2001)

Networks are, according to the literature, particularly suited where:

> *there are high levels of uncertainty, a need to co-ordinate multi-professional and multi-site teams and where simple solutions of outsourcing or vertical integration fail to address the problem of how to co-ordinate complex activities.* (Griffiths 2001, p.10, citing NHS Confederation 2001)

However, a series of seminars in 2004 (Griffiths *et al.* 2005a) demonstrated that for public health networks the uncertainty encompasses perceptions of the role, organisation and functions (*see* Box 37.3).

Box 37.3 Networks

Networks are characterised by diversity in:

- managerial format
- formality of the business plans and workload
- staffing levels
- levels of commitment from the locality in which they are based
- financial standings.

The public health network is a geographically variable concept, with models evolving on a spectrum from the highly organised and well-coordinated managed network with a formal business plan, to informal information sharing without any specific infrastructural support (*see* Box 37.3 [NHS Confederation 2001]). However, despite this variability, there is a tendency to refer to networks as a single entity (Fahey 2003), which the responses from the specialist workforce made clear was neither true, nor necessarily desirable:

> *There should not be a national model for networks – each area is very different and networks should develop to meet local needs.*

This view reinforces the findings of a National Workshop in 2003, which suggested that in practice there were two discrete forms of emergent network – those which 'shared to survive', particularly prevalent where public health capacity was poor, and those which sought to 'add value' and undertake work not possible in a single organisation (PHRU 2005).

Networks: the core functions

> *Networks should be about relationships, connections and mutual help.*
> (Carlson and Wright 2004)

The NHS is only one component of the public health system, albeit an important one – many other organisations play a role (Adshead and Thorpe 2005). This is recognised in the 'stages of maturity' model, which highlights six stages, and four levels within each stage, of development (*see* Box 37.4).

Box 37.4 'Stages of maturity' model

- Membership.
- Accountability.
- Resource coordination and administration mechanisms.
- Organisational structure.
- Communication.
- Risk management and arbitration.
- Relationships with other statutory and voluntary organisations and clinical networks.

(*Source*: NW Regional Office)

Networks, by facilitating connections between 'grass roots' (PCT) public health and the other key organisations in the system, are a vehicle for robustness and the maintenance of organisational memory. They are not, nor should they be, a 'comfort blanket'. There is a price to pay for corporate involvement and that price is the demonstration of a purposeful element, whereby networks show that they add something to the system which would otherwise be lacking. The National Public Health Network Action Learning Set identified a series of five core functions which networks bring to the system.

Public health workforce development (Carlson and Wright 2004)

A cross-sectional survey carried out by Fahey *et al.* (2003) suggested that there was popular support for the role of public health networks in continuous professional development (CPD) and education of the workforce. Recent reports (Carlson and Wright 2004; PHRU 2003) suggest that there are four key dimensions to this:

- supporting education, training and development
- empowering public health practitioners
- mapping local skills
- engaging with other sectors in education, training and development.

But public health is a dynamic occupation, with a dynamic workforce. Public health workforce development is, and has been, undergoing something of a revolution with:

- new policy contexts, i.e. *Modernising Medical Careers* (Department of Health 2004c) and *Agenda for Change* (Department of Health 2004a)
- new concepts, i.e. multidisciplinary public health
- the introduction of a multi-sectoral, multi-level skills escalator approach to workforce development, which sets out the concept of a workforce continuum at all levels and links public health more firmly to mainstream workforce development (Department of Health 2004b).

The skills escalator model for workforce development brings with it its own challenges for development of the workforce at all levels, from the basic level to the specialist, and across sectors. Networks need to be able to adjust to this changing climate if they are to support the public health workforce in the delivery of the public health agenda. New 'communities' are opening up, for example, with the development of the health trainer role and flexible training packages. These processes will broaden considerably the basis of public health practice both within the health service and in the wider workforce. Public health networks need to be able to respond to this by creating an infrastructure of appropriate communications and a framework to engage with the field in this wider conceptualisation.

While the role of the network within this changing context is at present undefined, they are in a unique position to facilitate the creation of a shared learning environment for their locality. There can be structural barriers to the development of inter-sectoral working; however, networks offer the potential to reach out to local authority, acute trusts and voluntary sector colleagues around shared interests in the public health agenda, providing access to formal and informal learning opportunities. This could be through providing opportunities for sharing intellectual capital in the form of reports, organising opportunities for shared learning (such as seminars and workshops) and by facilitating electronic networking for network members, offering 'real-time' support from their peers.

While capacity issues may undermine the extent to which networks can, at the present time, take on this challenge, the potential to facilitate shared learning and contribute to the strengthening of professional development across organisational divides is inherent in their nature. Working within local systems, promoting the best use of existing frameworks and resources, and engaging in quality partnerships (for example, with public health observatories and local education providers), networks could become an integral part of the sustainable system articulated by Walters *et al.* in 1999 whereby personal and professional development of individuals is linked into organisational and service objectives. This could demonstrate visibly the 'added value' to PCTs and other organisational members of the network, as supported by 84% of those who responded to the *Choosing Health* specialist survey, while simultaneously supporting the workforce development needs of their individual members. As one respondent commented, '*networks need to demonstrate clear and precise added value to those (potentially) populating the network*' – be they individuals, or employing organisations. Demonstrating this value by developing appropriate communication strategies and a cross-cutting framework for linking in all the levels of the public health workforce continuum will be a challenge for networks – but particularly in those areas with an existing capacity deficit.

Public health knowledge management (Carlson and Wright 2004)

Enock suggested that: '*The key to successful networks is knowledge management, without which we cannot function effectively*' (Enock 2004).

Knowledge management, fundamentally, is about proactively utilising communication strategies and opportunities to disseminate knowledge in order to facilitate improved practice, outcomes and efficiency (*see* Chapter 35). Fahey *et al.* (2003) found that 72% of their survey population saw a network role in providing a database of public health information and knowledge, with 82% in favour of a national network. Work on this area has led to the development of PHeNET (the Public Health electronic Network), a national, interoperable electronic software package, which facilitates electronic communications between networks using the same software. For more information, the website is: www.phenet.org.uk/.

However, electronic networks are not the whole story. The *Choosing Health* surveys found that 84% of responses supported the suggestion that networks could set up alliances with academic departments and public health observatories. The role of PHOs in particular excited considerable interest:

> PHOs need more and better communication and information sharing with PCTs.

> They have not realised their full potential in terms of supporting networks and PCTs.

This view is reflected in the subsequent *Choosing Health* white paper, which suggested that PHOs, while not replacing the need for PCTs and local government to have their own information systems, were '*a key contributor towards partnerships and network*' and had a role in '*augment[ing] and complement[ing] this intelligence network*' (CH. Annex B, No80) (Department of Health 2004b).

In this way, *Choosing Health*, together with its explicit commitment to establishing a public health research consortium and to providing additional funding for public health research, addresses Wanless's call for action on improved use of information on the population and its health status. By engaging with this process, networks can have a key role in this.

PCT health protection (Carlson and Wright 2004)

One of the key changes to public health's structural organisation was the separation of the health protection function heralded by *Getting Ahead of the Curve* (Department of Health 2002). Health protection is a core component of an effective public health delivery system, and one of the three core domains of public health practice (Griffiths *et al.* 2005b). *Choosing Health* suggests that the general public health infrastructure must be able to support delivery on key national challenges such as influenza, SARS and chlamydia, etc. Networks are a key mechanism to support public health delivery and would therefore have a role within this sector in building effective links to and robust relationships with the HPA. The National Action Learning Set for Public Health Networks (PHRU 2003) identified six areas where networks could have a role in health protection:

- emergency planning
- screening
- on-call arrangements
- vaccination and immunisation
- resilience planning
- chemical incidents, pollution control, statutory consultation and decontamination.

Examples of this process in action can be seen through the various international networks set up as a result of the SARS epidemic. Networks provide a way in which information can be disseminated in a timely and efficient manner to ensure that communities of practice are working on the most up-to-date and relevant information towards a common goal, providing informational and professional support to colleagues as and when required.

Delivery of local plans and public health programmes (Carlson and Wright 2004) and input into health service planning, provision and evaluation

The need for partnership working, via public health networks, to deliver the public health agenda has been explicitly mandated in many policy documents over the years. With the continuing move towards a primary care locus of control for health service commissioning, networks have the potential to facilitate the sharing of common approaches between PCTs for issues which are best addressed across larger populations, to avoid duplication of work and maximise scarce resources (Fahey 2003; Griffiths *et al.* 2005a) '*by working to a robust business plan consistent with the work of constituent PCTs*' (quote from DPH).

Arguably, there is also a need to make links between the different population levels – from the local PCT, to the intermediate tier, and to the centre. The changes in health service structures which are imminent open up new vistas and challenges, not least around supporting commissioning and ensuring that engagement in health improvement agendas is maximised. How this impacts on network development in practice remains to be seen, but there would seem to be an opportunity for development, and for demonstrating the added value of networks as an integral part of a robust public health delivery system.

The issue of sovereignty is central to this process (Scottish Office Department of Health 1999). Achieving shared objectives can mean surrendering organisational sovereignty over staff, funding and the project. Resources are not currently equitably distributed across PCTs, with some experiencing difficulties in recruiting to Director of Public Health posts, high mobility of the workforce and large variations in the size of public health teams from single-handed practice to large specialist teams operating across multiple PCTs. This has implications for the ability of the network to deliver on the operational agenda.

Local capacity determines the possibilities for local networks.

There is no way that a single-handed DPH can play a full role in their local network, and bullying them won't make any difference.

Networks cannot plug capacity gaps which need further public health capacity development ... There are so many opportunities and requirements within PCTs that I am reluctant to pull people out for network activities unless it is really essential ... it is better to keep a strong PCT base. (Quote from DPH)

These quotes, taken from the responses to the specialist survey (Griffiths *et al.* 2006), highlight a fundamental conundrum in the organisation of public health: PCTs which have larger teams have the capacity to be self-sufficient and therefore do not need to network to deliver local objectives, whereas small teams and single-handed DsPH need network help to deliver on the public health agenda, but cannot contribute the time and resources to the development of the network (Griffiths *et al.* 2005a). The ability of the network to support operational delivery in the face of a fragmented workforce is directly linked to the critical mass of the public health function within its locality. As Shanks (2001) notes:

When the total pool of resources is inadequate, the tendency is to revert to fighting the local organisational agenda at the expense of the greater good ... A feature of networks [is] the tension between localising forces (which tend to push forward the agenda of the separate units) and integrating forces (which promote the shared agenda of the whole network). (p.108)

In many areas of the country, this minimum capacity level has not been reached, which in turn impacts on the scope of activities for the local network (*see* Box 37.5).

Box 37.5 Challenges and opportunities for the future

The favourable policy context for public health adds its own challenges:

- supporting delivery
- being seen as relevant
- supporting the wider workforce
- keeping an eye on the end goal – health of the population.

Conclusion

This chapter has suggested that public health networks can facilitate delivery of common professional goals by:

- systematically and purposefully seeking out and providing a forum for 'meeting' with people – either by email or in person

- articulating shared values, understanding and goals to build relationships which cross organisational and cultural barriers for mutual benefit
- building and maintaining professional relationships to underpin a wide variety of professional activities, including continuing professional development
- providing a forum for sharing raw data, collaborating on projects, etc. (Agre 2003)
- providing a forum for sharing scarce expertise across a wider geographical area
- providing a forum, often managed by the DPH or public health specialist, to input into health service planning, business continuity programmes and delivery of health services through providing professional expertise and a stabilising influence throughout periods of structural change.

The chapter has focused on the domestic uses of public health networks – but the concept has much wider applicability, as the professional reaction to SARS demonstrated. Networks have the potential to support and advocate for evidence-based interventions in very different political and geographical environments – supporting professionals by transmitting ideas and encouraging debate both locally, nationally and internationally.

In England, *Choosing Health* further reinforces the need to develop public health networks as key mechanisms to support partnership work and organisations by providing highly specialised and essential public health skills, charging PCTs in partnership with their local organisations and local authorities, to proactively manage specialist public health services and functions across the whole community. The potential for structural change is, as ever, both an opportunity for and a threat to public health delivery, but networks could provide a stabilising influence in any future service re-design. With the positive policy context and the new regulatory frameworks, public health is increasingly becoming recognised as mainstream. Public health specialists need to take best advantage of this opportunity to demonstrate that sustained and focused public health action can and does improve people's health.

Networks are a fundamental part of this process, but it is only by addressing the issues of capacity, and promoting recognition of the value of network involvement, that the true benefits of the approach will be realised. At the current time, one of the key challenges to networks will be their ability to respond to the dynamics of structural change, providing support to the profession and to the delivery agenda. This will require a focused approach to delivery, supporting, managing and facilitating links across the profession. The potential for networks to impact positively in all aspects of public health development (both at a local level and beyond) is huge – the challenges are equally huge.

References

Adshead F and Thorpe A (2005) Delivering *Choosing Health*. *Public Health*. November. **119**(11): 954–7.

Agre P (2003) *Networking on the Network: a guide to professional skills for PhD Students*. 11 June. http://polaris.gseis.ucla.edu/pagre/network.html#section2 (accessed 17 February 2005).

Carlson C and Wright J (2004) *Enabling the Development of Public Health Networks: National Public Health Network Action Learning Set Programme: summary report*. March. Oxford: PHRU.

Connelly J and Emmel N (2003) Preventing disease or helping the struggle for emancipation: does professional public health have a future? *Policy and Politics*. **1**: 565–76.

Connelly J, Macareavey M and Griffiths S (2003) *National Survey of Working Life in Public Health after Shifting the Balance of Power: results of Wave 1 Survey.* Presented at FPH conference.

Department of Health (1997) *The New NHS: modern, dependable.* London: DH.

Department of Health (1999) *Saving Lives: our healthier nation.* London: DH.

Department of Health (2001a) *Shifting the Balance of Power: securing delivery.* London: DH.

Department of Health (2001b) Speech by Lord Hunt to Faculty of Public Health, November.

Department of Health (2001c) *The Report of the Chief Medical Officer's Project to Strengthen the Public Health Function.* London: DH.

Department of Health (2002) *Getting Ahead of the Curve.* London: DH.

Department of Health (2004a) *Agenda for Change.* London: DH.

Department of Health (2004b) *Choosing Health: making healthy choices easier.* London: DH.

Department of Health (2004c) *Modernising Medical Careers.* London: DH.

Department of Health (2005) *Commissioning a Patient Led NHS.* London: DH.

Enock K (2004) Networks or not works? *Public Health News.* 7 June.

Faculty of Public Health, National Public Health and Primary Care Group and the Health Development Agency (2001) *Consensus Statement on Managed Public Health Networks.* London: FPH.

Fahey D (2003) *The Public Health Network: a systematic and model-based approach.* MSc in Health Informatics dissertation. City University London. Submission 18 September.

Fahey K, Carson ER, Cramp DG *et al.* (2003) User requirements and understanding of public health networks in England. *Journal of Epidemiology and Community Health.* **57**: 938–44.

Griffiths S (2001) *Public Health Networks: where are we now, where do we want to be, and how might we get there.* London: FPH.

Griffiths S, Thorpe A and Wright J (2005a) *Change and Development in Specialist Public Health Practice.* Oxford: Radcliffe Publishing.

Griffiths S, Jewell T and Donnelly P (2005b) Public health in practice: the three domains of public health practice. *Journal of Public Health.* **119**(10): 907–13.

Griffiths S, Thorpe A and Wright J (2006) Public health in transition: views of the specialist workforce. Submitted to *Pub Health Med.*

HSC 1999/065 (1999) *Clinical Governance: in the new NHS.* London: DH.

NHS Confederation (2001) *Clinical Networks – a discussion paper.* London: NHS Confederation.

PHRU (2003) *Enabling the Development of Effective Public Health Networks.* Report from National Workshop held at Avonmouth Centre, London, 2 March. www.fph.org.uk (accessed 21 March 2005).

Scottish Office, Department of Health MEL (1999) *The Introduction of Managed Clinical Networks Within the NHS in Scotland.* Edinburgh: Scottish Office.

Scottish Partnership Agency for Palliative and Cancer Care (2000) *A Framework for the Operation of Managed Clinical Networks in Palliative Care. Report of a Working Party of the Scottish Partnership Agency for Palliative and Cancer Care.* February. www.palliativecarescotland .org.uk/publications/clinicalnetworks.htm (accessed 19 April 2005).

Shanks J (2001) Managed Public Health Networks: squaring the circle in London? *Public Health Medicine.* **3**(3): 107–11.

Walters R, Choudhry N and Illingworth R (1999) *Strengthening the Public Health Function: review of potential for shared learning.* April. London: LHEC.

Chapter 38

Health and wellbeing promoters of the future: skills for leaders and practitioners

Steve Feast, Jean Penny and Helen Bevan

In order to predict new roles and associated skills for those responsible for promoting health and wellbeing in the future, we need to think about the context of tomorrow and the issues that contemporary practitioners will be focusing on. There will still be certain familiar drivers from today such as more user involvement and the need for flexible, decentralised, non-hierarchical teams working across functional and organisational boundaries. There will also be other factors which are less easy to define which will have tremendous effect on future roles, responsibilities and required skills. These include the impact of innovations and technologies linked to the increasingly sophisticated contracting processes that deliver choice, contestability and plurality of provision of health and wellbeing services. All these factors raise very real challenges for health and wellbeing professionals dedicated to ensuring quality, equality and equity of access across a multitude of services with implications for the design and functions of the organisations of the future. Issues include:

- What will be the focus of the work?
- What will be the priorities?
- What will be the key activities for those involved in health promotion?
- What will be the range of the work?
- How will the work be allocated?
- How will health and wellbeing promotion be organised?
- Across what boundaries will practitioners operate?

Only when we begin to explore and predict these issues can we begin to think about different roles and skills required in promoting health and wellbeing and how jobs will be different (Armstrong 2003). One thing is certain: those involved will definitely require different skills sets from those of today. Specialist roles will be blurred with many different people involved and responsibilities allocated according to local priorities. Frontline empowerment and decentralised leadership may be the norm. To reflect this and for consistency throughout the chapter, we have chosen to use the term 'health and wellbeing professional', which we use as a generic term for everyone, including from those with senior strategic responsibilities to those with frontline operational and health-promotion roles. The names of specific roles are not important at this stage; it is the work and the associated skills to promote health and wellbeing we will discuss.

A vision for the future: a prediction of need and leadership skills

Predicting future needs is not an easy process. Health promotion in the UK may be operating in an environment dominated by perceived and real community safety risks, related to environmental and terrorist instability. Reforms may have achieved a system where 'joined-up' health and safety services, as well as a diverse array of primary care providers, increasingly champion improvement of local environmental, physical and psychological wellbeing of populations. A future may exist where commissioning by the NHS and partner organisations ensures the population experiences a wellness service in addition to its role in ill health. This is a future where safety, health and wellbeing are explicitly aligned with the environment, workplace and community health and local investment drives furthering improvements in the lifestyles of the population. A patient-led NHS changes the role and function of existing health service organisation (DH 2006). The role of health-promoting practitioners and how these are effected across systems will change to reflect this.

What follows is speculation. It is a vision based on the perspective of the user, their needs and a future general public who are more aware and inquisitive. In this vision are assumptions that there will be major differences in the structure and organisation of services with the traditional divide between health, social care and local government removed, witnessing staff jointly employed across these sectors. In addition mutual, not-for-profit, community-led initiatives, building on social capital and enterprise, will have added further complexity to the potential user experience.

The Patient Led NHS makes clear that the purchasing and commissioning of services will be very different. Plurality of provider will place increasing reliance on and input from health-improving practitioners linked to a closer political accountability with local communities. There will be a continued drive to empower frontline staff within practices or groups of practices to lead commissioning decisions on behalf of communities. In some areas, patient-led commissioning will have evolved with patient collectives commissioning 'years of care' for themselves from a wide variety of providers. With the traditional NHS provision as only one part of a complex web of patient-focused care, services will be competing for contracts that are negotiated through payment by results (PBR) in a fixed-price environment, with negotiations centred on the maintenance or development of choice, added value, quality, accessibility and reduction in inequalities.

To coordinate and orchestrate this environmental complexity, the health service will be managed across regional units with senior health and wellbeing leaders developing advanced skills that operate in a business-focused environment. There will be close monitoring of the 'NHS standards' set to ensure an equivalence of population provision and experience similar to equivalent 'industry standards' whatever the provider's size, generating a wealth of data as they are reported and excepted. A much closer relationship between health promoters and commissioners will ensure that organisations are assuring equity of access, have an overall strategy to reduce inequalities and improve the quality of services used. Health and wellbeing leaders of the future will need to be skilled in business and quality processes with highly developed brokering and negotiation skills in order to lead these system-wide developments, reflecting both the social and commercial environment locally.

Health and wellbeing leaders of the future will operate across multiple systems characterised by the generation and collection of real-time data. The wealth of day-to-day locally derived information linking community resources with all local healthcare providers referenced to national information sources will allow leaders to spot trends and anticipate potential problems. They will need the skills to analyse and understand business, disease, patient safety and outcome data that indicate where organisations are not fulfilling their functions. There will be a focus on community improvement and locally agreed targets linked to broader cross-sector local targets that report success or otherwise. Longer-term strategies linked to community planning will operate across smaller community units as health and wellbeing leaders act as the local executive brokers to ensure cohesion of effort and investment. In response to problems rapid response teams will focus their efforts on areas of concern using highly developed improvement and innovation techniques, ensuring that commissioners and providers are supported in maintaining quality and healthy outcomes for both current and potential service users.

The successor bodies to primary care trusts (PCTs), as the intermediate tier of community management and commissioners, are to be charged with ensuring that all the providers are operating at maximum efficiency, assuring optimal use of public funds, while undertaking much of the day-to-day invoicing and business processes. Most of the traditional health and wellbeing promoting skills sets will have been devolved to frontline provider organisations. Consequently PCTs will focus less on direct health promotion themselves, moving their business to drive health promotion through the decisions that link investment in local targets to population outcomes. As the 'parent body' to many smaller organisations, they will agree strategies that are explicitly linked to longer-term investment gains. The link between the healthy populations and the use of facilities owned and maintained by the local health services, the use of medical technologies and therapeutics investments will be more explicit.

Current local strategic partnerships (LSPs) will have matured to oversee and ensure linkages between the local population and the workforce. Health and wellbeing leaders will develop skills to link community purchasing decisions to a breadth of providers, matching local population demographics to those of the employed NHS workforce. They will utilise the purchasing power of the local NHS promoting its role as a corporate citizen, developing policies and commissioning templates to maximise the impact of any local purchasing or supplier decisions.

Through extensive communication and consultation, local communities will be much more aware and engaged in where their local health services are investing and deploying resources. Leaders at this level will be engaged to ensure local health services are responding to the population's needs and desires. They will need to:

- oversee communications strategies that operate as models of empowered community activism
- liberate the untapped social capital linked to non-traditional use of the local resources and infrastructure

- lead community-wide initiatives focused on empowering self-care, health risk reduction and the creation of health and wellbeing choices that are delivered in less complex, lower cost environments
- link measures of community engagement and performance to assess how well they are engaging the total community resources in health-promoting activity.

In general, health-promoting leaders will need to develop new skills, ensuring closer links to those who hold the purse strings, in order to help empower others engendering a widespread systemic effect to improve communities' health and wellbeing.

A vision for the future: changed roles at the frontline

Common skills sets will develop, encouraging cross-sector and new ways of working, moving traditional role definitions towards common skills sets for health and wellbeing in whatever role and organisation the employee is currently engaged. Common community aspirations, goals and needs will facilitate a mobility of the local workforce, further reducing organisational boundaries and ensuring the best employees remain in the local system. Recruitment and retention strategies will allow local 'churning' of employees, maintaining the local workforce within agreed high-quality working environments.

Through local leadership development initiatives linked to devolved budgetary responsibilities, frontline delivery teams will actively prioritise and target team expenditure to deliver added health and wellbeing gains where possible. The provision of real-time health data and better understanding of high impact interventions will empower health and wellbeing professionals to set local goals linked to community interventions evidenced by better measures of success.

The GP surgery will cease to be the main port of call for most communities who wish to engage in health and wellbeing related activity. As well as pharmacies and other health providers, education, social care, local government services and the voluntary sector will be engaged in the core business of improving health and wellbeing and reducing inequalities. Traditional healthcare leaders such as GPs and senior nurses will work across complex care teams through many new roles embracing the health-promoting agenda. Staff in larger group practices or health providers will be encouraged to develop incentives that reduce demands upon local services developing lower-cost local solutions for identified healthcare needs. As a result of these role changes different tiers of health and wellbeing professionals will emerge delivering through different roles, responsibilities and grades.

A dramatic increase in the use of technology will engage the whole community in lifestyle issues. Local cable TV services will develop alongside internet and web-based services and through careful branding the local primary care organisation aspires to be the premier health-promoting agency across the community. The contracts that employing organisations hold with the NHS commissioner will require staff to act as health and wellbeing champions at work and in their natural communities. Many may be accredited health trainers. It will increasingly be the norm for staff to engage directly in community wellbeing initiatives with neighbours and colleagues. They will require skills to:

- lead proactive collective initiatives and community-wide strategies in order to jointly manage health-related issues

- lead wellness activities both within and across communities, utilising the local web and cable resources
- work with local schools and commerce to encourage the use of their community links and infrastructure to provide facilities and resources for voluntary and activist groups to lead local change
- work with local employers and suppliers, ensuring they are committed to the improvement in the physical and mental wellbeing of employees, such as operating no-smoking environments
- draw communities together across a spectrum of activities and local campaigns including:
  - weight awareness, linking exercise opportunities to employment
  - tobacco consumption reduction
  - sensible drinking.

A vision for the future: the citizens' role in health promotion

Citizens will also be taking responsibility for their own health and wellbeing. Through the empowered activist model and building upon community social capital, direct delivery of core health and wellbeing services will be by the community members themselves, especially in areas such as exercise, tobacco consumption and alcohol reduction strategies. Building on the health trainer model, communities will engage with local services to develop their members as local 'wellbeing champions'. Drawn from the local population, cadres of activists will promote and signpost opportunities and raise local awareness of self-care in conjunction with an expanded expert patient programme. This will deliver health-promoting opportunities to the front door. Wellbeing co-operatives will trade products and activities across communities to maximise available funds and to ensure that local communities achieve maximum benefit from NHS investment.

Better understanding of genetic profiling and the impacts of self-inflicted environmental challenges, linked to a sophisticated use of this data by employers and the financial services industries, will create a market for personalised improved health. Personal responsibility and genetic make-up will be linked to wellbeing with direct financial consequences if these are ignored. Discounts will become available to those who are able to demonstrate improved lifestyles. Local smart cards will offer citizens the ability to use savings accrued through reduced use of ill-health services on free or reduced-rate health-promoting activities delivered via local amenities. Citizens will expect help in achieving these goals.

Health and wellbeing professionals will work with employers to develop model employer status that includes supporting staff in managing their own health, diversifying and generating income either as private organisations or as profit-making arms of the NHS. The services developed will continue to be supported by the NHS in areas of inequality or deprivation, ensuring that all populations are allowed the opportunity to better manage their own individual health profiles.

A vision for the future: underpinning knowledge and skills

In order to be capable to fulfil these requirements, the health and wellbeing professionals of the future will need continual development of their care delivery knowledge, as well as a wide range of additional skills, knowledge and techniques that drive improvement and innovation across organisational boundaries. These include:

- strategy development
- working across boundaries
- purchasing and commissioning services
- brokering and negotiation
- industry standards of quality as related to healthcare
- real-time data collection and analysis
- workforce development
- empowerment of frontline staff
- community engagement and facilitation
- application and impact of technological innovations.

Many of these are skills are currently being discussed in the literature in terms of transformational and transactional leadership: two quite different aspects of leadership (Alimo Metcalfe 1998; Collins 2001; Rainbird *et al.* 2004; Storey 2004).

> **Transactional leadership** *commonly known as management in dealing with the given, organising, planning, objective setting, monitoring performance and producing patterns of reward and punishment to influence the behaviour of followers.*

> **Transformational leadership** *is about possessing qualities and competencies of transforming individuals' self interest to take on the interests and needs of the group and to transform individuals' self belief, motivation expectations and self efficacy such that they produce outstanding performance.* (Alimo Metcalfe 1998)

However, implied in transformational leadership are the skills of improvement of health and wellbeing professionals of the future. No matter what their role or responsibilities, they will need to be actively involved in continuous improvement. Current thinking recognises the required skills set described in terms of the Discipline of Improvement. The Discipline of Improvement draws together a group of ideas and skills based on the experience of quality and service improvement in many health systems over the last two decades. While some of these ideas are well established, the way in which the Discipline of Improvement makes connections between them offers a new framework to our understanding of change in the complex world of health and wellbeing provision (Clarke *et al.* 2004; Penny 2002). It focuses on four interconnected themes (NHS Modernisation Agency 2005).

- Effectively involving all stakeholders across the system: users, carers, staff and the public, in improving health services, recognising that their experiences and needs should be at the heart of all improvement work related to health and wellbeing.
- Using process thinking and a 'whole-systems' approach to the provision of health and wellbeing services, rather than focusing on individual departments, or organisations. It is about the application across care of industrial concepts such as capacity and demand, flow and waste reduction and involves process measurements to gain insights into variation and flexible, innovative redesign of processes and system.

- Developing individuals and organisations in a systematic way by using the principles and thinking from psychology and organisational development. This will raise awareness of different styles and preferences and recognise and value the differences in others. Health and wellbeing professionals can then work constructively and communicate more effectively with everyone involved, colleagues and users, and build a culture that is supportive of improvement, innovation and learning.
- Initiating and sustaining improvement in daily work and making improvement a habit. Health and wellbeing professionals need to manage the local improvement initiatives with the development of aspirations, goals, measures and evaluation processes as well as linking it into the local and national context, politics and strategies.

Frameworks of knowledge and skills, such as this, must not be allowed to become static. Health and wellbeing professionals in the future will need to form close alliances with experts in leadership and improvement or develop the expertise themselves to regularly scan and comment on the latest thinking, best practice and emerging underpinning theories. They need to be aware of the high leverage points for change and get those who hold the budgets, and have the power, aligned, involved and responsible for the delivery of health and wellbeing initiatives. This may be in terms of 'technical' approaches to providing services in the most efficient way, or in the way key stakeholders can be empowered. Underpinning theories worthy of exploration and consideration include:

- social movement theory
- complexity theory
- design theory
- adult-learning theory
- psychodynamic theory
- sense-making, post-modernism and social constructionism
- contingency theory
- quality improvement theories.

Learning opportunities

However, it is recognised that the leadership, improvement skills and knowledge required is not alone enough: it must be put into practice in everyday work (Storey 2004). Users and staff at all levels of the future organisations need help to raise their awareness to the knowledge and skills that currently they may not have experienced. They need easy access to the range of theories, principles and models that will help them develop their services. Local education providers will need to co-develop with the NHS to create educational opportunities that are aligned with the needs of the local health providers and linked to future employment as we begin to understand it. This will create a closer match between future needs and supply. Training will become routine to enable community activists, including professionals and champions, to engage with and lead local programmes influencing commissioning decisions.

There is also a need to identify and invest in existing people engaged in health and wellbeing promotion who already have these skills helping them to develop further and become the experts of the future. They will need to be confident in being able to share their skills by teaching and coaching others, facilitating improvements.

As the social capital and enterprise of communities is liberated, new devolved and diffused leadership models will develop. Those who are currently charged with developing and supporting improvement and innovation for health and wellbeing will face new challenges and will need to change their focus or attention from many of the senior top-down leadership approaches and developments currently observed, to a focus on the environment and culture that allows distributed leadership across communities.

A vision for the future

As was said at the beginning, this is speculation; however, we know the practice and promotion of individual and community health and wellbeing is continuously changing. Society's expectations, technological and environmental changes are linked to central health policy drivers of choice, contestability and plurality of provision. In response to these challenges future health and wellbeing professionals will need to structure and organise across organisational tiers and teams supporting involvement and change across organisations and communities in different and more innovative ways. Information and its analysis will be key. Understanding the tools and techniques that facilitate community engagement and the diffuse leadership of change will need to become routine, empowering a cadre of health and wellbeing activists of professionals and champions. If this is achieved, it will lead a real, live dialogue and debate with local populations about their own health, the health of those less fortunate and the future health risk reduction of the whole community. The future healthcare practitioner may witness unparallel levels of engagement with communities and those who are charged with supporting them.

References

Alimo Metcalfe B (1998) 360 degree feedback and leadership development. *International Journal of Selection and Assessment*. 1 January. **6**.

Armstrong M (2003) *A Handbook of Human Resource Management Practice*. London: Kogan Page.

Clarke C, Reed J, Wainwright D *et al.* (2004) The discipline of improvement: something old, something new? *Journal of Nursing Management*. **12**: 85–96.

Collins J (2001) Level 5 leadership: the triumph of humility and fierce resolve. *Harvard Business Review*. January.

Department of Health (2006) *Our Health, Our Care, Our Say: a new direction for community services*. London: The Stationery Office.

NHS Modernisation Agency (2005) *Improvement Leaders' Guide: improvement knowledge and skills*. London: Department of Health.

Penny J (2002) Building the Discipline of Improvement for health and social care: next steps for NHS improvement, the early vision and way forward. *MA Management Board*. November (unpublished paper).

Rainbird H, Fuller A and Munro A (eds) (2004) *Workplace Learning in Context*. London: Routledge.

Storey J (ed.) (2004) *Leadership in Organisations*. London: Routledge.

Part 6

Looking to the future: what next for public health?

Siân Griffiths and David J Hunter

In keeping with health policy generally, public health is a fast moving field and we fully recognise that we have not been exhaustive in covering all the emerging themes and issues, notably ethics, law and social marketing. When we embarked on this second volume of essays on public health we sought not to provide a full contemporary history but to present a cross-section of views and opinions on the state of public health. From the response of our authors a number of key themes have emerged, many of which recur throughout the volume:

- globalisation and its impact on health and health behaviours
- challenges of creating a public health system when subject to continuous organisational change
- acceptance of multidisciplinary practice and the need for new models of practice
- an increasing awareness of public health challenges at all levels, from the individual to the global.

Underlying each of these themes is a further cross-cutting one – the growing marketisation of public policy which has major implications for public health policy and practice and for what we mean by, and want from, the public realm in contemporary society (Hunter 2005; Marquand 2005).

Globalisation and its impact on health and health behaviours

In the introduction to Sach's *The End of Poverty*, Bono writes:

> *Every morning our newspapers could report: more than 20,000 people perished yesterday of extreme poverty. The stories would put the stark numbers in context – up to 8,000 children dead of malaria, 5,000 mothers and fathers dead of tuberculosis, 7,500 young adults dead of AIDS and thousands more dead of diarrhea, respiratory infection and other killer diseases that prey on bodies weakened by chronic hunger.* (Sachs 2005)

It is easy to forget this wider perspective and the suffering of many communities in such dire circumstances through no fault of their own. The impact of war, corrupt government, and natural disasters all contribute to global health problems. At the same time, the Millennium Development Goals (www.unmillenniumproject.org) remain elusive. They amount to an ambitious programme to:

- eradicate poverty and hunger
- achieve universal primary education

- promote gender equality and empowering women
- reduce childhood mortality
- improve maternal health
- combat HIV/AIDS, malaria and other diseases
- ensure environmental sustainability
- develop a global partnership for development.

We might wish it were otherwise, but the pursuit of health is not always at the forefront of economic policy. Social disparities are reflected in the increasing gaps in health status. Statistics such as one in six African children die before their fifth birthday, half of these from diseases preventable through vaccines, and that in Africa one woman dies every 2 minutes from complications of pregnancy or delivery, cannot be ignored by those for whom maternal death is a rare though tragic event (Dare and Buch 2005).

But it is not only the differences *between*, but also those *within*, countries which are stark. The factors behind the well-known statistic of a boy born in the poorer part of Manchester living 8 years less than a boy born in leafy Surrey are reflected differently in the Chinese statistics. The infant mortality rates in poorer rural areas is 37/1,000 live births comparing badly with rates of 11/1,000 in urban areas, and *'Perhaps most shockingly in some poor areas infant mortality has increased recently although it has continued to fall in urban centres'* (Blumenthal and Hsiao 2005).

The widening inequalities within and between countries are a result of new patterns of consumption and communication, commercialisation, rapid urbanisation and degradation of the environment. The accompanying economic and demographic changes affect working conditions, learning environments, family patterns, and the culture and social fabric of communities. A vivid example of the dynamics of disparities comes from Ukraine which has the highest per capita rate of HIV/AIDS infection in Europe (1.4%) (DeBell and Carter 2005). The economic collapse that followed transition has left a legacy of high levels of poverty and inequality and poor investment in the development of the country's health system. HIV carries severe social stigma and public awareness of risk is low. Pregnant women are the only ones to get antiretroviral treatment. Young people are at highest risk of new infections and there is an urgent need for a strategic approach for information, prevention, treatment, and care with improved in-country surveillance.

Against this background, during the course of compiling this book many countries have signed up under the aegis of WHO to the Bangkok Charter (World Health Organization 2005) with its key principles of:

- globalisation as a positive force for health improvement
- promoting health as a core government responsibility
- health promotion as good corporate responsibility
- environments empower individuals and communities to improve health
- regulation and legislation to protect citizens and promote their health.

In promoting these principles, drawn from the Ottawa Charter, signatories are recognising the requirement for investment and partnership across governments, international organisations, civil society, and the private sector. This approach moves the debate from the global market as the enemy of good health and the corporate sector as unengaged, to recognising that pragmatic approaches to seeking win:win solutions will be needed and in doing so new models and ways of working are also needed. This is not a case of governments abdicating their responsibilities for exercising stewardship. Far from it. The need for leadership from governments has arguably never been greater. But what is required is a new approach which seeks to work with a range of different stakeholders whose priorities and objectives may well differ, and remaining resolute when the going gets tough, as it surely will.

This is evident when considering the challenge of non-communicable disease. While the world's newspapers focus on the risk of avian flu, chronic diseases are and will remain the major cause of death and disability worldwide, many occurring in low and middle income countries. Over 35 million people will die from them in 2005, double that from all infectious diseases (including HIV/AIDS, tuberculosis and malaria), maternal and perinatal conditions, and nutritional deficiencies combined (Beaglehole and Horton 2005). Without action to address the causes, deaths from chronic disease will increase by 17% between 2005 and 2015. Risk factors, as identified in the English public health white paper, *Choosing Health* (Secretary of State for Health 2004), are modifiable and the same in men and women: unhealthy diet; physical inactivity; tobacco use.

Other identified risk factors contributing to the burden of disease include harmful alcohol use which contributes to a wide range of problems, among them injuries. Over five million deaths worldwide annually are due to injuries which are largely predictable and, therefore, preventable. Psychosocial stress also plays a role. Mental disorders account for 5–10% of the burden of disease in developing countries. Vulnerable populations, such as the poor and those affected by disasters, are at greater risk. Effective and affordable treatment is available. However, in many developing countries most of those in need do not receive any treatment either because care is inaccessible or because it is unaffordable while in developed countries their problems are inadequately treated (World Health Organization 2002).

A further disease burden is related to environmental factors, such as air pollution, which contribute to a range of chronic diseases, including asthma and other chronic respiratory diseases. Chronic diseases and poverty are interconnected in a vicious circle. The poor are more vulnerable for several reasons, including greater exposure to risks and decreased access to health services.

Against this background, and as described in many chapters in this book, public health can and must be placed within its global context. No single country's public health system can remain exempt from the impact and influence of global developments regardless of whether these take the form of terrorist attacks, natural disasters, or the effects of global warming and the geopolitical developments around the depletion of oil supplies with their implications for population health and economic development.

Challenges of creating a public health system when facing continuous policy and organisational change

Another key theme to emerge from the contributions has been the complexity of practice, demonstrated both by the stimulus of devolution and regionalisation and by the need to adapt to a continuous cycle of policy and organisational change. Many of the chapters refer to the English changes heralded by *Shifting the Balance of Power* (Department of Health 2001) and subsequent developments but this is largely because the churn and turbulence have been so much greater in England than in other parts of the UK.

As we go to print significant change is taking place in the policy and organisational landscape although most of this is confined to England. By comparison, the other countries making up the UK appear to be enjoying a degree of unprecedented stability – at least for now. The thrust of government policy has become clear through a series of policy statements over the past year or so. These have culminated in the lengthy white paper published in early 2006, *Our Health, Our Care, Our Say: a new direction for community services* (Secretary of State for Health 2006). The white paper reaffirms the government's commitment to prevention and early intervention in order to ease demand on acute and, for the most part, hospital-based services. It also heralds the end of the government's preoccupation with hospitals since building new ones through the private finance initiative has been a central plank of policy in recent years. No longer it seems. There is also concern, expressed in the Prime Minister's Foreword, that health inequalities remain 'much too stark – across social class and income groups, between different parts of the country and within communities'.

Echoing proposals presented in earlier policy statements and white papers, the government wants to see joint commissioning for health and wellbeing between primary care trusts and local authorities. Much of the white paper directly builds on the 2004 English public health white paper, *Choosing Health*. The desire to see more joint posts in public health, from DsPH down, is clearly stated so that in future there is much closer joint working between the health service and local government.

The organisational changes underway are every bit as far-reaching as the policy pronouncements. These will impact significantly on public health, including the base for public health specialist posts as the tiers of the health services are reorganised and the nature and role of the work environment of specialists shift yet again. Such organisational change is often a costly diversion which leaves the population health challenges untackled. Experience from the last reorganisation in England provided many lessons (Griffiths *et al.* 2005b). Yet, despite a ministerial commitment to listen, these lessons remain to be learnt. And, as noted above, the organisational turbulence shows no signs of slackening if local government is included. Major change in this sector is being planned for a public announcement later in 2006.

The need to be responsive to external factors both in structures and in effective and prompt action has been demonstrated by the events of 9/11, SARS and other natural disasters such as the 2004 Boxing Day tsunami and 2005 Hurricane Katrina. In his introduction to *Getting Ahead of the Curve* (Department of Health 2002), the Chief Medical Officer for England, Sir Liam Donaldson, wrote:

> Standing at the beginning of a new millennium and trying to place the problem of infectious disease in context, it is difficult to escape the conclusion that it must be viewed as a global threat. A threat not just to health, survival and well-being of populations but to the economies of many countries, to social stability and to security in some parts of the world.

The factors he identified as adding risk were:

- adaptations of organisms with increasing virulence or resistance
- the impact of technology

- the increased number of people with weakened immune systems
- human behaviour
- changes in the environment
- global travel.

Recognising these, he formulated a new organisational response in the shape of the Health Protection Agency (HPA). Thus, since the first edition of the book, the language around communicable disease control and environmental health has changed. We now talk about health protection, with a greater awareness of the need to respond to emergencies and disasters. The practice of public health now extends to cover the breadth of communicable disease control, emergency, planning for disasters, preparedness to respond to biological, chemical and radiological emergencies as well as environmental health issues.

Organisationally there is now a vertical system in England extending to all levels of the NHS and linking to key partners at each level. The new structure relies on having an effective system which can communicate, coordinate and respond appropriately. As described elsewhere, for public health the vertically organised HPA needs to interface with the more horizontally organised local public health services. These relationships rely on networking, another recurring theme of this book.

Such changes have emphasised the need for public health systems which address health needs in the longer term rather than constantly diverting the existing systems to respond to structural change. Population-based public health programmes can achieve this through utilising the different levels of skill and a wide range of contributions within communities. While organisational bases may change there will be people whose skills provide them with the expertise to address important public health issues, be it preventing falls in elderly people, smoking cessation, support for reducing teenage pregnancy, improving the uptake of the winter fuel allowance or reducing the risks of HIV/AIDS. A public health system delivering public health programmes addressing these topics brings together key players with knowledge, skills and experience. We have suggested elsewhere that the characteristics of the public health system are (Griffiths *et al.* 2005a):

- a national policy framework
- a network of public health specialists working at all population levels: local, regional, national, international
- providing comprehensive public health programmes for populations, including vulnerable groups, to improve and protect health
- as an integral part of primary care, working with all partners
- led in each locality/geographic area by a Director of Public Health
- working through locally organised multidisciplinary public health teams made up of specialists, practitioners, clinicians and interested people in communities including voluntary and community groups, community advocates and the corporate sector.
- who are all part of managed public health networks.

To be effective, such a system needs a robust infrastructure supported by timely, accurate and accessible public health information. The creation of Public Health Observatories has been a significant step in this direction. Strong partnerships with communities, local government and the voluntary sector are needed, and local influence can be secured through DsPH framing and monitoring activities through their annual reports to provide an independent assessment of the health of the local population. The public health effort needs to be an integral part of the health, social care and local authority systems and to be reliant on partnerships created across communities. As demonstrated in Wales, a framework constructed along these lines can form the basis for delivery, audit and governance in all three domains of public health practice.

Acceptance of multidisciplinary practice and the need for new models of practice

Recent years have also witnessed the development of multidisciplinary public health practice. Since the first edition there has been increasing recognition of the need clearly to identify skills and competencies. One contributory step in 2002 was that the Faculty of Public Health agreed that specialist status should be dependent on acquisition of competencies and qualifications that did not necessarily rely on having a medical degree (www.fphm.org.uk). This meant that those with relevant public health skills and who met the established standards set can be formally recognised as specialists. The move was supported by the establishment of the UK Voluntary Register (www.publichealthregister.org.uk) and has paved the way for a truly multidisciplinary specialist profession, enabling specialists from backgrounds other than medicine to take up post as Directors of Public Health. In parallel, healthcare professions, including nursing and pharmacy, have developed their public health professional standards and educational pathways.

The increasing emphasis on the bridges between primary care and public health as the means to improve population health underscore the need for local leadership, often worryingly weak. Joint posts (*see* Chapter 25) are one way of creating the profile needed to lever change, particularly as they provide the opportunity to engage with locally elected leaders and move away from NHS bureaucracy.

Since there will be more pluralism in service provision in the future, public health practitioners will need to be able to work in more complex settings involving new forms of public–private partnerships. The government is intent on moving to an arrangement whereby public services, like the NHS and local government, move from being provider organisations to commissioning ones. The aim is to encourage greater plurality and diversity in respect of service provision in the expectation that greater supply-side competition will raise quality and improve efficiency.

Public health is unlikely to remain immune from such developments although it is not possible to anticipate their precise impact since the changes may well be modified in the face of opposition from the government's own supporters. However, it could be that services such as public health nurses could be contracted out or could be organised by nurses buying themselves out of the NHS and setting up in business and selling their services back to the NHS in the form of social enterprises. It is also likely that services for a local population or community in respect of particular chronic disease entities such as diabetes may be provided in future by private companies set up for precisely this task. Their service package would include a strong preventive component. Whatever the details of the new models of service delivery, public health practitioners will require new skills and new understanding of the context and environment in which they are operating.

Increased awareness of the importance of public health issues: but is the response up to the challenge?

Since the first edition of our book the profile of public health is higher – but we remain unconvinced that enough has been, or is being, done to address the root causes of many of the preventable problems of ill health in society today. We welcome the vote for a comprehensive ban on tobacco smoking in public places uniformly across the UK rather than the piecemeal approach which was occurring in the constituent countries.

The systems which govern the levels and profile of research have not shifted sufficiently to recognise the relevance and importance of qualitative research and policy development, and academic public health is now in a parlous state.

Furthermore, continual reorganisation hampers the capacity to develop public health practice in a sustainable and consistent manner, not only because individuals are destabilised by the absence of work security but because communities become confused about who is their local leader and how their engagement can be effective if bureaucracies are inward-looking and obsessed with structures rather than health outcomes. The role of the media remains complex and paradoxical. Rather than simply reporting events, they are significant players in shaping the news in the first place.

But while the glass can appear half empty, it can also be half full – if not fuller! There has been growing engagement with the issues of obesity, environmental pollution and unhealthy lifestyles as well as with the risks of communicable diseases and the devastation caused by failure to contain diseases such as HIV/AIDS. Child poverty has fallen and there have been real economic shifts towards reducing health inequalities. The indices for major killers such as cancer and heart disease have shown dramatic improvements – not just from improved evidence-based clinical care promoted through good public health practice but also through a greater awareness of prevention at all points along the care pathway. Primary care has a far higher level of engagement in public health, particularly through community engagement and increasing recognition of the need to work with local government colleagues and social care providers to add not just years to life but life to years.

However, there is no room for complacency. If there have been some important public health gains in recent times, arguably progress has not kept pace with the forces making for growing inequalities and, in particular, a widening income gap. We opened with the government's special adviser, Derek Wanless's overview and assessment of policy developments and progress in implementing his 'fully engaged scenario'. It is fitting to end with his wise counsel.

> *A step change will be required to move us on to a fully engaged path. In practice, full engagement will mean achieving the best outcomes that individuals in aggregate are willing to achieve with strong leadership and sound organisation of all the many efforts being made to help them.*

References

Beaglehole R and Horton R (2005) Chronic diseases of adults – a call for papers. *Lancet.* **365**(9475): 1913–14.

Blumenthal D and Hsiao W (2005) Privatization and its discontents – the evolving Chinese health care system. *NEJM.* **353**: 1165–70.

Dare L and Buch E (2005) The future of health care in Africa. *BMJ.* **331**: 1–2.

DeBell D and Carter R (2005) Impact of transition on public health in Ukraine: case study of the HIV/AIDS epidemic. *BMJ.* **331**: 216–19.

Department of Health (2001) *Shifting the Balance of Power: securing delivery.* London: The Stationery Office.

Department of Health (2002) *Getting Ahead of the Curve: action to strengthen the microbiology function in the prevention and control of infectious diseases.* London: Department of Health.

Hunter DJ (2005) Choosing or losing health? *Journal of Epidemiology & Community Health.* **59**: 1010–12.

Griffiths S, Jewell T and Donnelly P (2005a) Public health in practice: the three domains of public health. *Public Health.* **119**: 907–13.

Griffiths S, Thorpe A and Wright J (2005b) *Change and Development in Specialist Public Health Practice.* Oxford: Radcliffe Publishing.

Marquand D (2005) Monarchy, state and dystopia. *The Political Quarterly.* **76**: 333–6.

Sachs J (2005) *The End of Poverty: economic possibilities for our time.* New York: Penguin Press.

Secretary of State for Health (2004) *Choosing Health: making healthy choices easier.* Cm 6374. London: The Stationery Office.

Secretary of State for Health (2006) *Our Health, Our Care, Our Say: a new direction for community services.* Cm 6737. London: The Stationery Office.

World Health Organization (2002) *The World Health Report 2002 – reducing risks, promoting healthy life.* Geneva: World Health Organization.

World Health Organization (2005) *The Bangkok Charter for Health Promotion in a Globalized World.* Geneva: World Health Organization.

Index

Page numbers in *italic* refer to boxes or figures.